DATE DUE

BE 4'00		
MY 2 6 01		

DEMCO 38-296

UNDERPINNINGS *of* Medical Ethics

UNDERPINNINGS of *M*edical *E*thics

Edmond A. Murphy, M.D., Sc.D.
James J. Butzow, Ph.D.
Edward L. Suarez-Murias, M.D.

The Johns Hopkins University Press
Baltimore and London

This book has been brought to publication with the generous assistance of the Carroll House, Inc., Baltimore, Maryland.

© 1997 The Johns Hopkins University Press

ı on acid-free paper
5 4 3 2 1

Library of Congress Cataloging-in-Publication Data

Murphy, Edmond A., 1925–
    Underpinnings of medical ethics / Edmond A. Murphy, James J. Butzow,
Edward L. Suarez-Murias.
        p.   cm.
    Includes bibliographical references and index.
    ISBN 0-8018-5568-3 (hc : alk. paper)
    1. Medical ethics—Philosophy.   I. Butzow, James J.   II. Suarez-Murias,
Edward L.   III. Title.
    [DNLM: 1. Ethics, Medical.   W 50 M9778u 1997]
R725.5.M87   1997
174′.2—dc21
DNLM/DLC
for Library of Congress   97-1405
                                                                                              CIP

To Dr. Walter T. Gouch, C. S. P., the presiding genius
with admiration, gratitude, and affection

First old gentleman: Is this Wembly?

Second old gentleman: No, Thursday.

First old gentleman: Are you? Let us go and have a drink.

Contents

I Overtures   1

II Some Important Structures   109

Preface

Recent years have seen a mounting interest in what has come to be called Medical Ethics,[1] prompted by several factors: (1) the rapidly increasing scope of possible Medical procedures that make a vast difference to the diagnosis, management, and care of disease, at the price of some loss of privacy, temporary disablement, and increased expense; (2) a mounting public interest in disease and the benefits and abuses of Medical intervention; (3) an increasing litigiousness; (4) the flood of publicity; and (5) commercialization. These preoccupations have been intensely practical. They are driven by the clinical applications of science—they may be fairly described as technology rather than scholarship.

In parallel with this technical change, and largely causing it, there have been vast upheavals in the basic sciences on which clinical practice draws. They mostly deal with topics in which the resolving power is high: biochemistry, biophysics, pharmacology, neurological sciences, and such quantitative studies as psychometrics, statistics, genetics, and epidemiology. The harvest has been rich, and there is no hint of slackening. Inevitably, technical advances have shifted interest from the whole-thickness issues of bedside Medicine to reductionistic sciences; and more and more the contributors have been scientists rather than clinical practitioners.

There is no quarreling with the successes. Nevertheless, the clinical stalwarts will note that while all branches of genetics, immunology, metabolism, endocrinology, and infectious disease, among others, have made immense and conspicuous strides, the problems of mundane clinical practice have not; and the basic science of common disease is little changed. Naturally there have been some concerns as to why there should be this disparity. There are abroad hints of a belief that, by and large, health and disease are essentially complicated matters; that the palpable triumphs of high-resolution science of pure and simple mechanisms are not the whole story or even the main part of it. We, the authors, have substantial involvement in genetics and the pathogenesis of genetic disease, and are only too painfully aware of the public image of geneticists as purveyors of the exotic and often

---

1. This term, like several others used in this book, is capitalized according to a set of conventions described in the section titled "Capitalization of Terms."

the trivial. From this constraining image we may hope to escape by a combination of scientific boldness and renewed allegiance to the true concerns of clinical practice. An authentic clinical science that addresses real clinical challenges certainly exists; but it is both fragmented and rudimentary.

Unless the new Medical Ethics is to be either an insouciant concern with the exotic, on the one hand, or a mixture of preventive medical jurisprudence, diplomacy, humanistic compassion, and marketing techniques, on the other, it must have a concern with the analysis of true clinical matters. It is of the very first importance that Medical Ethics and the adjunct field of bioethics should be the scholarly study of adequately analyzed phenomena properly formulated. For this reason our exclusive interest in this book is with safeguarding the supply of Medical knowledge as raw material to be delivered to the Medical ethicist. Of the many books on Medical Ethics, this book is the first we know of to take on that task as its sole objective.

It would be a thankless business, and make monstrously dull reading, to list all the topics that this book is not attempting to address. We are not concerned to provide an Ethical system, not even at the most abstract level. We are not trying to expound Medicine or psychiatry or Medical jurisprudence or forensic Medicine. We propose no system of values or method for devising them. We do not review the standard epidemiological concerns about reliability, accuracy, precision, sensitivity, or specificity of tests or the challenges and problems of misclassification. We are attempting no Medical Philosophy (although we find it convenient to use some of the vocabulary of Philosophy and to borrow some wisdom and analogy of method from it).

The goal, as we shall repeat from time to time, is to explore some of the major areas of confusion that exist in the no man's land between scholarly clinical Medicine (in the tradition of Harvey, Sydenham, Hunter, Charcot, Sherrington, MacKenzie, and Lewis) and the professional ethicist, typically nurtured in Philosophy. There is little hope of constructive dialogue between clinicians who have little patience with Philosophy and Philosophers who have no mud on their boots. It is a fatal error to take for granted that the clinicians know what they mean when they use words like *normality, disease, suffering, pain, human, responsibility, act, action, probability, proof,* and *decision.* We have not found them easy matters, even without any strategic commitment to the needs of Ethics (Murphy 1997). In this difficult endeavor we draw much strength and comfort from H. W. Shaw ("Josh Billings")—a Philosopher who may not have read the masters but had plenty of mud on his boots: "It is better to know nothing than to know what ain't so" (Bartlett 1962: 594).

We would rather perform an unpretentious task well than a sophisticated one badly. So we have given ourselves the role of caterers of clinical theory to Medical Ethics. We have been reluctant to stray beyond what we see as our area of competence. Nevertheless, even in so simple an encounter as shaking hands, one must at least make a guess where the other person's hand is. We cannot wholly escape the task of defining what we perceive as the operation of Ethics. But this is not our main endeavor, and we would welcome suggestions.

These writings have grown slowly and deliberatively from many years of discussions. The authors see themselves as the principal, but by no means the entire, source of the ideas presented; we are as much as anything a group of spokespersons undertaking to sort out the contributions of many and bind them into a coherent whole. Those taking part in the discussions have at one time or another included members of a wide range of Christian sects from Catholics to Quakers; Jews; Buddhists; those with no formal religious beliefs; and frank agnostics. They have included men and women of all ages from twenty to eighty, mostly students and faculty at the Johns Hopkins University, at the East Baltimore Campus (Health Sciences). This diversity has been a valuable corrective against any unconscious tendency on our part to insinuate private and inappropriate beliefs: beliefs that (in our perception and definitions, at least) do not fall within the domain of Ethics proper or that of the concerns here.

We appreciate the participation of all those who took part in those discussions, which grew up around the Carroll House in Baltimore. We especially acknowledge the participation of Drs. James Murphy, Juan M. Baertl, and Salvatore Raiti.

We acknowledge with pleasure the helpful and constructive comments on the finished manuscript from Drs. R. W. Sherwin, Helen Abbey, and B. E. P. Murphy, and Chester J. Jakowski, who must in no way be held responsible for its shortcomings or the invincible ignorance of the authors.

Mr. Henry J. and Mrs. Marion Burk Knott, through their generous endowment of Carroll House in the 1960s, provided a rich social environment in which the Ethics discussion group took root. In the writing of this book we have undertaken to make use of the light and understanding that emerged. The result, this book, is a wholly separate enterprise.

Arrangement of Topics

In the interest of coherence, the matter in this book has been arranged with the most fundamental ideas and terms first (Part I), followed by particular topics in order of complexity: basic structures of Medical Ethics (Part II), and, finally, the involvement of the human person (Part III). Readers anxious to get quickly to the meat of the book might choose to read the Preface and Chapter 1, and then jump to Part II. The Glossary should help in smoothing out any difficulties encountered as a result of skipping Chapters 2–5. However, to follow the arguments in detail, it would probably be necessary to refer back to the appropriate portions of Part I.

Capitalization of Terms

Because of the particular need in this book for precision in terminology, some few nouns and their derivatives are capitalized to denote a special, technical meaning, where the ordinary demands of grammar would leave them lower-case. This practice is used sparingly but strictly. Thus we avoid intruding much new vocabulary to differentiate these terms from words of identical spelling used in their ordinary meaning, or worse, coining new terms to replace them. Even if the reader initially finds the capitalization itself somewhat intrusive, it does provide for clear distinctions that, we trust, will come to be appreciated. An alphabetical list is appended, with the distinguishing meanings briefly defined; fuller definitions are to be found in the text and in the Glossary. Generally, adjectival and adverbial forms of capitalized nouns are themselves capitalized.

act: A coordinated muscular movement. **Act:** A discrete deliberative action by a human being.

agent: (1) One who acts. (2) A chemical participant. (3) A representative. **Agent:** A responsible human being who participates in a transaction.

certitude: Total assurance. **Certitude:** A state of total personal assurance that is not formally warranted by the data and their analysis.

chaos: A state in which there is no discernible order that admits of assured general principles. **Chaos:** A state in a dynamic process characterized by three properties: a sensitivity to initial conditions; topological transience; and having at least one region in which the periodic points are dense.

diagnosis: The inferred state of the patient. **Diagnosis:** The diagnostic process.

ethical: A term of approbation applied to behavior. **Ethical:** Pertaining to analysis of the relationship of facts and arguments to courses of action.

ethics: (1) An informal code of behavior. (2) A particular explicit application of Ethics. **Ethics:** The formal study of the relationship of facts and arguments to courses of action.

law: An arbitrary judicial prescription imposed by the political system for the governance of social or moral behavior. **Law:** A necessary or empirical relationship among distinguishable components of any system.

legal: Lawful. **Legal:** Juridical.

logic: (1) A reinforcing term used rhetorically to bolster up a point of view. (2) A logistical component. **Logic:** The formal study of the legitimate inferences from the relationships among propositions.

medicine: A therapeutic concoction. **Medicine:** The professional care of health and disease among human beings.

moral: Seemly, virtuous, chaste, etc. **Moral:** Pertaining to the role of conscience.

objective: Applied to that body of knowledge or inference that appeals only to evidence available to all. **Objective:** Applied to inference or knowledge that appeals to explicit data and arguments free of idiosyncratic values and judgments.

philosopher: A benign, contemplative person of equitable temperament. **Philosopher:** A scholar who studies values and reality by speculative rather than empirical means.

philosophy: An informal set of perspectives, values, principles, etc. **Philosophy:** A formal system of perspectives, beliefs, judgments, and speculation that appeal to reflective analysis rather than empirical fact and experimentation.

probabilist: One who follows a reputable opinion. **Probabilist:** One who casts formal statements about the outcome of an event in stochastic terms.

probability: Plausibility, probity. **Probability:** The measure on the scale (0–1) of the chance that a particular outcome from a homogeneous Random event will take place.

psychology: An informal interest in the working of the human mind. **Psychology:** The formal study of the operation of the human or animal mind.

random: Confused, haphazard, chaotic, of wholly unknown or indescribable provenance. **Random:** A quality of samples, estimates, and propositions drawn from a set or population, the corporate behavior of which can be sufficiently described by a Probability distribution.

statistician: One interested in statistics and figures in general. **Statistician:** One expert in the theory and practice of formal inferences, estimation, testing of hypotheses, models, and optimizing decisions from data that are at least in part stochastic.

statistics: Measurements or denumerable data. **Statistics:** The theory and application of formal and manipulative analysis of qualitative or quantitative data perceived as in some sense stochastically representative of a population of reference.

subjective: Applied to knowledge or inference that is wholly or in part idiosyncratic. **Subjective:** Applied to inference or knowledge that incorporates data and arguments not available to all.

thing: A noncommittal object of experience, manipulation, or discourse. **Thing:** An abstract, arbitrary interfacing between the human mind and reality.

I Overtures

There is some risk that the intent of this first part will be misunderstood; and we would like to practice a little preventive diplomacy. We start from the viewpoint of clinical Medicine and Medical science. Like many of our kind, we meet Ethical problems. In our appeal to expert guidance, we are dismayed, not that the opinions available are incoherent or incompetent, but that they seem to be entirely irrelevant and probably bear little similarity to what any applied ethicist would do in clinical practice. We hope to see this hiatus effectively diminished and smoothly bridged and are anxious to improve the Medical input into Medical Ethics and Medical Philosophy. However, having much interest in these latter two subjects but no expertise, we can at best guess at what exactly the experts would like to know about our fields. In this we feel we must impart *some* guidance or the undertaking may end up, as before, with expert advice that has no domain of application in Medicine.

To hope to establish authentic contact, we must try to identify what structures in Ethics and Philosophy may be related to, and commensurable with, authentic Medical practice. Part I of this book breaks the ground. We find that we must start at the very beginning, examining assumptions and agenda. In Chapter 1 we confront what the scope may be, culminating in a definition of Medical Ethics, to be used throughout this book. We next explore what a system of Medical Ethics comprises: principles, empirical experience, inchoate intuitions, the momentum of conventional practice, surmise, and the creative dialogue among them. To a professional ethicist Chapter 2 (and the backlash it generates in Chapters 14 and 15) will doubtless seem naive. But at least it is a scheme involving matters we regard as fundamental in Medical science. Chapter 3 takes on a number of paradigms that are implicit in the organization of Medicine. Finally, in Chapters 4 and 5 we deal with problems in disciplined speculation at the interface between Medicine and Philosophy: ontology, epistemology, and semantics. The special problem of ontological cohesion, addressed in Chapter 5, pervades much of the rest of the work.

1 Introduction to Medical Ethics as a Discipline

The term *Medical Ethics* conveys a wide range of meanings, from the most pragmatic to the most abstract. There is an enormous and rapidly growing literature on the topic, which we cannot hope to review or to compete with here. The topic of this book is rather different: it is to explore, not Ethics itself, but the Medical prerequisites, the raw materials, of a discipline of Medical Ethics. This approach is unusual, and if it is to be coherent and intelligible, we shall have to devote this first chapter to setting the scene and even to breaking with some traditions. The result may be unfamiliar but is not arcane. Almost all our illustrations will be so commonplace as to require a few lines of exposition only, mostly for the benefit of those unlearned in clinical detail. We also make a limited appeal to scientific illustrations, usually because they provide cleaner and better-established illustrations than we can find in Medicine proper. But they too are mostly the common matter of premedical education. (As a simple, if utilitarian, criterion, such illustrations are of the sort likely to be used in FLEX and National Board examinations, by consent the standard benchmarks of clinical competence.)

The misgivings of the reader are likely to be not so much "Do we need to know about all this material simply to deal with Ethics?" as "Do we need to think about all these things that we already know?" Needless to say, if we did not believe that the answer is yes, we would not have written this book. But the reason why is not easy to state concisely, and we think that a brief history of our own experiences may help.

THE ORIGINS OF THIS BOOK

We note at the outset that excruciatingly precise definition of disease, for instance, has not been an ordinary concern of clinical Medicine. However, those of us interested in the analytical (mathematical) aspects of non-Mendelian genetics became concerned about the nature of what are commonly called normality and disease. Formal analysis of empirical data on hypertension (to mention one classic example of ferocious debate) is highly sensitive to how *hypertension* is defined. Darwinian and genetic theories of selection, in particular, may be made or broken by such manipulations and change in the allocation of patients.

Quite separate from that topic of research, there existed a discussion group, of which we three authors were members, that undertook to explore various practical issues in Medical Ethics. It soon became clear how much of Medical Ethics centers on one aspect or another of anomaly, disorder, or disease or their prevention. There seemed to be no satisfactory source or even criterion established to which we could appeal for enlightenment. What is more, we became progressively aware of a much deeper defect. To define or identify the field that has suffered this neglect is not easy; nevertheless, it is not wholly without history or content, as the writings of, say, Sydenham, Bernard, Sherrington, Trotter, and Cannon make clear. But the cohesion of that field was eroded by physiologists, pathologists, psychologists, Philosophers, and others who undertook detailed, although fragmentary, studies and abandoned responsibility for the corporate demands of a comprehensive fundamental Medical theory. To try to call attention to some of the void, one of us was impelled to write a text, *The Logic of Medicine* (Murphy 1997 [2d ed.; 1st ed. 1976]). (That book, however, was much narrower in scope than the current text.)

The more the discussion group on Ethics debated, the more apparent it became what catastrophic gaps there are; and although there is a modest but excellent literature on the theory of special topics (e.g., pain and suffering, insanity, responsibility), to say nothing of the pertinent Philosophical literature, it was difficult to find writings by those undertaking to analyze systematically the Medical data and what purport to be their Medical merits. Unfortunately, the contents of the clinical textbooks (on which Philosophers rely, often to a perilous degree) are cast in ruthlessly pragmatic terms rather than in terms of radical analysis, and—as Pellegrino and Thomasma (1993) point out—they look to phronesis born of robust, pragmatic, common sense to grapple with any shortcomings or inconsistencies. Yet in the long run, makeshift devices do no good to scholarship. It is not so much that they are untidy as that they leave the profound misgiving that we are driven to make do with botched solutions because the issues concerned have been inadequately analyzed and imperfectly understood. As a consequence, they are unlikely to help in bridging gaps where, for one reason or another, adequate empirical data and the wisdom of experience are denied us.

Now, our first concern is that whatever is to be made of Medical Ethics, as distinct from general Ethics, we must ensure that there is an authentic input from Medicine qua Medicine. We have been dissatisfied in bioethical debate with how much well-established and pertinent Medical science never surfaces at all. Moreover, we have our pride. We do not want Medicine to be cast in the role of a poor relation or of a Third World nation to be colonized by experts from advanced civilizations bartering raw clinical materials at a trading post of academic law, or Philosophy, or theology. Medicine should undertake to put its own house in order and then do sophisticated business enjoying something like parity with Philosophy, just as physics, chemistry, and mathematics have done and continue to do. This preliminary refinement of Medical ideas should enhance, rather than undercut, the productiveness of professional ethicists. This belief amounts to demanding that Medical Ethics is to come not solely from a docile consultation of clinicians operating under judges' rules or the canons of Philosophy but from an authentic dialogue among the disciplines in which all participants bear a symmetrical relationship to one another. The dialogue is to occur under procedures agreed on by all, with rights of cross-questioning; and if there are to be formal depositions, *all* participants are to be "sworn in" and held to account for competence, truth, and fairness of argument. It is to be a true dialogue and not a judicial inquiry. Our preparatory task, then, was to set about preparing a proper and fitting Medical brief.

Needless to say, this task has had its price. The unfamiliarity of the analysis will make for some misgivings as to whether it is all really necessary.

GENERAL ORIENTATION

There is a widespread notion that Medical Ethics is a good, earthy, practical subject born of common sense and experience. We shall have something to say about these claims later. However, to anticipate, we have found repeatedly and from much frustrating experience that when, going beyond naive rules of thumb, we try to deal with the Medical substrate of Medical Ethics in deeper and more enriching terms, sooner or later we come up against three relentless difficulties that will not go away:

1. the lack of precision in the Medical aspects of the terms of discourse;
2. confusion over the rules governing the interpretation of Medical evidence; and
3. deficiencies in the structure of germinal ideas to which, in discourse, casual appeal is often made by physicians, lawyers, sociologists, and professional ethicists (among others).

For all practical purposes, these defects are the fault of the field of Medicine, and the remedies to be sought are the responsibility of Medicine. Our book is written from this perspective. We shall have failed if we end up by drifting off into amateur philosophy and neglecting to do a searching examination of how the matter of Medicine should be analyzed. In this sense of our task, the Philosophers are treated as onlookers, not participants— but only in this sense. For we shall also have failed if as a result we do not enhance the raw material on which the latter may work their skills.

At the outset, we lack technical vocabulary to denote the areas of study needed for addressing these pre-ethical questions, although under various disguises they are the subject of a modest literature (Feinstein 1967; Ingle 1976; Schaefer, Hensel, and Brady 1977; Elstein, Shulman, and Sprafka 1978; Albert, Munsen, and Resnik 1988). Discussion and analysis of the three vulnerable areas bear a kind of rough analogy to what in traditional Philosophy would be termed *epistemology* and *ontology*. We appropriate these very words, preceded by the actual or implied qualifier *Medical,* to our own uses in a kind of metaphorical sense. However, it must be understood that in using them we are not attempting Philosophical pronouncements, and accordingly we claim a diplomatic immunity from the technical criticisms of Philosophy. Nevertheless, we are sensitive to the demands of Philosophy, and in Chapter 4 we deal with these terms in some detail.

It is not even our goal to address Ethics, even when the term *Ethics* is to be understood in an unfashionably abstract sense. Rather, we shall try to identify and discuss some of the more persistent gaps in our knowledge and understanding, in the hope of promoting a clear communication with Ethics.

Thus, anything we shall have to say about rights, values, prescriptive laws or case law, moral doctrine, or the other traditional paraphernalia of Ethics will be at an ontological or epistemological level only, with no attempt whatsoever to explain how they would actually be used in Ethical discourse. From time to time we may appeal to illustrations that arise from the structures of Ethics proper, but only to point up the implications that appealing to these illustrations may have for the fundamental analysis with which we are concerned.

EXAMPLE 1.1. Arguably the XYY karyotype (Borgaokar and Shah 1974; Hook 1975; Hamerton 1976) has an impact on aggressiveness and hence has a bearing on the forensic Medicine of judicial mitigation. But in searching out what the implications of that argument may be, we find that in some cases, at least, the decision may rest on the measurement in some test of psychopathic behavior. The latter test is on an arbitrary scale of assessment that has been devised in historic time; and it holds its warrant from the good sense of those who devised it, and from practical experience of its application. It is well to realize that the measurement has the advantage over the broad impression of the psychiatrist (dealing with the ill) in that it contributes to the overall collective experience of the test and, at least retroactively, helps to standardize the content and terms of the assessment. Nevertheless, however indulgently we may view it, the epistemological standing of such a measurement is not at all the same as that of the measurement of height or weight. Perhaps in the nature of psychometrics it never could be. One cannot take for granted that this distinction in the soundness of the measurements is made by every particular ethicist. It is not merely that weight is a much simpler and more restricted measurement and that centuries of inquiry and experience have gone into perfecting it. Weight is a simple and restrictive means of measuring mass, but the precision of the measurement is bought at the price of narrowness in its meaning. Much of preventive Medicine has centered on the weight of the patient. But there is a growing feeling (in the light of ill health, even tragedies, in overconditioned athletes, notably gymnasts) that the bearing of weight on health is perhaps poorly understood.

We perceive at once what a slippery term *meaning* may be. In any Medical context it comprises a hierarchy of analyses that are not to be airily discussed in brief and impatient footnotes. Penetrating understanding and judgment are not to be fully attained by shibboleths and battle cries about objectivity and reproducibility and unbiased sampling. This theme of caution will be a recurrent one throughout the text.

THE SCOPE OF ETHICS

At the outset and to redress the balance, we must try to rid our approach of what we may call a false perception of credentials and competence. Medical Ethics proper has been explored by scholars of two main groups: Philosophers, theologians, and related humanists; and members of the clinical professions. Both approaches are illuminating, but neither is quite satisfying to us. The former experts have tended to stress the use of formal systems at the expense of the authentic particularities of the world of sensible experience, or the actual state of living Medical knowledge. Clinicians have tended to consolidate a well-entrenched code of conduct for meeting certain classes of cases. We have become concerned that the content of so-called Medical Ethics (in the United States, at least) has become more and more identified with the principles of what has traditionally been called *forensic Medicine:* the judgments of the law courts in both civil and criminal issues. It seems to us that a major function of academic Medicine should be to instruct and inform the discipline of the law under the rules of symmetrical dialogue (in the sense in which we used the term above) and mutual cross-questioning on both fact and meaning, and not under the one-sided patronage of the law court. But that viewpoint has faltered for lack of advocates.

For the most part, clinicians have provided no system and no principles of Ethical argumentation; hence, no criticism is possible, and there is no basis for extending or improving the code. The advent of cardiac transplantation and of in vitro fertilization caught both the clinicians and the ethicists almost totally unprepared. The often thankless task of imparting cohesion a posteriori to pragmatic customs has devolved on a broad class of ethicists who go about the task in various ways—some prescriptive, some historical, some reconstructive, and some intensely practical (Engelhardt and Callahan 1976; Reiser, Dyck, and Curran 1977; Veatch 1981; M. Cohen, Nagel, and Scanlon 1981; Jonsen, Siegler, and Winslade 1986; Vandeveer and Regan 1987; Loewy 1989; Beauchamp and Childress 1989). We recognize these writers and their goals. But if we appear to slight them, it is because they are engaged in a task that has almost nothing to do with what we are about at the stage of development of Medical Ethics presented in this book.

More fundamental criticisms could be leveled against many writings in Medical Ethics by physicians. Two major defects stand out.

First, there is a temptation—no doubt often provoked by the immediacy of some imminent decision—to pronounce solutions where the real nature of the problem has ontologically and epistemologically been inadequately explored.

EXAMPLE 1.2. One of many such instances arises over the Ethics of dealing with a diseased organ. Little thought is ever given to what is meant by *diseased* and by *organ*. The major impediment is the great reluctance on the part of either ethicists or clinicians to acknowledge that there is any problem whatsoever over these terms. But those caught in the toils of high-resolution science (e.g., Medical geneticists) cannot afford to brush these definitions aside as pedantic exercises. Even the smallest ambiguity over what is meant by *disease* may deprive of all formal cogency analyses of such topics as what regulates the frequency of schizophrenia or how a tissue type or blood group is related to the etiology of ankylosing spondylitis or peptic ulcers. We have something to say on this topic in Chapter 8, on normality and disease.

Second, there has been a prodigality both in the principles and in the values that various writers have invoked to defend some position: esthetics, purpose, common sense, religion, revelation, even mysticism. It is not our thesis that the complete clinician in practice should be indifferent to any of these considerations; but here we ourselves have exercised the greatest parsimony in appealing to such structures, and this for two reasons.

We hold these elements to be, not discredited by, but foreign to, the true field of Ethics. The bearing of the demands of state, though real enough, is not a matter of Ethics but of Medical politics; the bearing of the rulings of the law courts is not a matter of Ethics but of forensic Medicine; religious writings and practices are germane to Moral theology but not to Ethics.

Moreover, we hold that even if such evidence were admissible in Ethical discourse, there is little hope that it would be given the same weight by all reasonable thinkers. To plan for an Ethics that only a small proportion of the population accepts would be to win the battle and to lose the war.

EXAMPLE 1.3. We trust that all reasonable physicians believe their functions to include the relief of suffering,[1] and this would be a sound Ethical principle. On the other hand, to invoke the Ten Commandments in order to decide whether or not euthanasia is Ethical would be unnecessarily restricting. Many of the most upright and compassionate physicians would attach no authority whatsoever to the Ten Commandments. This statement is in no way to belittle or to slight apocalyptic theology. In order to prove the isoperimetric theorem or to understand the working of the hemoglobin molecule, no sensible person will quote Homer or Samuel Johnson or Tolstoy, however revered their wisdom.

Our project is to lay out some fundamentals that have some reasonable chance of contributing to a consensus. But *consensus* is not (as might be too readily supposed) a euphemism for a compromise of some sensitive ideal; nor (a common abuse) should a minimal consensus be advanced to dissuade or restrain some individuals from abiding by stricter principles in their own practice.

Traditional arguments in Medical Ethics have been often more or less hazy, largely because there has been ascribed to the terms of discourse a spurious definiteness that may evaporate on close inspection in concrete situations.

EXAMPLE 1.4. Thus, it is far from obvious what a *thing* is. A dozen people may use the term in a dozen different senses. What results from long discussions may merely create the illusion that they are communicating among themselves with some precision. To be sure, an impressive list could be assembled of previous writers who have tackled the question of what a thing is, Heidegger (1967) and Lonergan (1957) among them. The reader might wonder what more there is to gain from further analysis. But the clinician has the uneasy feeling that many discussions are dealing not with the properties of *Things* as connected to reality but rather with the properties of abstractions of things as noncommittal objects, a kind of constructive idolatry. They leave untouched the issues of how (if at all) their deliberations are to be translated into concrete clinical terms. (If this concern is in turn met with the very same criticism, that the clinician's notion of a thing is merely an analysis of the properties of a different abstraction

1. We are on treacherous ground here. Writers (Cassell 1982, 1991; Fordyce 1988; M. L. Cohen 1991) have distinguished with some care between pain and suffering. We are arbitrarily taking the stance that suffering, at least in the severely ill, serves no useful clinical purpose. See Chapter 12 for a detailed discussion.

of things, so be it; there is, no doubt, room for many abstractions and many analyses. But at least any absolutist notion that (say) Heidegger's model of a thing is the only one worth considering will have been demolished.)

EXAMPLE 1.5. Is the adrenal gland a Thing? Or is it two Things, a cortex and a medulla, that have different phylogenies, ontogenies, functions, and histologies, but that gross anatomy does not define nearly so well? Or does it become one Thing again because its two components are both concerned with addressing stress—in the sense of Selye (1936, 1956)—from environmental challenges? Here lies a gap between the Philosopher and the practitioner that is not to be bridged by a little casual adjustment.

EXAMPLE 1.6. There is a widespread sentiment that the mentally defective should receive special care and protection. That sentiment, however admirable, is too vague to be of any utility in making decisions in concrete cases, and much too vague to be worthy of the title *principle*. How exactly are "the mentally defective" to be defined? Some would see them as those who are at the bottom of the scale of intelligence. But at once two satellite questions arise.

First is the ontological problem of whether at some point a cutoff may be set, on what basis that point is to be chosen, and whether it has any virtues that may be sustained or is forever condemned to be nothing but an arbitrary or even a capricious choice. It is not utterly unthinkable that the components of intelligence below that point represent a function operating in a quite different region of the brain (as the autonomic respiration from the respiratory centers in the pons and medulla differs from the sigh of the bored or the singing of the diva); or have different provenances (as hard-wired instinctive behavior differs from that learned by experience or teaching); or have different vulnerabilities (as epilepsy differs from tremor or hyperactive reflexes). But it seems on general experience most unlikely either that there is a completely sharp separation at any particular point or that the point should be hit upon by a capricious choice.

Second is the epistemological question of what the scale is on which intelligence is rated, and what grounds there are for believing that this scale faithfully reflects society's special concern about the fitness of the individual (namely, the capacity to make sound judgments). It may well be true, but it is far from obvious, that the criterion of (say) whether or not subjects can solve puzzles of analogy or repeat numbers backward (which are among the abilities the psychometrician tests) is a sound measure of whether or not subjects are able to look after themselves (which is what the social reformer has in mind). There are further promptings (which we shall later address under the term *provenient*): Who devised the psychometric tests? What were their motives in doing so? How far were the tests they devised colored by the personal experiences of these psychologists?

What groups of subjects were these tests validated against? What was the sampling scheme, and how faithfully was it applied? And much more of the same.

There seem to be two approaches that can be taken in the face of this kind of difficulty. One approach is to develop a fully explicit criterion *that is to be distinct from the components of the immediate problem*. This criterion then must be deemed reasonable by consensus of the informed. The term *fully explicit* excludes any appeal to ill-digested arguments from other fields. Such illegitimate arguments include statements like "Statisticians have shown that the normal range lies within two standard deviations from the mean" or "The law defines mental deficiency as an IQ of 80 or less." The second approach, which we ourselves prefer wherever possible, is to recast the principles (and develop them further, if need be) so as to embrace and accommodate the intrinsic indefiniteness of the idea.

EXAMPLE 1.7. In the narrow context of Statistical analysis, we mostly prefer to use, where appropriate, the methods of multivariate analysis rather than those of categorization. This Statistical policy of appealing to the assumption of continuous, rather than discrete, variables must not be confused with the fact that some decisions based on the analysis may be categorical. Also, of course, continuity is a quality to be discerned, not an edict to be imposed. Whatever the narrow experts may say, it is not, for instance, an exaction of science that gender shall be represented on a discrete scale. (We shall have more to say about that problem later.)

In this primordial approach we think it wise to remind the reader from time to time that we deal exclusively with the nature of the terms, making no appeal to the paraphernalia of Ethics whatsoever, still less proposing courses of action.

EXAMPLE 1.8. Such a statement as "It is normal for boys to go through a homosexual phase" has no precise meaning until the words *homosexual, boys, normal, go through,* and *phase* are clearly defined, if then. This semantic and ontological analysis has to be done at some stage and is a worthwhile activity even if finally there is no attempt to arrive at any Ethical pronouncement about it. Indeed, the example of other scholarship is that a basic theory, to be sound, must be coherently developed in its own right and not in a haphazard collection of ad hoc judgments under the pressure of some concrete example.

The fundamental concern of the authors is with neither the truth nor the value of any proposition, although that is not to dismiss or even belittle the importance of either. Rather, the concern is with the proposition's meaning and whether or not valid inferences may be coherently made about or from it. If a proposition is meaningless, of course, then predications about it will be meaningless; and more generally if the proposition is ambiguous, the predications will also be ambiguous. It is surprising, indeed disturbing, how much need there is for this kind of analysis and how much work must go into the shaping of an Ethical system before we even think of introducing values at all (Murphy 1978a). Often analysis will recast obscure problems in terms such that the clinician may feel the conclusions are obvious.

Concrete Ethical problems will be of the most interest to the clinicians, but their analysis will also be the least complete. An Ethically acceptable solution to a problem will involve empirical fact such as what the course of a disease may be; and it will also require methods of probing and measuring impacts (pleasure, pain, fulfillment, etc.). When we appeal to either of these fields, knowledge of empirical fact or assessment of the patient's response, embarrassingly many deficiencies come to light, not always because they are difficult to grapple with but often because they have simply been neglected.

In this dire need, sound clinicians will do what the wise have always done: suspend judgment where they see no virtue in speed, and in other cases do the best they can with what is available. The one course they will not take is merely to allay the anxiety that occurs to all who must act in doubt, by erecting a brazen false certitude. The imperatives of what purports to be knowledge extend beyond the immediate deliberations of the clinician.

The deficiencies in our corporate knowledge are in large part due to lack of interest in, and commitment to, these evident goals among the scholars and the investigators. There results a dearth of the (to us) self-evident moral commitment to remedy every pertinent item that is lacking in our knowledge and understanding. While the blame for these persisting deficiencies may not fall on any one person, one must surely feel that there are corporate responsibilities that belong to scholarship as a whole. There must be some distortion in the climate of opinion if there is no concern to meet a pressing Ethical need (Murphy 1981c). The right that particular physicians have to devote their lives to basic scientific research does not absolve the responsibility of the Medical profession as a whole to meet the needs of the sick. Arguably, the same judgment applies to Ethical scholarship.

THE MOTIVE FOR MEDICAL ETHICS

We return to our starting point, the naive complaint about the scope and utility of Ethics: that these deep discourses are time-consuming, dry, tedious, and exacting; that a sufficient Ethics is a matter of common sense, compassion, and experience; that clinical professions have little or no need of deeper reflections on their commonplace daily acts, and still less need of interference from outside. What is it that all this bothersome Ethics is supposed to be adding to this natural equipment?

Wherever Ethics is a coat of varnish laid on a body of de facto clinical knowledge from outside, clinicians have every reason to be unmoved, even suspicious. The idea of a kind of foreign power, uninvited and unversed in the language, customs, and gritty realities of clinical practice, proposing to colonize Medicine and presuming to regulate it after a little supercilious analysis, can generate little but enmity. If the prescriptions should be in a foreign language, so much the worse. By "a foreign language" we mean not merely that Ethical discussion is too often laden with obscure jargon (often invented ex parte for the purpose) and impenetrable allusions, but also that, vocabulary aside, it is not cast in the authentic terms of clinical practice. It is like a theoretical particle physicist intruding his theories about quantum electrodynamics on a builder of small cottages. Any soothing rejoinder that detachment is a valuable quality in deeper understanding and delicate deliberations, and that there is nothing that promotes dispassion like distancing oneself from irrelevant detail, will be coldly received by the clinician on the firing line. Such a casual and arrogant dismissal of certain features as "irrelevant" overlooks the fact that what is to be regarded as relevant is, likely as not, the very point at issue.

Yet this confrontation over power, over who is to adjudicate, however much it may have arisen in the past and continues to persist, is a parody of the authentic relationship among scholars. Ethics is indeed a fitting companion of Medicine. But that statement does not mean that the exigencies of clinical practice must willy-nilly be fitted into some Ethical theory manufactured, with however much erudition, in a propertyless void. The theory, to command respect, must be ponderously and faithfully rooted in the quiddities of clinical practice.

On the other hand, clinicians may just as arrogantly and complacently deny to Ethics any toehold even under the conditions of fidelity and modest self-effacement by the ethicist. Such clinicians may be answered by pointing out the inadequacy of the very terms in which they produce their homely makeshift solutions to Ethical problems. If the principles of Medical conduct are indeed to be "common sense, compassion, and experience," are there, then, no ways worth seeking of discerning what common sense prompts? No way of distinguishing compassion from sentimentality? No systematic way of distilling the true wisdom out of the multitudinous individual and collective experiences of clinicians so that, for instance, it would be readily accessible to the inexperienced clinician? No way in which to define and optimize the qualities required of decisions?

But further, are not all clinicians from time to time in doubt as to how they should act? Even when they are sure in their own minds what they ought to do, do they not consult other clinicians, perhaps to tap their knowledge and professional skill, but also for reassurance? There is always a risk that an Ethical system may constrain the practitioner; but we suspect that such constraint would be an abuse of the primordial purpose of Ethics. The utility of Ethics is akin to that of science: it provides a kind of flywheel that is powered by countless individual experiences. The flywheel will lend stability to the judgment of a clinician overwhelmed by the bizarre aspects of some atypical or personally distressing case. There is nothing very new about this idea of a flywheel; it is precisely how collective experience is turned into sound Medical theory. There is a growing sense that the procedures for establishing Medical knowledge need to be articulated and provided with a set of rules of evidence. Competent clinicians never feel threatened by sound knowledge: they never feel that their freedom is being compromised by reliable information, but rather the contrary. The fact that so many clinicians readily accept this relationship to knowledge and yet do not adopt a comparable attitude to Ethics suggests that too often the role of Ethics has been distorted.

THE PRINCIPLE OF CONTERMINALITY

At this stage we confront a principle that is invoked often throughout this book. Its importance is twofold. First, identifying it by name reinforces one of the great strengths of science and the operation of the scientific method: wherein science differs from the humanities and why the two approaches differ so widely. Second, it smokes out what we perceive as a frank abuse by bolstering up arguments of dubious provenance. It is based on the idea that Ethics (or any other systematic scholarly field) necessarily deals with facts and relationships that in some sense can be more compactly stated than an exhaustive list of particulars. A compact statement might, for instance, be a set of rules by which income tax is to be computed. There is not a special set for each taxpayer (which not only would be unworkably cumbersome but also would raise the strongest doubts about fiscal justice). In contrast, a telephone directory is by nature a wholly individual statement in which it is of the essence that every subscriber have a unique designated number. At an empirical level we may point to the distinctive character of fingerprints.

Now, compactness has a price but also enjoys a virtue, and they are embedded in the same perception: that the individual case be in some degree at least subordinated to a more general recipe. The price is that (as in a class action at law) there is an actual or at least some perceived loss of sovereignty. The virtue is that the individual case may draw on the wisdom, the information, and the authority of the general principle and in turn lend weight and wisdom to it. The freedom of the individual case to appeal or not to an Ethical principle involves precisely this quid pro quo. From these considerations we construct the following principle:

• The boundaries and domain of an Ethical principle may not coincide with the domain of its application.

The notion of a *principle* means that it must not be constructed ad hoc. If it were, then there would be no larger body of wisdom, fact, or authority on which it could draw. Then the principle is contributing nothing that is not exhaustively represented in the individual merits of the case.

EXAMPLE 1.9. One may not usefully argue that euthanasia is wrong on the principle that euthanasia is never lawful. The conclusion may in some sense be quite correct, even compellingly so. However, the principle (as a principle) is quite useless. By its very terms, *it has no domain of application to anything other than the topic* (euthanasia) *it was invoked to address.* It is like saying that all those over sixty years of age are senior citizens because all sexagenarians are senior citizens. The conclusion is sound, but the argument, although formally correct and indeed harmless, is void. The conclusion contributes nothing that is not contained in the major premise. In contrast, in the context of euthanasia, appeal to the principle "The killing of human beings is always wrong," while by no means self-evident, at least does not violate the principle of conterminality, because it encompasses many instances of killing that would not be put forward as euthanasia. It has some claims to being a broad principle and not like one expressly invented to deal with this particular case.

Some clinical matters such as hereditary cancer may involve many people. Likewise, infectious diseases that are transmitted implicate more than one person. There are more subtle problems.

EXAMPLE 1.10. One such area lies in the domain of human sexuality. There are aspects to sexuality that are distinctive. Leaving aside autoeroticism, sexuality, unlike many other activities, is a reciprocal relationship, characteristically involving two people. But sexuality also commonly involves the offspring as well. In Medical genetics there are typically at least three people involved in some problem ("the nuclear family"), and often many more. The necessary dimensions of sexuality differ from those of appendicitis or common emphysema, where only one person is intrinsically involved. But that does not mean that sexuality is so totally other that addressing its Ethical problems warrants the intrusion of a mass of conterminous principles about sexuality that are generated out of thin air.

———

There is a deeper principle involved in Ethics that may not be quite so readily accepted. It may be thought of as standing behind the principle of conterminality. The notion of *science* is that a vast array of individual data may be usefully and faithfully condensed into a more compact, coherent structure that may be stated concisely. However suspicious scientists may be about metaphysics, and however reluctant to give final consent to a proposition, they nevertheless suppose themselves to be pursuing in some sense a cleaner, more rational representation of reality that lies behind the multitudinous particularity of actual personal experiences. In this respect, most of scientific endeavor is incurably Platonic. A scientific discovery is not merely a useful fiction, a mnemonic device that helps overtaxed memories to grapple with individual facts. Even if a scientific principle is only an approximation, scientists (except for certain Bayesian statisticians) would hold that at least there is some kind of true state of nature to which a scientific datum is intended as an approximation. In principle (as the logical positivists and some of the more extreme Bayesians would have us believe) it may indeed be meaningless to talk about approximations where the true answer is unknown and perhaps unknowable; but, exotic opinions of theorists notwithstanding, few scientists would make such a nihilistic stance into a normative principle.

So let it be with Medical Ethics. If even in principle it cannot be supposed that there are better and worse ways of acting in a particular case, then clearly Ethics has no authentic content; practitioners had better get on with their tasks and dismiss all misgivings. It seems as if some physicians suppose that the main function of Ethics is to help the clinician to steer clear of lawsuits. But that view (which we expressly excluded in our conception of Ethics) is by no means universal, and preoccupation with it would do nothing to enhance the standing of the clinical professions in the eyes of the public, or the law in the eyes of clinicians.

But if Ethics is something more than a kind of preventive legalism, who shall decide on its structure and content? In principle there is no reason why Medicine itself should not be its own client, its own scholar and counselor, its own last court of appeal on Ethical matters. But just as even the most self-reliant homebuilders may learn from others without compromising their freedom, Medical Ethics too may model its approaches and solutions on those that have been developed in other fields, without being hidebound by them.

A DEFINITION OF MEDICAL ETHICS

We have now perhaps cleared the air sufficiently to define what we mean by *Ethics*. In doing so we are not arrogating to ourselves any authority to prescribe how others should use the term. Our task, remember, is to establish a point of contact between Medicine and Ethics, and to organize Medical theory accordingly. Such a confrontation must needs involve arbitrary choices, and it is to impart coherence to that process of choice that we formalize the discussion.

So the word *Ethics* will be used in a strict, even narrow, sense. In particular, we distinguish it from *Morality, Legality,* and *custom.* By so doing we do not, of course, categorically dismiss these other topics as irrelevant to Ethics. At the least they act as touchstones to detect those errors of reasoning that may creep into Ethics as they may into any other discursive field. But we imply that they have no right of veto over the conclusions of Ethics.

Morality

Despite their wider etymology, the words *Morality* and *Morals* will be used to denote norms of behavior that are derived from authority, whether or not they involve social custom, religion, or an appeal to divine revelation. This narrow meaning we give to *Morality* is perhaps unusual, although by no means unique or original. Accommodation of Moral principles of this kind within Medicine may conveniently be termed *Medical Morality.* It will clearly not sway those persons who do not believe in social or transcendental authority; and even among those who do, its content will vary widely from one religion to another. *Christian Ethics* or *Jewish Ethics* would, in this view, be terms as empty of meaning as *scientific poetry* or *hexagonal soup.*

• We may state once for all that *we shall not be dealing with or catering to Medical Morality;* and readers are expressly advised not to make from this silence any inferences whatsoever about the private opinions of the authors or their associates.

Legality

Legislation is an arbitrary embodiment of the will of a governing body into laws. (It is irrelevant to these distinctions what the political system and the distribution of power may be, whether democratic, oligarchic, or tyrannical.) Legislation has an arbitrary quality with considerable appeal to the legislators; and where unworkable, it can be revoked or amended. Arising out of legislation there is a higher quality that we term Legality, which sets a tone of civic behavior by transcending the technical details of the law. Holmes wrote:

> It is something to show that the consistency of a system requires a particular result, but it is not all. The life of the law has not been logic; it has been

experience. . . . The law . . . cannot be dealt with as if it contained only the axioms and corollaries of a book of mathematics. We must alternately consult history and existing theories of legislation. But the most difficult labor will be to understand the combination of the two into new products at every stage. (Holmes 1881: 1)

The fragmented quality of legislation leads, from time to time, to inconsistencies that the Legal theorist, in developing notions of Legality, may be at a loss to reconcile even with the most contrived principles (as Holmes illustrates repeatedly).

Most reasonable scholars would agree that what is true is something external to themselves, not an invention of their minds and not something to be arbitrarily controlled. Legislators may turn to other fields, including Ethics, for guidance in framing laws. Nevertheless, however wide their backing, the legislators are not necessarily equipped to decide what enactment conduces to professed goals, any more than they are competent to discern scientific truth.

EXAMPLE 1.11. The massive evidence on the impact of smoking tobacco has been systematically compiled and evaluated by an expert committee of long standing, appointed by the surgeon general of the United States Public Health Service. On that authority, both the federal and state governments have passed many laws. But however noble their purposes, legislators as a class are unfitted to decide from scientific evidence whether smoking causes cancer or whether it is beneficial to health to prohibit smoking.

It can be argued that Ethics, which deals with a kind of idealized behavior, is something to be discovered, not invented. Granted that some end is desirable, the best means of attaining it is decreed by the nature of things and the limitations of our understanding and knowledge (which are not to be supposed the same constraints). The price of efficiency is a restriction in freedom of choice. If houses are to be kept warm, then the effective methods must conform with the rules of thermodynamics. If economy is a goal, then one burns old newspapers to keep warm rather than ten-dollar bills.

Custom

Conventional behavior may decree what is thought fitting, respectable, decorous. It is an intuitive and informal expression of the common standards of the society. It has diverse origins, many of them highly reputable. For the most part, customs have been the fruit of much experience. One does not "put the knife in the mouth," as Herbert Pocket so tactfully pointed out (Dickens 1860: chap. 22), "for fear of accidents." But custom furnishes at best a rough-and-ready Ethics.[2] Empirical studies may show that one's fork is even more dangerous. Then presumably there would be a change in the custom, however reluctant.

Nevertheless, in principle, the weight of somebody's expertise has little evidential merit *beyond the accessible facts and the explicit arguments from which it has been derived.* The claim, however disinterested, by a world-famous athlete that his speed of foot is due to rubbing his feet with raw onions every night should raise doubts in the minds of the discerning scientist. Does the athlete know anything about the rules of scientific evidence? Has he applied them in establishing his claim?

EXAMPLE 1.12. The opinions of expert obstetricians about the circumstances in which abortion should be lawful will be informed by their actual experiences of the authentic detail of many individual cases. But while they may have much compassion and wisdom, their conclusions about what *ought* to be lawful do not flow inexorably from these experiences. Their opinions (though probably more valuable than most) remain only opinions and, like everything else they or other experts may say, are more or less subject to error. Ethics would at the least require that the experts marshal the evidence—obstetrical, sociological, psychological, or other—for their views; and that they convey a precise idea of what they mean by *lawful.*

But we are ascribing idealized attributes to the obstetricians in the example. Much less weight would be given to the opinions of any experts, however eminent in other ways, who unreflectingly develop habits that they then seek to endow with qualities that stand beyond the ordinary rules of evidence and its interpretation. This specious practice may be found among those who construct Ethical arguments about "the best standards of clinical judgment" without giving any statement at all about the evidential warrants for their claim that these standards are the best available. The Medical profession has too often, even within living memory, been corporately and emphatically in error over points of plain verifiable fact to encourage uncritical belief in the infallibility of their views about conduct (consider the therapeutic use of bleeding in fever; laudable pus; the vigorous use of potassium phosphate to promote diuresis in anuria; the absurdity of cleanliness in obstetrics; high-protein diets in hepatic failure; the futility of open-heart surgery; the perils of light anesthesia combined with muscle relaxants in abdominal surgery). Of course, this reservation about the corporate Medical judgment of conscientious clinicians is not to be pushed to absurd extremes. Whatever its shortcomings, in default it is still the best opinion available and should be weightily respected. It is not

2. The ingress of custom as part of corporate wisdom of practice in the constitution of Ethical systems is discussed in Chapter 2.

to be supposed that the end of Ethics is to destroy convention; its end is rather to refine convention and give it greater coherence.

We are then led to the following statement:

DEFINITION.   *Medical Ethics* is the systematic study of the processes whereby the making of decisions in concrete clinical cases may be optimized, with respect to certain goals identified as desirable, by rational analysis in the light of accumulated experience.

CONCLUSION

We close with several comments.

First, *Ethics* is commonly used in two main senses: (1) as a system of conduct in a class of cases, as in a code of Medical Ethics for the profession; and (2) as a scholarly discipline by which this code is arrived at. The distinction is one between content and scholarly methods. The same distinction arises in the word *diagnosis*. "The diagnosis for Mrs. Jones is sarcoidosis" is a statement about the categorization of a particular patient (content). "Professor Brown has devised a new method of computer Diagnosis" is a statement about the means of categorization in general (scholarly method). In this book we use the word *Ethics* predominantly in the latter sense (i.e., Ethics as scholarship). That is, our concern is not to arrive at explicit decisions in individual cases or even in individual classes of cases; rather, we explore the nature of the Medical and scientific contributions to the task of doing so.

Second, the object of Ethics is human behavior; the investigator is human. The study of Ethics is thus incurably reflexive. In this respect Medical Ethics is radically different from veterinarian Ethics. Human beings are both the judge and the judged, and this relationship presents problems that are, by analogy, well known in Philosophy and mathematics. We quote Bronowski, writing from a purely physical standpoint: "Once it was enough to think that the world keeps still and distant while we painstakingly carve it into sections. . . . We have reached the stage where . . . the gap between the observer and the fact cannot be kept open" (Bronowski 1951: 83 ff.). Still less can the gap be preserved when the *fact* is human behavior. We have much more to say about the reflexive nature of Ethics in Chapters 14 and 15, on responsibility.

Third, reason, like Logic, deals with the relationship between ideas that are in some sense arranged. Then, insofar as Ethics is reasonable, it has component parts. There must be aims or objectives or ends; and there must be means to these ends. We might apply the term *Major Ethics* to the study of the relationship between Acts and their consequences. The study of the application of means to broad classes of ends might be called *Minor Ethics*.

(The terms are taken by analogy from Major Logic, or epistemology, and Minor Logic, or the formal devices of argumentation.) Note that we do not mean by this distinction that (for instance) Major Ethics deals with whether in eclampsia, abortion is desirable, and Minor Ethics with the appropriate way to do the abortion. Major and Minor Ethics both deal with arguments for arriving at conclusions about conduct; but Minor Ethics is a narrow, often a formalistic, application to particular kinds of problems (e.g., diseases) of the grand perceptions devised by Major Ethics. These purely analytical activities may be extended in two main ways: (1) Minor Ethics may be further adapted to some individual case and all its particulars and mitigations, a practice that is usefully called *casuistry*. (2) Into the purely dispassionate Ethical discussion may be introduced components of Moral obligation, and it has become the custom to refer to this development as *deontology*. The only one of these topics with which this book engages is Major Ethics. No Moral or deontological component is addressed, except occasionally to point up relevance and pertinence in some otherwise rather abstract and unmotivated analysis.

Fourth, there is nothing in the definition that implies that Ethics is the last court of appeal on behavior. In the eyes of some readers, Ethical considerations may conceivably be overtrumped by arguments from other fields such as politics, Morals, or esthetics. The objective of the definition is to state *the scope of the evidence and argumentation used in arriving at the answers inside the domain of Ethics.* Just as it may not be possible to prove by mathematical arguments that Rembrandt was a great painter (a judgment that falls inside the domain of esthetics), so it may not be possible to prove by Ethical arguments that for motorists to exceed the speed limit is always wrong. Against the charge that our definition sets too high a value on human reason, we answer that, to the contrary, it is merely setting tight limits on the scope of Ethics. Note also that the criterion is human reason, not formal argument alone.

Fifth, so far as possible, the empirical evidence used in Medical Ethics is to be derived from purely formalized, mostly scientific, experience. But lines are not always so easily drawn. Psychology, which in the classical theory of knowledge was a branch of metaphysics, is now treated as a more or less secure scientific discipline. But the distinction among *mind* (which is the subject of Psychology), *soul* (which is a matter for Philosophy), and *spirit* (which is in the domain of theology) is not an easy one; and it seems (to say the least) a trifle arrogant to dismiss summarily certain considerations (such as the esthetic quality of life) for no better reason than that they cannot be studied inside the framework of authentic empirical science.[3] Psychiatrists are concerned with the data of Psychology and psy-

---

3. We say "authentic" because analyses that do not meet the standards of sound empirical studies may nevertheless put on the trappings of scholarship and masquerade as scientific or mathematical or esthetic studies.

chiatry, which must perforce grapple with many nonscientific phenomena. Medicine as a whole is scientific, but not exclusively so. Physicians must concern themselves with compassion, happiness, responsibility, and the like, not all of which have been (or perhaps can be) soundly formulated in scientific terms.

Sixth, narrowly Philosophical problems will be avoided entirely. Nevertheless, if any useful contact is to be established at all, matters touching both Philosophers and clinicians must inevitably be considered fair game. Indeed, there is serious risk that even purely scientific statements will be misconstrued in their Philosophical dimensions; and then disclaimers are necessary. But again, the clinician trying to decide what is authentic Medical knowledge demanding the attention of the Philosopher may be unaware of some express Philosophical reason why the clinician's supposition is mistaken. The clinicians then must withdraw that demand in good grace, but in doing so they will revise somewhat their perception of the scope of the Philosophers' responsibilities, and act accordingly.

EXAMPLE 1.13. Medicine may (in the spirit of Chapter 9) seek expert Philosophical help to resolve the notion of normality. Philosophers may see fit to regard normality as a topic that they are neither equipped nor concerned to explore. Or perhaps (a less improbable outcome) Philosophers may furnish their own concepts of normality but decide that there exist no methods, no vocabulary, no principles, by which their concepts may be translated into possible Medical terms. This view clinicians may acknowledge, perhaps against their better judgment. But then one of two adaptations is available. Either the clinician will decide that the Philosophical usages have abdicated all bearing and weight in Medical Ethics; or, the more devastating adaptation, the clinician may decide that rational negotiations between Medicine and Philosophy have broken down. (This deplorable breakdown would then readily extend, in principle, to all contacts between Medicine and Philosophy.)

Finally, behavior comprises inaction as well as action. There are at least occasional situations in which suspension of judgment is itself a form of behavior and may impinge on Ethics.

2 Ethical Systems

W e cannot afford to treat in isolation from each other Medical Ethics as such and the Medical ideas and structures on which it draws. If *normality* is an idea invoked in Medical Ethics (without perhaps any Ethical apparatus for exploring what the term may mean), then equally so, normality is a notion addressed in Medical ontology that may have a *point d'appui*[1] in Medical Ethics. Without mutual recognition that both fields have broad scope, useful cooperation is doomed. We note further that Ethics is a topic that raises ontological problems that cannot be brushed aside. Let us take up a problem that has arisen in a purely ontological context.

EXAMPLE 2.1. If a person *feels* happy, does that mean the person *is* happy? As an Ethical *point d'appui,* suppose that the question arises as to whether the feeling of happiness is due to the euphoric phase of a bipolar mood disorder, which the psychiatrist proposes to treat. If so, by what right may the psychiatrist cut short that happiness? There is a subtlety here. Although point and focus are being added by raising an Ethical question, the issue that we raise here is purely ontological. Setting aside completely the matter of whether or not happiness is good, to be promoted or not, and so on, what is the nature of happiness? Is it a matter of feeling and of mood? That would certainly be the common way of using the term (*Webster's* 1988: senses 2 and 3). Psychiatrists may well see fit to give *happiness* a technical meaning that allows them to talk about false happiness, or incongruity of affect, or pathological euphoria. But then they must accept the responsibility for taking a step that is certainly intrusive and defend it by an appeal that at least implicitly involves a proper ontological analysis.

---

1. We apologize for this exotic term but can find no satisfactory English equivalent not already overloaded with the wrong connotations and associations. It means literally a fulcrum (or, in a derivative sense, a base of military operations). Unfortunately, by widespread metaphorical use, in English the word *fulcrum* has acquired overtones of coercion, unscrupulous political and diplomatic pressures, and so forth. We mean the term to designate a point of legitimate unforced engagement between fields that are distinct and (as here) traditionally rather isolated from each other. It is to be seen as like an embassy rather than a center of subversion; or (in military terms) as a "military presence" rather than a beachhead.

The reader might call to mind Dickens's sketch of the First Meeting of the Mudfog Association:

> Dr. Kutankumagen (of Moscow) read . . . a report of a case which had occurred in his own practice . . . of a virulent disorder. He had been called in to visit the patient on the 1st of April, 1837. His frame was stout and muscular, his voice loud, his appetite good, his pulse full and round. . . . He laughed constantly, and in so hearty a manner that it was terrible to hear him. By dint of powerful medicine, low diet, and bleeding . . . in the course of a month he was sufficiently recovered to be carried down-stairs by two nurses, and to enjoy an airing in a close carriage, supported by soft pillows. . . . It would perhaps be gratifying . . . to learn that he ate little, drank little, slept little, and was never heard to laugh by any accident whatsoever. (Dickens 1839: 637–38)

Now, of course, both aspects of happiness, ontological and Ethical, require to be treated by the experts concerned. It seems to us likely that the ontologist and the ethicist would gain from communication and collaboration. But that neither involves nor implies any infringement of the sovereignty of either's expertise.

EXAMPLE 2.2. Is it possible to compel a person to be free? The Ethical *point d'appui* is that society compels children to be educated, on the grounds that education enhances their intelligence and skill, which will give them more freedom in life. We express no opinion here about how the ethicist should answer, but broad common sense would concur with education, compulsory if need be.

The apparent paradox of the notion of *compelling freedom* raises questions about the ontology of freedom and how it may differ from *liberty*.

We pursue the matter no further at this stage but trust that the reader will get from these two examples the spirit of this chapter. There emerges the clear need for an ontology of Ethics. Indeed, it will soon become evident that we take for granted that Ethics is an orderly process of making decisions and acting on them. This chapter is concerned with the possible kinds of interplay there can be between the various components of Ethics. This discussion is not at all an attempt to impose any particular system of Ethics; rather, it is an imposition on our system of ontology in the context of Ethics. We would welcome enlightened comment.

POSSIBLE SYSTEMS OF ETHICS

Analogies from the structures of mathematics and science suggest that we should recognize three pertinent elements in an Ethical system: *prin-*

ciples, consequences, and *existential custom and behavior.* Each one may be viewed as a contributor to the Ethics, as we shall try to show.

The *principles,* which are often cast in the form of *axioms (A),* are commonly viewed as an important guide to behavior; and since Ethics must always be somewhat concerned with the promotion of good, the *consequences (C)* of action are also germane. Rather less obviously, there is a third important component that resides in unexamined *practice* or custom *(P),* the kind of primitive pattern that grows up in the pragmatic and unsophisticated stage of development in a practical field. Since practice is somewhat loosely defined (if indeed it can be said to be defined at all), we could certainly subsume under it those many factors that are not amenable to either the hard discipline of cogent Logic or the solid basis of empirical fact. Keane (1984) strongly argues that there must be some ingress for this aspect of human action.

By analogy, at law, the judge may draw on three main sources: (1) jurisprudence and the principles of justice (many traceable to Moral Philosophy); (2) prudential appraisal of the effects on some policy of justice ("If I rule in such and such a way, it will act as a deterrent"); and (3) appeal to some proverb or other form of folk wisdom ("When in Rome, do as the Romans do") or some sentiment ("An Englishman's home is his castle") to which the layman is most liable to turn (McHugh and Slavney 1983).

We may suppose that in a particular Ethics, each one of these three components may conceivably be represented at a minimum of three levels:

1. *Overriding:* Fully and inalienably built into the system. It may not be overruled, and any conflict between two such states will be a stalemate. In what follows, overriding components will be indicated by the corresponding symbol in upper case *(A, C, P).*
2. *Accommodating:* Weighty and respected but apt to be outweighed by other components or overtrumped by an overriding component. An accommodating component is indicated here as a lower-case letter *(a, c, p).*
3. *Void:* Totally unrepresented. The state is indicated by a dash (–).

Theoretically, then, there are at least twenty-seven possibilities ($3 \times 3 \times 3 = 27$), but in practice the main interest lies in whether the source is overriding or not, so that there are seven main classes (Figure 2.1). We may add an eighth class in which the degrees of representation of all components are partial, and a ninth in which the system decays into a dimensionless void so that none is represented.

We shall first briefly enumerate these nine classes of Ethical systems and then analyze the implications of each system: what may be viewed as the strengths and weakness of each but with no judgment as to whether

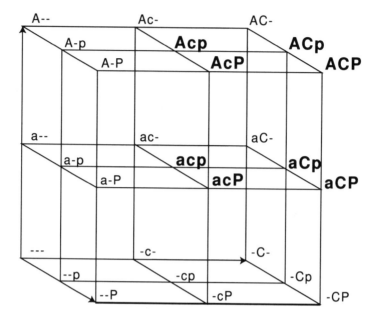

Figure 2.1 This diagram depicts twenty-seven possible Ethical systems defined in terms of three components: axioms, consequences, and practice. Each component is represented on a separate axis, with magnitude increasing with distance from the origin. Each Ethical system is identified by a trinary code that denotes the relative importance of each component in the system, with an upper-case letter *(A, C, P)* indicating that the component has a dominating role; a lower-case letter *(a, c, p)* indicating that it is considered but does not dominate; and a dash (–) indicating that it is ignored. The codes appearing in boldface and the one consisting of three dashes correspond to the nine systems of chief interest analyzed in the text. Confrontational Ethics, which neither affirms nor denies the importance of any of the features, has no representation in this system.

these terms are commendable or not. The discussion is to be seen as addressing the ontology of Ethics. It has no concern with the Ethics of Ethics, except for the primitive comment that it is venal to declare one system better than another simply because it saves on the amount of thinking required. Subject to that general attitude, we shall proceed as impartially as we may.

PRIMARY SYSTEMS

Axiomatic or a Priori Ethics (Type *Acp*)

Traditionally, the Ethics of Aristotelian (and particular Catholic) writers has been mainly based on deductions from particular principles that we may conveniently treat as axioms.

EXAMPLE 2.3. Take the axiom "It is a function of the physician to relieve suffering." From it certain rules of conduct may be inferred: it is important to acquire knowledge, be compassionate, be judicious in the use of drugs, and so forth. Arguments from practice and benefits are at best a subsidiary consideration, modifying a conclusion, perhaps, but never overriding it.

Consequentialist or Prudential Ethics (Type *aCp*)

The shape of the Ethical system may be dominated by its effects, not by its antecedents. Stated in the familiar epigram, it is the principle that a (sufficient) end justifies a (proportionate) means. The test of the justice of the means is the end to which the means is directed.[2] It is arguable that without some experience, no Ethics would be possible.

COMMENT. We must carefully distinguish consequentialist Ethics from Ethical impotence or Ethical agnosia. Any Ethical decision necessarily supposes that there is some connection between an explicit Act and the outcome. That in itself does not make the Ethics consequentialist. If nothing that one can do makes any difference to the outcome, there may be Moral problems, but the problems are Ethically void. Likewise, one is sometimes aware that there may be, perhaps must be, an outcome, but there is no way of predicting it or anticipating it. (Such a problem arises in Chaotic systems.) Again the case is Ethically void, and no such Ethical

2. This statement is made recognizing that there may at times be genuine difficulty in deciding which is the end and which the means. Flew (1989: 22–24) has put his finger on a vital feature of deductive arguments, namely (in his phrase) their reversible character: that in a valid syllogism the premises and the conclusion may be permuted without loss of validity, although the sense of the conclusion is reversed:

All insects have six legs.
A spider is an insect.
Therefore a spider has six legs.

This syllogism is valid *modus ponens*. But the conclusion is false: spiders are not insects (spiders have eight legs). However, we may then use the falsity of this conclusion as a valid syllogism *modus tollens* under the Flew principle to prove that the minor (second) premise is false.

decision can be consequentialistic. We shall have more to say about this phenomenon later.

Popular or Traditionalist Ethics (Type *acP*)

The third term in the system is the overriding factor. It proposes to canonize what has come to be "good practice." A code of principles can then be generated out of these practices.

COMPOUND SYSTEMS

We may mix the three primary types in various proportions.

Pragmatic or Holmesian Ethics (Type *AcP*)

Pragmatic Ethics is one of several composite systems. The requirements of these systems are that should any clashes between the components occur, each is to be given a full and fair hearing; overriding factors must be fully reconciled to the complete satisfaction of both, under pain of a deadlock. In the present instance, the Ethics is to be fully axiomatic, but it is also to square with accepted practice. The actual practices function in this Ethical system much as the totality of empirical experience does in science. The axiomatics is required to embed this collective wisdom in solid terms that can be expounded. The analogy that comes to mind is Holmes's notion that the multiplicity of rulings in the law court *(P)* must be welded together into a coherent system *(A)* from which judgments are to be formally deduced (Holmes 1881).

Commonsense Ethics (Type *aCP*)

An Act is to be judged right if it conforms to the best practices of the profession (which may be seen as a kind of corporate judgment of those qualified, in some arbitrary sense, to judge) *and* if the consequences, or the foreseen consequences, or the probable consequences, are evidently good.

EXAMPLE 2.4. According to commonsense Ethics, it might be argued that abortion is warranted if the mother is in danger of death and that entails death of the fetus, because the death of the fetus alone is a preferable outcome to the death of both mother and fetus; moreover, this is the way most obstetricians would act. Arguments about the rights of the fetus (which, whatever the decision, is doomed not to survive) are in this context trivial.

Consistential Ethics (Type *ACp*)

We use the term *consistential* to denote an Ethics in which there is a demand that both axioms and consequences be fully respected. Since both these areas are cast in exacting terms, reconciliation is by no means always easy. There is to be no surrendering of either, but there is room for negotiation and refinement between the two. Flew's principle (1989: 22–24.) will be frequently in play. The method of reconciliation needed, which involves endless traveling backward and forward between the two demands, is commonly termed *iteration;* it is a topic of some complexity and will be discussed later.

The spirit of this approach is that the clash between the axiomatic and the consequentialist components is due, for instance, to error in the data; or to error in the interpretations of the data; or to some flaw in the precise way the claims of the two components have been stated; or to some flaw in the way in which they are apposed; or to a deficit in the dimensionality of the model in which they are embedded; or to some confusion as to what the word *good* may mean. It is the business of the Ethical system to do what it must to resolve the discrepancies.

No doubt critics will object that this method is slow and difficult; that it asks too much and for no good reason; that there is nothing in the nature of things that demands that such a reconciliation be possible. But it is evident that these critics have confused the ontological analysis of Ethics with partisan advocacy. Ethics, we have agreed, is *not* a set of invented rules to be implemented juridically but a search for authentic relationships. There is (by analogy) nothing in the nature of things that scientific theory and empirical scientific data should give the same answer. But the canons of science demand that that be so; if it is not, then either the theory or the empirical methods are defective, and one or both must be amended (e.g., by amending the complexity of the theory, improving the resolving power of the empirical methods, etc.). The fact that conflicts between them may take hundreds, sometimes thousands, of years to resolve has never dismayed the true scientist. The demand on consistential Ethics that it fully respect axioms does not mean that the axioms may not be changed, even radically changed; but the same is true for the ontological analysis of the consequences. What is demanded, however, is that the principle of conterminality (see Chapter 1, Glossary) must be scrupulously maintained for both. No scientific Law or experimental method can be held reputable or be in a position to advance science if every clash between them is resolved by putting a patch on one or the other. The inalienable governing principle both in consistential Ethics and in science is that conflicts must be equitably explored with no preference (as there is with *Acp* or *aCp*) as to which will have an ultimate casting vote *on the basis of priority rather than on the basis of content.*

Consensual Ethics (Type *ACP*)

The consensual system of Ethics involves full satisfaction of all three components and a reconciliation of all their demands. In the fullest meaning of the word it implies a *consensus* of the conflicting theories. By a strict consensus we do not mean a majoritarian action, or any kind of a compromise of absolute demands, but a united system in which *all coherent demands are heard and either shown to the satisfaction of all (even the proponents) to be empty, or else fully incorporated into the system and conserved in it.* The criticisms and the issues here will be precisely the same, *mutatis mutandis,* as in the previous system.

Situational or Existential Ethics (Type *acp*)

In its less extreme forms, situational Ethics draws on the traditional sources of principles, consequences, and custom but is not dominated by them. If the conclusions to which they lead are in some sense unreasonable or unsatisfactory, the ethicist reserves the right to reject them all and to do so without any special pleading. There is no imperative of due process. This view is sometimes expressed under such nominalistic principles as "No two cases are the same." However, deeper analysis suggests that most decision makers making this claim are not quite so extreme as they may sound. Invocation of this principle of radical uniqueness commonly stems from a confusion of *dimensionality* and *cardinality,* a topic we shall discuss later. The principle that no two cases are the same is not equivalent to saying that all cases are utterly other, which in extreme form would imply that the ontology is so disrupted that no amount of evidence or past experience would help at all. Moreover, while there is in practice likely to be a region in every ontological space that is treated as nonexistential, there is some part of the space that is treated as existential.

Ethical Nihilism (Null Ethics, Type – – –)

Ethical nihilism may be viewed as an extreme form of situational Ethics in which the three standard sources are wholly abandoned. It may be understood in two senses: Ethical solipsism and individual Ethical denial.

In *Ethical solipsism,* the individual person is capable of elaborating a personal system of Ethics by one means or another but in general cannot communicate it to another person. The structures are such that cross-questioning by others serves no purpose. The lack of communication might be ascribed to various factors: the conceptualization of the terms of a problem, the notions of the good, the means of argumentation, the emphasis on the importance of internal consistency of argument, and so forth. Apart from the traditional courtesy in discourse, it is wise to ascribe such failures in communication to perverseness, arrogance, or dishonesty *only in the face of the most severe provocation.* Much discussion convinces us, for instance, that even in the cognitive domain there are great and genuine differences in the way in which minds view gestalts, some using them freely, others having great difficulty in seeing them at all. To some, meaning is of the highest importance; to others, proof; to yet others, empirical data. There may be much dispute over the merits of abstraction. But all the more so, we may perceive why there may be failure in the coherent and orderly communication of other matters, either because they are in a less articulate domain, like affect, or because they involve much more subtle judgments.

One form of Ethical solipsism would be a personal, unstructured system that, for instance, puts all the weight of adjudication on feelings or strivings (affective or conative), assessed at the moment of decision. But if the basis for decision is truly conative in character, such a system, it seems to us, does contain structure.

EXAMPLE 2.5. Cannibalism would be abhorrent to almost all sane people in the civilized world. It is not easy to bring oneself to explore either why it is abhorrent or what the essence of the complaint of its abhorrence may be. It is difficult to see how this abhorrence would accommodate simultaneously the benefit of supplementary amino acids in the diet. The chemical point of view would be that amino acids are pure, or at least purifiable, chemical compounds; and once in that pure form it is difficult to see how the provenance of (say) tryptophan has any bearing at all on what is, and is not, acceptable food. Or, within the bounds of chemistry, we might achieve a critical division, according to whether or not there is a secondary structure present. But on what grounds do we decide to treat the gravamen of cannibalism as a chemical problem? For that matter, on what grounds do we decide that it is not only a cognitive problem but is to be solved cognitively?

Of course, we may make the arbitrary decision that Ethics should be made more cognitive and pay less attention to such considerations as affect, conation, sentiment, and so forth that open up the risks of nihilism. Relaxation of this rigor may indeed tend toward nihilism. But such a concern invites the rejoinder that broadening the basis of Ethics is demanded by a very real complaint provoked by an abuse of reasoning and an arrogation by only one aspect of the discussion.

This is not the last time we shall encounter this *infinite Chinese box* problem: the unbounded set of processes of a system endlessly trying to get outside itself. The only practical recommendation we have at this stage is to preserve the most punctilious courtesy in detaching structured Ethics from idiosyncratic Ethics.

Individual Ethical denial represents a yet more extreme example of nihilism: the view that nobody can devise an Ethics that is even personally satisfying. Needless to say, if this claim is true, there is no point in trying to communicate to others what does not exist even idiosyncratically. This stand would, of course, make Ethics quite featureless: not only would there be no principles, but there would be no useful discussion with others, and no appeal to experience. Ethics would in fact be quite useless, although the problems to be solved might still be perceived as real enough.

Confrontational Ethics (Ethics of Zero Dimensions, No Representation)

For completeness, we include a species of Ethics outside all these categories. According to this confrontational view, the only mission of Ethics is to solve problems that are the result of inadequate analysis; that is, if the issues were clearly presented and analyzed, their solution would be known immediately. This view would argue that Ethics neither has nor needs any special structures proper to it. It is tantamount to collapsing the diagram in Figure 2.1 into a void. It has analogues in speculative Philosophy, such as the extreme positivist position of Ayer (1946), who denied that metaphysics meets any authentic need of thought; and the stance taken by Wittgenstein in his early writings, that the function of Philosophy is to show that there are no Philosophical problems (1969). However, an Ethics may be confrontational without being excessively positivistic; it will be argued that juxtaposing Acts and their consequences (for instance) produces considerable clarification. In this view, axioms of behavior may be artifacts that arise because the Laws of science are not understood; consequential arguments are unmanageable because they are incomplete (i.e., they lack the vision that complete data would provide); and custom varies because bewildered clinicians huddle together for warmth. To know all would be to rise above any specifically structured Ethics. This characterization of confrontational Ethics is in no sense a condemnation or a belittlement. *But to many readers it may seem to be ominously deconstructive and to throw a heavy burden on the use of phronesis and illation* (which we shall be discussing in some detail later). *For this reason, it is dangerous to ignore the other systems we discuss here.*

Commentary

The more one reviews these various possible systems, the more difficult it is to make a single choice among them. Our own approach is one of the utmost dispassion: we are in no hurry to reach a conclusion. Indeed, there is no deadline at all. A spirit of scholarly detachment in Ethics is not to be discarded because of some wholly mistaken sense of the urgency of the answer, any more than the deliberations of science are to be abandoned because of some urgent technological demand. In emergencies, more than likely, casuistry will supervene. To take an ironclad, irrevocable position prematurely will almost certainly mean some betrayal. To be sure, one may view some particular perspective as the most profitable line of inquiry; but it is precisely by keeping weaknesses as well as virtues in mind that the richest advances will be made. That very state of mind must demand that Ethics be treated as a dynamic field of inquiry, not a topic that must be formulated in terms that thenceforth are to be treated as inalienable. There are some who would see Ethics in inflexible terms. They should learn from the rather bumpy fortunes of physics. Even now there are scientists who cannot imagine that we should ever have to abandon relativity physics (any more than their forefathers could imagine that we would ever abandon Newtonian physics). But history suggests strongly that this premature hardening of ideas always impoverishes in the long run.

However, to suspend final judgment indefinitely is not the same as to say that one is wandering in a featureless desert, or is incapable in concrete cases of making judgments that are at least approximately sound. To anticipate later developments, we remark here that even where ideal judgments exist, it may not be feasible to use them because of issues that are of the essence and in conflict with the idea (e.g., urgency).

Perhaps a brief critique of the present strengths and weakness of each of these main types of Ethics may serve better than further generalities. It will become evident that many of the difficulties have little to do with Ethics itself and a great deal to do with our patchy and distorted understanding of Medical facts and principles.

STRENGTHS AND WEAKNESSES

Axiomatic Ethics

Axiomatic Ethics starts out in a privileged position. Not only has it had a long history (at least as far back as the Greeks), but it also is the embodiment of popular, somewhat outdated middle-class sentiment. The man of principle is regarded as the most admirable;[3] his chief rival, the consequentialist, is dismissed as a villain of expediency. The reasonable man is regarded as the superior intellect, the man who knows his own mind, the man not swayed by facile tears and sentimental tricks. The scholar, scientific or humanistic, looks up to those who try to hold a rational outlook on life. As Keane (1984) pointed out, it is only belatedly that there has emerged

3. In view of the Victorian sententiousness of the sentiment, the word *man* is here used advisedly.

some sensitivity to the coldness, even brutality, of a narrowly rationalistic Ethics. Indeed, Keane insists that "the rational" properly embraces all that is human, and not merely the abstract operation of the intellect.

But leaving aside the criticism that axiomatic Ethics is cold and incomplete, how well does it measure up even by its own chosen criteria? Axiomatic Ethics is not exactly the same as Logic; but we might borrow analogous wisdom from history. The virtues of deductive Logic are narrow but highly successful, whereas induction is rich but, formally speaking, in a much more precarious state. We might expect much the same to be true for Ethics. But the difficulties are vastly greater for Ethics than for Logic. Flew's principle (1989: 22–24.) can always be used as a safeguard in Logic, but formal statements in Ethics forfeit much of the natural symmetry to which the Flew principle appeals. The problem is discussed in Chapter 3. Those who have no axe to grind will always wonder where the axioms of deductive Ethics are supposed to come from. Insofar as they come from some revelation, they will be suspect to those who do not believe in transcendental authority. On another front, we have learned, if not to mistrust, at least to be chary about what is "obvious to all those of good will."

Of course, it is unwise to make too much of the contingent nature of the axioms. Theory of genetic counseling (A. C. Stevenson, Davison, and Oakes 1970; Murphy and Chase 1975; Emery 1976), for instance, enjoys the benefits of a deductive science, despite the fact that epistemologically it was originally derived (Statistically and ontologically) from experience, and thus technically comes under the rubric of induction. Popper (1959, 1963) has persuasively argued that the belief proper to systematic testing of a hypothesis transcends in certitude the purely inductive character of passive and casual observation of experiences.

Besides, many of the axioms are not matters of fact but matters of reasonable aspirations that would have wide acceptance. Killing for no purpose would get little support from reasonable people; pain that is in no sense useful would be widely deplored; there would be general belief that there are such matters as the good, the beautiful, and the true to be cherished, however much dispute there might be about details, or however much purely technical discussion might snipe at them. None of these informal statements is put forward with the weight of considered or demonstrated values. But a know-nothing stance can be pushed to absurd limits. It is difficult to see what is gained by trying to pretend that the inquiring mind starts out with a totally clean slate. Inchoate sentiments are neither here nor there in the formal arguments, but they at least color the prior judgment as to whether a proposed line of exploration is likely to lead to something of interest.

One feature that makes axiomatic Ethics suspect is the feeling—warranted or not—that it is put forward as a permanent structure, that there is to be no radical tampering with the axioms later on. We hesitate to pronounce on the point where the axioms are in the domain of Philosophy. But some of the propositions in Medical Ethics are squarely in the domain of science; and there the prudent have learned not to adopt adamantine attitudes about even the best-attested facts.

We quote one simple, even trivial, but nonetheless telling case.

EXAMPLE 2.6. Veatch (1981), in an example he deliberately selected as trivial, addresses the question of the need to get the mother's permission to do a chorionic biopsy during pregnancy. To be sure, her body will certainly be invaded, and that requires her consent. Now, why should the mother's permission be the *only* issue? We believe Veatch's analysis to be incomplete, for he overlooks an anatomical fact that is not scientifically in dispute. It seems from the example that the tissue being biopsied is at least in part fetal. Is the father (as de jure one of the guardians of the fetus's estate) not therefore to have an equal say in the matter of the biopsy? The issue arises only because scientific studies have shown that the chorion is at least as much a fetal tissue as a maternal one.

Whatever may be said about Philosophy, there is certainly a bewilderingly fast turnover of Medical data and facts. One would like to have a means of redressing an old opinion if it hangs on what subsequently turns out to depend on false information or on misinterpretation of sound facts.

Consequentialist Ethics

Extreme attitudes of the consequentialist principle are so easily demolished as to be hardly worth considering. Even the most fanatical consequentialist would draw the line somewhere, under pain of being excluded from all reasonable discourse; and even the most vehement anticonsequentialist would have to concede that there is some virtue to consequentialism, or have to take on the task of explaining away such principles as "By their fruits you shall know them" (Matthew 7:20) and "Greater love has no man than that he give up his life for his friend" (John 15:13). The extreme principle "Better that the whole world be destroyed than that a single lie should be told," if put forward as an Ethical principle without benefit of ontological modification, is one over which any reasonable person would choke. No amount of dedication to principle can leave one utterly unmoved by the consequences of an Act, however impeccable its axiomatic origins.

The very real force of the consequentialist view readily distracts one from the much deeper issues. Here we confine ourselves to what are Medical, rather than Moral, arguments. It is all very well to say that some procedure is a matter of unconstrained private choice provided that it does not harm anybody else. Waiving any objections to that principle, it is surely making a prodigious claim that one can be sure, or even reasonably sure, that anything done even in extreme privacy will harm nobody else. The concern is not with accidental consequences—the carelessly discarded banana skin on which a politician slips and breaks his leg, an accident that ruffles his temper and leads to the outbreak of war. We refer, rather, to results that are probable, perhaps inexorable, but so far removed from the original action that, through personal or collective ignorance, they are not foreseen. The point has not been wholly lost on the exponents of Chaos (Gleick 1987). That fact, of course, is operating in the domain of Ethical agnosia and does not in itself constitute an Ethical counterexample. It is merely a word of caution about the bold claims of the assumed harmlessness of private acts and the threadbare character of the "How was I to know" defense that may be used in exculpation. If through agnosia no positive claims can be made, by symmetry neither can negative claims be made.

EXAMPLE 2.7. The infamous influenza pandemic at the end of the First World War has ever since caused experts in public health to be alert to similar catastrophes. In 1976 there were some signs (including a relatively high mortality) that an epidemic of swine influenza was starting, and a strenuous immunization program was mounted in the United States. It was foreseen that, despite every precaution, the immunization was not without risk, and complications occurred, many of which were considerably delayed. The details do not matter here; the point of the example is that serious latent effects of a course of action must be reckoned with even when immediate circumstances make it necessary to take such risks. A recent paper (P. S. Moore and Broome 1994) explores the multiplication of variations within variations in the epidemiological pattern of the analogous condition meningococcal meningitis in central Africa, which in their complexity tax the prescience of even the most expert.

It seems to us doubtful that the more vociferous and intemperate consequentialism involves commitment to study anything but the most immediate consequences. Of course, one may analyze all the evidence and still decide that the particular course of action is, on balance, warranted; but, let it be hoped, there will be as much concern for the future as the axiomatics has for the past.

Popular or Traditionalist Ethics

The traditionalist approach has many desirable qualities. In the first place, it is readily available to the layman and those practitioners who do not enjoy the leisured exactions of scholarship. When compared with axiomatic and consequentialist methods, it presents a refreshingly whole-thickness, integral, approach to life. A danger with abstraction is that the abstracter can pick and choose the domain of discourse, rejecting any component, not on grounds of importance, but insouciantly because it is not amenable to some favorite process of analysis. The anomalies that may result can be dismissed, even callously dismissed, by conventional formulas often in flat contradiction with each other ("Hard cases make bad law" and "There is an exception to every rule"). The popular view will give this attitude very short shrift. Traditionalist Ethics is often quite inarticulate, even incoherent; on the other hand, like the proverb, it is often the "wit of many and the wisdom of one," which in itself became an anonymous proverb (Bartlett 1962: 1007).

Devotees of English common law would see much merit in traditionalist Ethics. There is force in the conservative principle of that great liberal, Chesterton: those who would change a custom would do well to try to understand its origin; it takes some arrogance to dismiss this pregnant but inarticulate vote. The main strength of the Ethics of custom[4] is that it is an embodiment of the will, conscious and unconscious, of a community.

Nevertheless, custom must not be mindlessly romanticized, and there are popular practices that no reflecting person would support. Furthermore, one must exaggerate neither the antiquity nor the corporateness of a practice.

This suspicion of spurious venerability must be active in the somewhat different case where the custom is not that of a community at all but rather that of a profession in that community. Members of a profession have all the advantages, but also all the disadvantages, of learning. Among the latter is contagion of belief, however rootless. The sword of the arrogant is not the weapon of democracy and hallowed by it; and the pen is mightier than the sword. One influential writer such as Galen can lead a profession astray for many years. And while our immediate topic is not Medical belief but Ethics, no doubt the same contagion infects Medical Ethics. One of the great perils of the guild or the professional society is that in ensuring probity in the short term, it may imperil that probity in the long term. Too often it is from outside the Medical profession that the greatest drive to reform and modernize has come (as penal reform, health care, the management of the insane, and slum clearance did).

Pragmatic Ethics

The pragmatic system may be considered a type of popular or traditionalist Ethics in which the collected wisdom is organized into principles of judgment. The border between traditionalist (acP) and axiomatized pragmatic (AcP) Ethics may be difficult to discern in operation. Distin-

---

4. A proponent might triumphantly point out that this term is a tautology that slips by unnoticed because of distortion. The word *ethics* is derived from the perfect tense of the Greek verb *ethizo* (to become accustomed).

guishing these two types depends upon how much appeal is made to an organized and reduced corpus of practice.

Commonsense Ethics

The commonsense scheme of Ethics is so popular and so attractive that to many there is no reasonable alternative. What more is there to take into consideration than what sensible people do and what science tells us will be the consequences? It is precisely those who see Ethics in this light who will be the least tolerant of interference from the outside. Indeed, if Ethics is nothing more than interference by people who have little knowledge of science, who have never been on the "firing line," and who appoint themselves as custodians of all the common sense, it would be difficult to defend its intrusion of axioms and principles.

Two major difficulties make the commonsense system difficult to operate. The more serious difficulty is that common sense does not naturally lead to due process, and whether we like it or not, in times of dispute we always look for a coherent system of arbitration. Arising out of what (for example) the Legal system will say or the penalties it imposes, there is a demand, however grudging, for at least forensic axioms and principles. We repeat the view expressed in Chapter 1 that these disciplines are not Ethics proper; but we may not deny that they are at least substrates for Ethics to work on. Whatever most people may profess, less and less do they hold ultimate loyalty to common sense; and since what professes to be common sense is often uncommon nonsense, we must be grateful that there is an escape hatch.

The other defect is that even among experts' experts there may be honest dispute over consequences. Moreover, the perceived consequences depend on the state of knowledge, which is continually changing. Those experienced in the practice of a learned profession will not be dismayed by this mutability. Apart altogether from disputed inference among professionals, understanding may be shaped and clouded in some individuals by a past experience of the disorder at first hand, in themselves or close relatives. They are apt to attach too much weight to that vividness and to overlook the fact that wisdom and skill are constantly changing with further development and experience. There is much idle chatter in the newspapers and on radio and television that implies that the wise professional lives on a diet of headlines from fashionable Medical journals. It is well to recognize that many of the professionals, for sound reasons, are reluctant to change their beliefs at every gust of wind; they suppose that their beliefs have a certain momentum of credibility that should be changed only by sufficiently sure accessions of knowledge. One can understand the concern that the wrong kind of axiomatization may petrify what is an unsound belief; but stone has the virtue of solidity that amorphous, ever-changing floodwater does not. Yet stone too may be lethal when attached around the neck. The field of healthy scholarship is surely best seen as dynamic, not static; and even when it is in equilibrium, it is a dynamic equilibrium. Unchanging views are unworthy of the word *ideas* unless their stability is sustained by unflagging critical review.

Consistential Ethics

The idea that Ethics should have the same kind of structure as science is a very appealing one: that the axioms (theoretical predictions) and the consequences (data) should be co-equal criteria, each respected in its entirety and neither allowed to override the other. These goals may seem incompatible, but they seem so only if Ethics is supposed to be a simple struggle for power and not a pursuit of complex truth and elusive equity. The notion that axioms must be respected in their entirety carries with it the imperative that such axioms are to be the best that the mind can currently grasp; as such, they are ever open to responsible amendment and refinement. In turn, the consequential aspect of the liaison carries its own drive to perfection. Unfocused reminiscences or vague inarticulate experiences are in no sense adequate. When both arms of the Ethics are arranged for the best possible effort, the system is then put together and constantly refined by a coherent *dynamic iteration* between them. The tactic is one, not of internecine struggle, but of mutual support. We call it *iteration* by analogy from mathematics, which we may illustrate.

EXAMPLE 2.8. It has been known for nearly two centuries that certain kinds of equations cannot be solved by any finite explicit recipe. The numerical solution is then attained by a system of improving approximations in which the mathematician tries one value and from the extent of its inadequacy systematically amends it to give an improved approximation. The goal is to reduce the inadequacy by the approximation, which is in turn improved by heeding the adequacy of the next attempt. There is to be no sense that either the accuracy of an estimate or the adequacy of the solution has a preferred status. Both must be satisfied.

In the Ethical context the most beautiful axioms are in some danger of being a crystallization of the wrong idea. The most extensive data, whatever their quality, may equally be irrelevant; and they will certainly not, of themselves, provide any system at all. As Popper (1959) points out, the touching belief in the power of unpolarized compilation of fact to illuminate is a system of knowledge that happily died with Francis Bacon.

EXAMPLE 2.9. Suppose that a society disapproves of killing. From this attitude one might abstract a first general principle that killing is unethical.

But then the consequential feedback: a strict constructionism would then infer that to slaughter, to swat flies, or even to use penicillin to kill bacteria is unethical. This excessively strict formulation would call for amendment, and the second version of the axiomatic statement would result—for example, "To kill human beings who are not harming us is unethical." And the second consequentialist feedback: X may feel that Y, a business competitor, does him harm, and therefore he may kill him. This conclusion would be too lax and call for a third statement of the Ethical principle. And so on. Eventually the scope of the principle is defined by testing the limits. Also, the Ethical (as distinct from a purely Legal) statement would include some principles of mercy and tolerance. Above all it would be dynamic: constantly awash with new insights, theoretical and pragmatic.

The difficulties with consistential Ethics are that progress is slow and time-consuming; and that it is unfamiliar or at least untrustworthy to many doctrinaire ethicists. There is an echo of this mistrust in the tendency of the less well educated empirical, and theoretical, scientists to belittle each other; but while no reputable scientist would approve of such polemics, comparable clear-sighted tolerance does not carry over into discussion of more personal matters such as behavior.

Finally, a pure consistential Ethics on these terms pays no heed to matters that do not lie within the domain of brute fact or austere reasoning. We shall consider this problem forthwith.

Consensual Ethics

The attraction of consensual Ethics is that it remedies the principal defect of consistential Ethics. Its ultimate criterion is the uniting of all three channels of input: formalism, fact, and custom and sentiment. It is perhaps the only system of Ethics that will ever really be trusted by all. Here the iteration employed in reconciling axioms and consequences is extended to cover custom and sentiment, which modify, and are modified by, the other two considerations; and the actual iterations may follow vastly more alternative pathways. Be it noted that the demand is true consensus, that is, a *thinking together*. It is not a clash among exactions any more than there is competition at the heart of consistential Ethics or mathematical iteration. If some serious body of opinion is not respected, then it seems that, however elegant in other respects, the system of Ethics is inadequate. But as before, each of the claims made by a body of opinion to be heard and respected exacts its own burden of responsibility for excellence. Just as bad axiomatics or incorrect science has no legitimate warrant, neither does shoddy custom or venal political pressure. However much we respect compassion and sentiment, we must recall that, under pain of nihilism, Ethics is to be a system; and the demands of coherence in a system, however much it may falter in the face of knowledge or understanding, must never be strategically abandoned. Needless to say, consensual Ethics is the most difficult of all and the one most slowly attained, for it is to respect and meet the needs of all constituencies. Consensus is more rapidly attained in some areas than others. But even so, it is not a static affair. Ethics is a dynamic state, not a petrified set of conclusions; and while it is not to be endlessly shattered at every whim, it must remain open to an orderly growth and enrichment as our understandings become deeper.

Situational Ethics

The notion that no contributing factor exacts inalienable respect raises some fundamental issues that we shall try to address, however inadequately. For those seeking an Ethics and intending to go on seeking it, *in principle* it is absurd for them to turn their backs on coherence. As the proverb goes, there is no point in keeping a dog and barking yourself. But having the instruments to overtrump injudicious conclusions from a theoretical argument is a redress against the only too real possibility that the Ethics is unsound or that the material on which the conclusion has been based is inadequate. Thus, to reject what one has concluded is not necessarily intellectual dishonesty: "A foolish consistency is the hobgoblin of little minds" (Emerson 1841). Any mathematician is familiar with facing an outcome that does not make sense and then hunting for mistakes first in the calculations, next in the algebra, then in the very axioms, and finally in whether or not the problem is "well defined." Such soul-searching lies at the very heart of science; once in a while it will lead to what Kuhn (1970) calls a scientific revolution in which some deeply entrenched system of thought is overthrown for a better, as Newtonian mechanics was forsaken for relativity physics. Good Ethics too can have no truck with propping up shoddy arguments. We have more to say about these special judgments in the next chapter.

On the other hand, an argument is not better because it is newer; quite the contrary. A fifty-year follow-up of the latest innovations—in art, in literature, in science, in theology—would show that very few fashions have lasting value, and that when the dust settles, the sum of human wisdom is little affected by them. Easy come, easy go. If some movement is motivated mainly by novelty, it is foredoomed; novelty is the quality above all qualities that does not last.

When a conclusion comes under question even though it is in accord with what is known of axiomatics, of consequences, of compassion, then it takes proportionate reasons for rejecting it. The image of physical inertia (or momentum, as some prefer to call it) is a highly apt corrective.

EXAMPLE 2.10. Suppose that an entirely new operation has been performed four times, and two of the patients have died. The conventional estimate of the mortality rate is 50%, and all in all that estimate can rarely be much improved upon by taking thought. But its implications may be probed. The occurrence of only one death might have been an unlucky freak accident. The occurrence of two deaths would surely strain that belief. But if the two patients who died were the first two who had the operation, we might wonder what impact those deaths had on the surgeon's skill. Perhaps all four patients were among the most severely affected and the operation was performed in the spirit of desperation. But whatever reason and imagination might urge, the data are few, so that the current belief does not, cannot, have much momentum. Ten more operations may produce striking differences for better or for worse. However, if the honestly estimated mortality rate were based on the first hundred operations, then there would be a far higher level of momentum, and it would take a much larger body of data to make much difference to that view.

There has been some attempt to construct an Ethics of exceptions that might have some analogy to equity in common law. However, there seems to be no justification for it in principle. Here we need to distinguish two kinds of cases.

One class of cases concerns idiosyncratic, wholly unforeseen, and perhaps unforeseeable combinations of circumstances that may perhaps never recur and certainly will be exceedingly uncommon. If there is genuine hardship, the ethicist might be disposed to mitigate the decision. But this course merits three caveats:

(1)   To convert the mitigation into a jury-rigged qualification (like an amendment to a constitution) is a violation of at least the spirit of the principle of conterminality addressed in Chapter 1. It is to be tolerated ad hoc only grudgingly and with profound professional embarrassment, if at all.

(2)   The special provision is indeed a mitigation, not a true exception; that is, it has to be seen as an exception not in judgment but in management.

(3)   The mitigation is not to constitute a precedent. Otherwise, the case should be dealt with under the second class (as follows).

A second class of cases involves crass defects in the Ethical formulation; here the term *exception* is really a misnomer. The remedy is to amend the formulation. The *cause célèbre* is then no longer an exception. It is to be noted that, even so, the amended formulation should respect the principle of conterminality.

Common law (in England, at least; less so in the United States) is encumbered by the principle that it is bound by its own decisions. But to our mind Ethics is not juridical but perpetually open to iteration. Moreover, the devices with which the law must rest content are not binding on Ethics and need not, indeed should not, be conserved. If there is a *coherent* system by which the anomalies of some system of Ethics may be righted, that is manifest evidence that the Ethics was improperly constructed—that the axiomatics of the system of exceptions should have been part of the axiomatics of the original Ethics. If that is the war that the situational ethicists are fighting, then we have the greatest respect for their honesty, but little for their Logic. Adding an annex to an existing building that would be cumbersome to replace may be tolerable if it is harmoniously done, but designing an annex in the first foundations of the building seems to make no sense.

One must, then, distinguish between rebellion against the system because it is inadequate and rebellion on principle. We do not imply that even those acting in the strictest morality are bound to adhere to any Ethics whatsoever. But we presume that those who are looking to Ethics for help are not attitudinizing but genuinely want help; and in proportion as they really need help, they are under some kind of at least intellectual imperative to abide by the results even if the results are of little help, just as whoever turns to mathematics is not merely looking for corroboration of prejudices.

Nihilistic Ethics

The position of nihilistic Ethics is (quite literally) unthinkable. One cannot think about what has been declared to be outside all articulated thought and coherent expression. We do not care to speculate about the moral position of the nihilist, except that to us it seems most unattractive.

However, yet once again, we may wonder whether nihilism is a true profession of belief or whether it is a rhetorical expression of revulsion against what its proponents see as shabby logic-chopping and dusty facts, just as dadaism in painting was an expression of revulsion, or the theater of the absurd. Are the proponents saying no more than that the defects they see in existing systems of Ethics are so gross that those who cannot see them would have no hope of understanding the concerns of the nihilists? Is the principal basis for their stance in effect a frustration over communication?

CONCLUSION

The foregoing discussion is intended as a reasonable working model of the possible structures of Ethics. It is put together in such a way as to include all the possibilities we can identify. However, it is not in any sense intended to be immutable. For instance, the rather loose category of custom is capable of much subdivision; so is that of consequences, although rather less freely; even axioms are not all of the same type. More or less extensive elaborations of these ideas will emerge in amplifying various topics in the chapters that follow.

We have a reservation to the foregoing scheme that we can hardly express without an extensive treatment. In brief, it resides in the problems and paradoxes that arise when we try to represent the idea of Ethics as an object of study by the ethicists whose thoughts, then, are to be supposed to occupy an ontologically higher position. We address this matter at greater length in Chapters 14 and 15.

3 Some Paradigms

I n this chapter we address explicitly some important, germinal, arbitrary ideas that may be unfamiliar to some readers. They are diverse, and (at this level, at least) the relations among them are only loose and often not at all obvious. Nevertheless, we shall be referring to them repeatedly, individually and jointly, throughout the book. We trust that the connections will become more evident in due course.

PARADIGMS

The original meaning of the Greek word *paradeigma* denotes a blueprint, a model, an example (Liddell 1889). The paradigm of a Greek verb comprises the stems from which the various tenses and moods can be remembered (more familiarly known in Latin grammar as the principal parts of the verb). Latterly the word has been used in many contexts in such a broad array of senses as to multiply confusions and ambiguities. We use *paradigm* here to denote at best a minimal set of germinal features in which Medical ontology deals. We hope that the following few paradigms, together with others we shall introduce later as needed, will reduce some of the misunderstandings about the scope of analysis of certain elementary problems submitted to Ethics. Discussing these components calls for delicate refinements; but they differ from the particular topics of later chapters in having greater fundamentality and broader utility.

REFINEMENT AND PRECISION AS A BASIC TENSION

There is a clash, which is not merely vexatious, between the more *structured* Ethical systems and the more *nominalistic* ones (i.e., those that propose to regard every case as wholly distinctive and utterly peculiar). Axiomatic ethicists *(Acp)* mostly prize simplicity and decisiveness. Situational ethicists *(acp,* or even – – –) are concerned with fidelity to authentic detail and are activated by a concern that axiomatic Ethics will not do it justice. These sound, but conflicting, demands have a parallel in sampling theory and in Medical nosology.

To set the scene for the proposed answers, we first turn our attention to sampling, because while it is epistemologically important, the issues are emotionally neutral and, in Ethics, noninflammatory.

Conflict in Sampling Strategy

The clash in finite sampling may be put in the following rough terms.

EXAMPLE 3.1. Suppose that the goal is to find out how best to judge the efficacy of vaccination in preventing influenza. Because of cost, the number of subjects is limited to one thousand. How are they best selected? In young healthy adult males, the estimate of the effect will be fairly precise because the subjects are similar and (as is well known to Statistics, and indeed to common sense) Random sampling error decreases with increasing size of the sample. By this argument, it is best to study a single well-filled class. However, such results tell little about the value of vaccination in children, or in elderly adults with chronic lung disease. To answer these wider questions also, more categories of subjects must be represented in the sample. So, the one thousand patients must be divided up among more categories with fewer in each; as a consequence, the estimate for each category will be less precise than it would be in one single homogeneous sample. The broader the question, the less precise any particular answer.

Is there some other approach that would enjoy the advantages of both precision and diversity? As we shall see later, there is: namely, regression analysis. But it involves making some rather subtle (although plausible) assumptions, treating input as a more serious matter and performing a good deal more computation.

Take a kindred topic, this time from clinical practice.

The Medical Problem

In clinical Medicine the burden on the memory is a major constraint. In principle, the desktop computer with a proper information base and good retrieval system has dealt with this problem. In practice, it is still used sparingly.

EXAMPLE 3.2. Routine Medical care for a child includes measuring the weight. Now, weight varies with age, which must be considered in interpreting the result. The pediatrician may work from a table or a graph based on empirical data on weight, each class being the result from a small number of readings in healthy children of rather wide age classes. Probably, most sophisticated pediatricians work with standard growth charts. But the use of charts merely shifts the problem further back. What methods were used to compute them? Again, if the sample is limited, then either narrow or coarse predictions will result, as we have just seen. It may not even be possible to include such niceties as whether the child had been born prematurely.

EXAMPLE 3.3. Some extreme physicians may feel that patients whose blood pressure is in question can without any ifs or buts be managed by dividing them into "normotensive" and "hypertensive." This policy is open to the same criticism. The clash can be largely resolved. But we shall first try to show (by analogy) how these examples bear on Ethics.

The nominalist complains that, to keep the Ethics workably simple, the categorizers force individual cases into a few crude (and often ill-fitting) categories. The axiomatist complains that the nominalists want to make every case so different that the very notion of guiding principles is (by definition) meaningless: this extreme individualism denies that experience contributes to the current case—a preposterous conclusion. So far as they go, both criticisms have merit. But they are hampered by two defects: (1) the patent falsity of both *professed* positions, and (2) the mistaken belief that the clash in these conceptual frameworks means that their views are irreconcilable. Our answer, in no sense a compromise, is that the dilemma is false.

First, the professed positions are distorted. Categorizers do not believe that nothing whatsoever is to be considered except a few coarse criteria laid down by their principles. They too have compassion and concern. They may even have an *Ethics of exceptions,* well meaning but misdirected because it is both botched and cumbersome. Many amendments become necessary, not because of circumstances that were unforeseeable, but for lack of attention to fundamentals that were merely overlooked.

On the other hand, the most nominalistic do not in fact propose that wisdom and experience should be utterly ignored, a policy wholly at variance with what anyone actually does. Neither in giving nor in taking advice do they for a moment suppose that the opinion of the beginner is as good as that of the seasoned counselor. It seems that ultimately both extremists aim to encompass *both* coherent Ethics *and* the uniqueness of the person. Because both have formulated their systems inadequately, they suppose themselves to be at loggerheads.

The remedy, Statistical regression analysis, exists (Murphy 1997). But its price, though harmless enough, may cause some concern. One problem is that it discourages, and may even exclude, criticisms that we have elsewhere (Murphy, Rosell, and Rosell 1982) termed *pentheric,* a term we now briefly address.

THE PENTHERIC

The notion of the pentheric is real and important, but it has not received the attention it deserves. Partly the reason is that it always brings to light what is a defect, even an embarrassing defect, in the way a proposition has been stated; and partly that it always calls for amendment that is more or less untidy. The flaw may be crass and obviously stated; it may be subtle and elusive.

EXAMPLE 3.4. In a trial at law, it is often the task of the *advocates* to assemble the evidence and perhaps enlist expert witnesses and solicit their opinions. It is the function of the *jury* to decide whether the depositions are believable and competent. The *judge* is the sole person to decide on questions of law. Now, due process demands that no evidence be used that is not stated openly in court; and the jury are explicitly barred from seeking evidence on their own. At first sight, the division of duties is quite clear.

However, there is an inconsistency. The jury is selected under certain principles, including the principle that the members represent the lay public. But the lay public itself includes experts. It is not at all impossible that a member of the jury may be a much better informed expert than one of the expert witnesses; or for that matter the jury may include a judge, and a more skilled and better-informed judge than the one presiding. The jury are not barred from using any knowledge or talents they possess, which may lead them to override the evidence of the formal experts, or the rulings of the presiding judge about (for instance) what is admissible evidence. Moreover, they would be doing so for reasons that are not made explicit in open court, and not available for cross-examination and the other safeguards (see Chapters 14 and 15).

We have no competence to judge how this problem is to be resolved. But it is only when it arises for the first time that an opinion will be expressed about what the original implicit intent of the jury system was in regard to such an inconsistency. That is, the commonsense formulation of the trial system is having a quasi-assumption imposed upon it *after the fact*.

Let us at this stage attempt a definition:

DEFINITION.   A *pentheric* criticism (or objection or protest) is one prompted by a condition not stated in an original agreement because, although important, it was not explicitly identified.

The interpretation of (for instance) epidemiological information is perpetually awash from pentheric conditions. They are perceived only *after* the fact but treated as if imposed *before* the fact. The whole idea of scrutinizing the data, not only to test a predetermined conjecture but also looking for adventitious evidence to sustain or undermine the answer given to the main conjecture, is difficult to justify according to the classical Neyman-Pearson theory of hypothesis testing (Murphy 1982: chap. 2). It is clearly pentheric. It imposes major problems on interpreting the result of the analysis. That does not mean that this practice is outlawed, uncommon, or misleading. But it is not codified.

Indeed, one of the difficulties in explaining to those unfamiliar with the clinical diagnostic process is just how large the pentheric component in clinical Diagnosis is. The clinician persistently and correctly claims that *a diagnosis is a statement not about a population but about an individual person.* This very proper claim is misunderstood and is being more and more ruthlessly ignored (e.g., by the more extreme proponents of the multiple-channel analyzer). Arguably the goal of Diagnosis is to construct the sample space for the patient that renders each of the pertinent diagnostic data either mutually independent or redundant (Murphy 1988, 1992). That view is perhaps extreme. But there is no escaping the importance of the pentheric. In the diagnostic process there is a priori no sample space at all. The crisis (as it were) of the process is the *differential diagnosis,* the listing of possible diagnoses and the prior probabilities of each, and the conditional probabilities of each of the data, and the combined merits of each hypothesis. It is not until this stage (which may not be realized until far into the Diagnosis) that even a provisional sample space exists, and the plan to acquire more data that will, in some sense, be more decisive. But even so, every item in the differential diagnosis may eventually be rejected and some other explanation sought, including (in extreme cases) that the diagnosis is some rare disease that has never previously been recognized, and therefore could not have been present in any previous empirical sample space. But an orthodox Probabilist would look upon this whole process with abhorrence. A scientist, while aware that this outcome is not without precedent, would be dismayed by the fact that (unlike the scientific challenge to establish the truth of general and not merely idiosyncratic events) there is no possibility of confirmatory experiments and—since the event under consideration is rare and obscure—no reasonable hope of encountering further spontaneous cases.

Example 3.5. Platt cites an illuminating case, presumably from his own experience (1965). A patient presented with the complaint that he was passing green urine. The most likely cause of that rare sign is that he was excreting some vegetable dye, such as methylene blue. However, the alert and precise reader will note that the complaint here is a *symptom* and not a *sign.* The eventual explanation was that patient had hematuria (blood in the urine) and also happened to be color-blind. This unexpected diagnosis could, in principle, have been foreseen. Yet the writer of a textbook stating that "a polyp in the bladder may present with the complaint of passing bright red urine except in the color-blind, in whom it may be reported as green," would be suspected by more sedate colleagues of facetiousness. Those grappling with computer diagnosis could not rescue themselves by any such disdain.

PHRONESIS AND ILLATION

The Greek word *phronesis* in nontechnical usage meant prudent, reflective, deliberative judgment. Aristotle uses the word *phronesis* in his *Nicomachean Ethics* (Thomson 1955: esp. bk. 6) to represent a rather more structured sense than that loose notion implies, but nevertheless with a rather practical domain of application. Newman (1870: 278–79) wrote, "It manifests itself, not in any breadth of view . . . not studious to maintain the appearance of consistency. . . . Properly speaking there are as many kinds of phronesis as there are virtues." We owe to Newman the invaluable but subtle term *illation*. It bears clear relationships with both the pentheric and Flew's principle (1989; see below). It is akin to phronesis, but Newman gives it a distinct technical meaning [1] to denote a tempering of conviction, to ensure that the literal consequences of arguments (however good) are not accepted indiscriminately and without reservation. He deals with it in what we regard as rather existential terms and offers no concise definition. So far as we have been able to assimilate it (Murphy, Rosell, and Rosell 1982), we propose the following definition:

DEFINITION.   *Illation* is a quality that transcends inference and allows the mind to reach a final state of acceptance or rejection regarding a proposition.

Pellegrino and Thomasma (1993) give a slightly different slant to the word *phronesis* with interesting possibilities. They write, "Phronesis is the intellectual virtue that disposes us habitually to attain truth for the sake of action as opposed to truth for its own sake which is wisdom or *sophia*." This definition hints, but does not quite explicitly declare, that phronesis is to be an Ethical rather than a cognitive idea, which in turn seems to imply consequentialism, or at least not axiomatic Ethics of the form *Acp*.

Illation might be regarded as the final step or steps in the Chinese box (q.v.). From it originates the pentheric criticism. It may be the only point of difference between two persons in full possession of all the facts and arguments. Newman (1870: 281) wrote that "in no class of concrete

---

1. The word *illative* is derived from that grammatical contrivance the irregular Latin verb of which the principal parts are *ferro, ferre, tuli, latum,* with the prefix *in-* which by assimilation becomes *illatum* in the supine. Thus, *inference* and *illative* are cognates and in ordinary usage are treated more or less as synonyms.

reasonings, is there any ultimate test of truth and error in our inferences besides the trustworthiness of the Illative Sense." Ultimately the most exquisite reasoning must be ratified by illation.

Clearly, illation may be abused, and no doubt it often is. But even apart from the courtesies of debate, to impute dishonest use of illation is a perilous tactic. Inability to grasp what the grounds for illation in others may be — or, for that matter, misgivings about one's own motives — is no warrant for leveling that accusation. These kinds of reservations about (in the very strictest aboriginal sense) the *integrity* of ethicists call for yet higher levels of illation. Grappling with, and criticizing, the upper regions of the Chinese box is always difficult and perhaps even in principle impossible. An illative veto may be the last stand of prejudice. It may also be the last bastion against absurdity. It is presumably the cradle of new and deeper insight.

The relationship to Flew's principle (1989: 23–24) is subtle but real. Flew writes that a valid syllogism "does not thereby force us, on pain of self-contradiction, to accept the conclusion. For it is another practically as well as theoretically important characteristic of such arguments that they are always reversible. . . . It always remains theoretically possible, and often practically correct to receive it rather as a disproof of one of the premises." The illative sense might be the principle of just such a reversal: the demand that there must be a flaw somewhere at a lower level in the argument or (by open extension) a chain of arguments.

Let us first, then, confront a very root of scientific conception.

THE BINARY PHENOMENON AND THE BINARY MODEL

The simplest possible descriptor of variable members of a class, the binary, is central to applied Statistics, genetics, epidemiology, and Medical Statistics. It radically proposes that members of a population, by their very nature, can be divided with respect to some characteristic (however trivial) into two unambiguous, mutually exclusive, and exhaustive groups; and that *further analysis can make no further use of the characteristic.* Now, this representation is an abstraction; and one must distinguish between the formal properties of the procedure and the faithfulness with which it is applied. A key, but usually neglected, question in any ontological analysis in Medicine is, What kinds of processes correspond, by nature and not by artifact or contrivance, to the binary model? In practice, the degree of fidelity varies widely. Some examples are given in Table 3.1.

EXAMPLE 3.6. Commonly, gender is seen as binary: every person is male or female, and for many practical purposes that is true. However, stringent epistemic and ontological standards tell another story. First, there are several possible ways of defining gender: anatomical, physiological,

Table 3.1.   Examples of Graded Ontological Appositeness of Binary Categorization

	highest	
Existence		Nonexistence
Positive electric charge		Negative electric charge
Hemoglobin type A		Hemoglobin type S
Alive		Dead
Male		Female
Right-handed		Left-handed
Clever		Stupid
Mad		Sane
Genetic Negro		Genetic Caucasian
Musical		Nonmusical
Employable		Unemployable
Friendly		Unfriendly
	lowest	

Source: After Murphy 1981a.

cytogenetic, immunological, hormonal, psychological, social. All these criteria conflict at one time or another. Second, the classification is not exhaustive because there are at least some few instances of true hermaphrodites who do not fall into either group.

We can construct a binary grouping by arbitrarily choosing one feature, the presence or absence of the Y-antigen, as the definition of gender. But in strict ontological analysis one aims for more than an arbitrary criterion as a deus ex machina—even one that in itself leads to ambiguity. If a few cases are misclassified, two conclusions follow. First, the definition may evidently be at odds with *ontological* gender, so the criterion is not the authentic binary trait but a fallible gauge of it. But second, there must be doubts as to whether *even in principle* there is a true dichotomy of gender. Certainly the existence of homosexuality (which, if the only purpose of sexuality is reproduction, has no evident Darwinian value) must fuel the doubts. Moreover, a third, neutral, gender is known in the insect world. (We stress that the object of this example is not to make any Moral or other judgment about homosexuality; we merely make the point that what at first sight may seem a simple, clean, binary variable, perhaps the most famous of all, proves on closer analysis to be much less clear.)

Such ontological problems are by no means a concern of Medicine alone. The dilemma of "the one and the many" (see Copleston 1948a: 57 ff.) is the oldest problem in formal Philosophy. The most enduring ambiguity in mathematics is over discreteness and the problems raised by continuity, which seemed to have been resolved early in the nineteenth century only to arise again at the hands of Kronicker (Bell 1937: chap. 25). Modern physics is still uncommitted over continuity and discreteness. In Table 3.1 we confidently dichotomize *existence* and *nonexistence,* since, at the present time at least, we find it difficult to imagine "slight existence" or to interpret it—except, perhaps, as a stochastic statement after the fashion of Schrödinger's cat (Schrödinger 1935; Penrose 1989: 290 ff.). But there are many cases where imposing an adamantine binary pattern leads to absurdity, injustice, even tragedy (e.g., in determining who is or is not eligible for military service).

We may add two brief notes on the binary classification. The first is that it leads naturally to the binomial and other binary distributions in Probability theory and Statistics and generalizations of it (e.g., the Lexis distribution, compound binomial distributions). The second is that binary classification may be generalized in another way, to other processes—such as ternary, quaternary, and generally manifold or n-fold—in which there are multiple, distinct, mutually exclusive, and exhaustive, categories, leading in their turn to multinomial distributions. We shall not discuss them in any detail; but they carry over the same ontological features and problems associated with the binary case. For instance, we might consider a categorization of gender into males, females, and hermaphrodites; or create an n-fold categorization by family size.

CONTINUITY AND DISCRETENESS

While avoiding formal mathematics, we address the idea of continuity insofar as it bears on Ethics. A rather simplistic test of continuity is that a sufficiently small step in one variable causes an arbitrarily small change in another. This notion is equivalent to saying that there are no gaps or sudden breakpoints, and hence that in some sense we can better understand what is going on at one point by knowing and taking into consideration what happens in its neighborhood.

EXAMPLE 3.7. The risk increases with increasing maternal age that a child will be born with Down's syndrome ("Mongolism"). The geneticist may need to know what the actual risk is in giving counsel to a woman of thirty-eight. It may be estimated simply from the data available from various studies such as Collman and Stoller (1962) of pregnancies in women of that age. The problem is that data for this age are scarce and the estimate imprecise. Pooling data on women aged thirty-seven to thirty-nine to increase the sample size is undesirable because even over that small range the rate changes; and the benefits from the larger sample are offset by heterogeneity, precisely the problem met in Examples 3.1 and 3.2. One solution is to use some kind of Statistical regression analysis.

However, regression demands that risk *be a coherent function of age.* That is, in every small age segment the risk either is fixed or is changing in a fashion that may be loosely described as small.[2] If the risk in the neighborhood of age thirty-eight is continuous, we may hope to enhance the estimate for all patients aged thirty-seven to thirty-nine. By extension, we may aim at a continuous estimate of the risk for all ages from (say) fifteen to forty-five: every datum at each age group contributes, however indirectly, to our knowledge about the individual risks for each and all. Ideally, we seek a formula that estimates risk just as there is a smooth continuous formula that converts temperature in degrees centigrade into degrees Fahrenheit.

The assumption that risk *is* a continuous function of age involves many well-known issues. In biological systems true discontinuities occur: there are critical stresses at which bones break, or critical concentrations at which kidney stones form. We acknowledge the contributions of Thom (1972) in the invention of catastrophe theory. We also recognize that (for instance) heart function in the individual patient may deteriorate steadily with age but punctuated by occasional abrupt deteriorations due to discrete myocardial infarctions (Murphy 1982: 178–79).

Deciding the appropriate mathematical form of the fitted function calls for subtle interactions among scientific theory, empirical evidence, and many technical details. We shall not attempt to discuss them here. Nevertheless, most people more or less explicitly appeal to continuity while recognizing that in many cases it is quite incongruous. Most physicians are happy with the statement that the victim of an accident has a slightly bruised leg, but not that the tibia is slightly broken. A person may be somewhat depressed but not somewhat married. A patient may be much more ill than he was yesterday, but not much more dead. We do not appraise these distinctions; we merely point out that continuity and discontinuity are widespread notions. To appeal to them is to introduce nothing foreign.

CRITICAL DISCONTINUITY

A continuously operating cause may be manifested as an interrupted effect, typically by comparison with some outside standard. This constitutes the threshold phenomenon. Well-known critical physical phenomena such as the freezing point of water, limits on the solubility of uric acid, or torsion fracture of crystalline materials may disrupt the survival of a cell. The disturbances of gas solubility in relationship to the depth and duration

---

2. To demand differentiability and higher continuity is too strict. The illative character of the discussion would make haggling over the status of Weirstrass functions (should they arise in some concrete case) absurd.

of scuba diving, the fracture point for bone on stress, and the rupture of a blood vessel are threshold phenomena on a larger scale that may threaten life. Thresholds are typically conspicuous in magnitude. Sometimes, however, there may even be doubt as to whether they exist, commonly for reasons that are epistemic rather than ontological.

EXAMPLE 3.8. The body is exposed to ionizing radiation, mainly from X-rays and radionuclides, encountered in Diagnosis, treatment, and physiological studies, and, more broadly, in industry. At first it was supposed that small doses are harmless, that there is a wholly safe threshold below which exposure may be ignored. Later it was argued by some that there is no threshold (Beebe 1981), that the risk is simply proportional to dose. Concern (much later politically inflamed by the irregularities at Three Mile Island and the frank disaster at Chernobyl) centered on assessing the risks and on trying to determine acceptable standards of control (U.S. Title 10, 1994). However, there is a root problem. If there is indeed no threshold, the minute risks from minute exposures will be very hard to detect. If the risk is (for instance) 1 in 10,000 in experimental studies in mice, it takes a prodigious size of experiment to establish with reasonable assurance that the number of mice affected is due to the effect of radiation and not merely a matter of chance variation from that in unexposed mice. Some ambitious studies to answer this question have involved a million or more mice, a scale of study at which there are perpetual problems in assuring satisfactory data that conform to rigorous standards of study. Of course, the demands of the notion of threshold are inexhaustible. But the Ethical question (which we shall not attempt to resolve) arises whether, threshold or no threshold, at some level of exposure it is proper to declare the risk "negligible," meaning not of no account whatsoever but something so small as to be "for all practical purposes" swamped by the risk from background radiation. This outcome may or may not be acceptable; but at least the precise ontological and epistemic nature of the proposition should be made clear.

CARDINALITY AND DIMENSIONALITY

Consider the impact of these notions of discreteness and continuity on our Medical ontology. The literal binary (or, rather more generally, n-fold) categorization means that *membership in a particular class comprises all there is to be found out about that individual datum.* The class is the ultimate and entire truth. All else is noise.

EXAMPLE 3.9. If patients each with a fractured scaphoid bone are a compact distinctive group—that is, if the patients do not have slightly, moderately, or badly fractured scaphoids—then their assessment, prognosis, and treatment are cleanly distinguished from those who do not have fractured scaphoids. A physician's management of a fractured scaphoid is not merely a quantitative variation from that for an unfractured one.

EXAMPLE 3.10. Obesity is not necessarily the same kind of problem. No doubt there is at least one ideal weight for each person; but there is no critical point at which the physician must suddenly change from complacency to urgent activity. An excess of ten pounds should be dealt with, although the earnestness with which treatment is given will differ from that for an excess of one hundred pounds or two hundred or three hundred.

Here, of course, there are two issues that are apt to be confused: (1) Surplus weight may be of concern simply because it may strain the heart and joints and interfere with social life. (2) Surplus weight may matter not only because of its mechanical effects but also because it is a symptom of some serious disorder of the psyche, hypothalamus, endocrine glands, liver, or heart. The prognosis in the latter case then may rest on a truly dichotomous diagnosis (namely, the presence or absence of a serious causal disorder). This caution points up the distinction (commonly overlooked) between *continuity in the effect* and *continuity in the cause.*

The Ethical *point d'appui* of this comparison is that some issues in Medicine are best dealt with as classes or (in the modern scientific sense) as *categories;* others are best seen as *measurements.* The distinction sets the scene for our paradigm:

DEFINITION.   The *cardinality of a set* is the number of elements in it.

EXAMPLE 3.11. The cardinality of the set of United States senators is one hundred.

EXAMPLE 3.12. The cardinality of the set of inpatients currently at the Johns Hopkins Hospital is equal to its current total number of inpatients.

EXAMPLE 3.13. The cardinality of the set of whole numbers (integers) is infinite.

DEFINITION.   The *dimensionality of a category* is the number of quantities or characteristics ascribed to the individual case in a particular context (e.g., Ethics).

EXAMPLE 3.14. In geometry, a single quantity (one coordinate) identifies a point on a line; two quantities (two coordinates), a point on a surface; three, a point in space; and so on. The respective dimensionalities are, then, one, two, and three. But the cardinality is infinite: the number of distinct points possible in a three-dimensional space.

EXAMPLE 3.15. The cardinality of the set of Ethical systems discussed in Chapter 2 is twenty-seven. The dimensionality of the category is three (namely, the axiomatic, consequential, and commonsense components of each).

If there are a few distinct and homogeneous classes, each abundantly stocked, then it may be best to treat each class as isolated and self-contained.

EXAMPLE 3.16. Animals may be two-legged (human beings), four-legged (horses), six-legged (insects), eight-legged (arachnids), and so on. This analysis does not appeal, really or by implication, to continuity of leggedness. The animals are so disparate that the data about them are best treated as quite unrelated sets. There is little to inspire hope that there is any continuity involved that is worth exploring. There is no interest in the properties of a five-legged animal, much less one with five and a half legs.[3] In contrast, there are systematic relationships in the structural properties of animals and their weights to which a paleontologist would appeal to infer the characteristics of long-extinct species.

IMPLICATIONS OF DENUMERATION IN THE ONTOLOGY OF ETHICS

Ethical decisions in accordance with *all* the circumstances command respect. Now, "all the circumstances" may be more numerous than what the axiomatist is accustomed to; but to the nominalist it will be far fewer than the number of individual cases to be considered which, though unique, are not totally unrelated. The uniqueness comes from cardinality; the number of pertinent features and circumstances is a matter of dimensionality.

EXAMPLE 3.17. The use of fingerprints as an identification of a particular person is justified by the principle that every person has a distinctive set: the (possible) cardinality of the set of fingerprints far exceeds the number of human beings. But to prove that claim, there must be a practical set of characteristics that make comparisons possible. The size of this set denotes

---

3. However, there is a curious instance of an ontogenic theory that a flower may sometimes have a nonintegral number of petals. There is a phenotypical counterpart (Pyeritz and Murphy 1989; Murphy and Berger 1991; Meyerowitz 1994).

the dimensionality of fingerprints, a vastly smaller number. Otherwise it is difficult to imagine how a manageable system for filing and retrieving fingerprints could be devised.

EXAMPLE 3.18. Consider the problem of setting up a fair system of food rationing in the face of famine in Ethiopia. Each person has claims to be considered. But the very number of different kinds of claims may make the task prohibitive. Arguably, needs (and therefore allocation of food) depend on *age, sex, occupation, state of health,* and *personal resources.* (Even that is a gross oversimplification, but it will do for our purpose here.) Age at last birthday would give perhaps eighty classes; sex, at least two, indeed three counting pregnancy, which would warrant special provision; occupation, perhaps twenty-five, some associated with heavy labor, some with exposure to particular infections, some (like lactation) requiring special supplements. States of health would number at least twenty; personal resources, perhaps four. The minimum cardinality of the set, then, would be 480,000. In contrast, the dimensionality is five: the terms in italics above. Another five factors to consider (e.g., vegetarianism, religion, food sensitivities, civic status, body weight) would make the dimensionality still only ten but the cardinality perhaps a billion.

A system of rationing involving a billion classes is unworkable. It would lead to so much error that the only alternatives are informal judgment and common sense, on the one hand, or a simple scheme in which details are ignored, on the other. Here the axiomatists and the situationalists are at loggerheads. Yet only ten facts are being considered in any individual case.

It is a common plea that rule by coarse principle must be, not merely tempered, but replaced, by exquisite judgment in the individual case. Thus, a rule that, though imperfect, is explicit, and therefore able to be tested, refuted, and corrected, is given up for an imperfect and implicit process of decision, usually merely masquerading as mature wisdom. Total Ethical nihilism argues that all cases are incommensurable, that Ethical formulations are pointless; and it proposes that every decision must transcend all possible formulations.

Yet it is not impossible to deal equitably with the problem. A solution lies in a quantitative relationship between claim and award; or, in less refined, more familiar, terms, the solution is a "system of points." In the penalty for driving offenses, the driver's license is suspended only when the driver has accumulated a critical number of points. In this way a comparatively minor offense does not in itself carry this penalty, but neither is it ignored. This policy is not the same as classifying offenses into all-or-none groups.

A parallel in Medicine is discussed in Chapter 10; in brief, decisions in Medical Ethics are not always dichotomous, instantaneous, or irreversible.

THE SLIPPERY SLOPE

Those who see discrete decisions as an indispensable part of Ethics, and categorical assertion or negation in ontology, are often uneasy about this latter kind of solution, in which the guiding principles are nearly all graduated. They suppose that the edges between the ethical and the unethical are as sharp as geological faults; softening the edge and admitting a no man's land is the thin end of a wedge that, as habit dulls the conscience, leads to progressive laxity. They talk of the perils of the slippery slope and see the worst of those perils as unawareness that one is on a slope at all.

Those wise and humble enough to learn from the corruption of the Nazis agree that this criticism has point. Like freedom, Ethics demands eternal vigilance and gives the most powerful motive for it. However, *motive* is no substitute for *reason*. That good people desire the good does not mean that they all have the same notions of what the good may be. In particular, we see two flaws in the concern with slippery slopes: (1) Fear, even when masquerading as vigilance, is no substitute for analysis of Ethical issues. Suspicion and recalcitrance toward changing do not prove good faith, a rule that applies equally to faithful adherence to ontological structures such as normality and freedom. (2) Perception of the good changes as knowledge and insight increase.

EXAMPLE 3.19. The belief that left-handedness is an abnormality to be amended even at the cost of distress or by frank cruelty, is now abandoned. (However, it is unjust to say that those who held that now-discarded view were necessarily malicious.)

LINEARITY

The course of many human issues that are rooted in common sense rather than formal theory follows from a more or less implicit assumption of linearity (Murphy 1979a). One example is the belief that if a hundred dollars spent on some cause will do good, a thousand dollars will do ten times as much good. (The economist's "Law of diminishing returns" denies this assumption, and so does the "Law of increasing returns.") The same linear assumption is commonly made about diet or vitamins or drugs in general, and the pharmacological notion of multiphasic response is again a corrective. A general scientific caveat about extrapolation in principle applies not only to linear models but even to models supposing continuity of any relationship.

The common empirical cause of this linear fallacy is that many relationships over a small distance may be scarcely distinguishable from a straight line. In other cases the discrepancies, though detectable, may be dismissed as trivial. Usually the discrepancies mount steadily as the use of the approximation is extended or the approximation is stretched over larger and larger intervals. This idea is so commonplace as to need no further elaboration. Nevertheless, it needs to be kept in mind, and illustrations of it arise in the next two paradigms.

INDEPENDENCE AND DISJOINTNESS

One instance of the linear fallacy is exposed by theory of sets, and hence of Probability. It calls for some attention to two phenomena widely confused even by professional scientists.

EXAMPLE 3.20. Consider two matters that are notionally quite unrelated: whether a patient has cancer, and the pattern that tea leaves form in the bottom of a cup. This unrelatedness is so widely accepted that to appeal to the tea leaves to diagnose cancer is summarily dismissed by scientists as superstitious. From such unrelatedness the Probabilist has developed the idea of independence.

Glossing over minor difficulties (Murphy 1982), we may state a simple principle:

DEFINITION.   Two events are *Probabilistically independent* if and only if the (joint) Probability that they will both happen is the product of their (marginal) Probabilities (i.e., the happening of each considered occurring in isolation).

EXAMPLE 3.21. Suppose that the (marginal) Probability is 10% that it rains tomorrow; the Probability is 51% that the first baby born in the world next month is male; and these two events are independent. Then the Probability that it will rain tomorrow and that the baby will be male is the product $(10\%)(51\%) = 5.1\%$ or, equivalently, $(0.1)(0.51) = 0.051$.

If the joint Probability takes some other value (say, 0% or 3% or 40%), then the events are not Probabilistically independent. If the joint Probability is 0% (i.e., it is impossible for both to happen), then the events are said to be mutually exclusive or *disjoint*.

However, in other fields there is a non-Probabilistic sense in which the word *independent* is used. To say that Robinson's food store is independent of Smith's means that they are separate enterprises that share no staff or property. Then the Probability that a particular person is employed by both companies is zero, which by the above definition means that the events "Tom Jones works for Robinson's" and "Tom Jones works for Smith's" are disjoint and that therefore *the two businesses cannot be Probabilistically independent.* This conclusion agrees with common sense. To know whether Brown works for Smith's changes our assurance of whether or not he works for Robinson's. So the term *independence* in the Probabilistical sense has a meaning different from the same term in the business sense. Confusion over this fact may have important Ethical consequences. The confusion is aggravated by the fact that in extreme cases the two senses are quantitatively very nearly indistinguishable. To find the Probability that *one or the other event occurs, or both,* one adds the individual Probabilities and (to avoid including the overlap twice) subtracts the Probability of both occurring.

EXAMPLE 3.22. In Example 3.21 the Probability that either it rains tomorrow or that the baby will be male *or both* (assuming independence) is

$$10\% + 51\% - 5.1\% = 55.9\%$$

But if they are disjoint (mutually exclusive), the term to be subtracted is zero, and the Probability of the one or the other is

$$10\% + 51\% = 61\%$$

However, if both events are rare, the product of their Probabilities may be negligibly small, and subtracting it will make little difference.

EXAMPLE 3.23. Suppose that one mature human being in ten thousand has a standing height exceeding seven feet, and that one in a million stands less than eighteen inches high. (The true figures are not critical to the Logic.) Obviously these events are mutually exclusive: standing height in any one person cannot be both over seven feet and under eighteen inches. Thus, the Probability of being under eighteen inches or over seven feet tall is a simple sum:

$$0.0001 + 0.000001 = 0.000101$$

There is nothing to subtract, because there is no overlap. If two subjects had been picked independently, the Probability that the first was over seven feet or the second under eighteen inches, or both, would have been

$$0.0001 + 0.000001 - (0.0001)(0.000001) = 0.0001009999$$

Such a difference is hard to detect empirically even in enormous samples. Clearly, in planning the size of a genetics clinic to manage these two groups of patients, the refinement would be ignored. In contrast, for people with arthritis and coronary disease, two very common disorders, the product term would no longer be negligible. Whether they are independent or mutually exclusive states would now be an important datum. The overlap may be as high as 100%. Moreover, there may be multiple illnesses that may call for Medical attention, and the Probabilities of two or more of them occurring in the same patient may be high.

The impact on Ethics of the linear fallacy (and the logical confusion) is greatest if a principle is first proposed when the approximation makes no practical difference, but the use of the approximation eventually leads to gross distortion.

THE BOTTLENECK

In a simple chemical system some ingredient is (in some sense) scarcer than any other and so sets limits on the maximum speed of the reaction. A small increase in the supply of it increases the maximum somewhat; but if the increase in supply of it is big enough, some other ingredient becomes the most scarce and hence takes over as the rate-limiting ingredient. Similar phenomena occur in more complex systems.

EXAMPLE 3.24. For instance, in the very early days of penicillin the treatment of patients was limited by the amount of the drug available. As the supply increased, the limiting step was the number of physicians skilled in its use; later still, the limit was cost; finally, the limit was the number of patients with treatable diseases.

EXAMPLE 3.25. Let us assume that it is desirable for pioneer populations to survive. In the early stages, in a benign and bounteous environment, the main threat to survival of the group is chance death or infertility due, perhaps, to a "run of bad luck" or some physical disaster or an epidemic. As the population enlarges, theory of branching processes (Fisher 1958: chap. 4) shows (what common sense hints) that the Probability of being wiped out by chance fluctuation falls. But the continued increase in population imposes other dangers, including scarcity of food. Hence, concern with survival imposes the precept "Go forth and multiply" in the early stages when the chances are limited by the number of people of childbearing age. However, in time the rate-limiting step in survival shifts to the resources of the community. Geometric (Malthusian) growth cannot continue forever in any finite environment, and then the best prospects for survival of the population are no longer served by unrestrained reproduction.

Even if the excess of that population could be accommodated by migration to other worlds, the duration of travel would no longer be negligible, and the rate of growth would be at most proportional to the square of time (the pattern of growth on a spherical front), which would not keep pace with a geometric increase of the nonmigrating part of the population.

It seems, then, that the applied Ethics of competition for resources is not immutable. Cost, for instance, limits the scope of renal dialysis (the "artificial kidney"). More recently, the diagnostic use of the MRI scanner has come to acquire a similar role (not, of course, Medically related in any way to renal dialysis). Examples 3.24 and 3.25 are pertinent but rather crude illustrations of finite resources from clinical Medicine. Their transparency stems from the fact that they involve a simple unambiguous bottleneck. It is scarcely surprising, then, that the examples that we know best are simple. The subject in general follows the pattern now so familiar in diverse fields: as the structure increases in multiplicity, the complexity mounts rapidly, and the reliable intuitions of yore prove no longer of benefit. There comes the need of the strategies for analysis of complexity that we discuss at length in Chapter 11. A fairly simple example may be used as a foretaste of the problems.

EXAMPLE 3.26. A chemical instance of some subtlety (Volloch, Rits, and Tumermann 1979; Libby et al. 1989) is a system of two parallel chemical reactions competing for a reagent. The first, biologically productive, reaction attaches a nucleotide to the growing RNA chain, A, to lengthen it by one unit. If the nucleotide presented is of type R, appropriate for transcribing the DNA chain, the reaction occurs easily and produces the new form AR. If the unit is not R but some other nucleotide, R*, it too may be incorporated to give the aberrant form AR*, but much less readily. According to the proposed mechanism for reducing the Probability of the aberrant form AR*, the inappropriate nucleotide R* is *specifically* degraded by the second, competing, reaction. Although R itself is liable to enter the second reaction and be degraded, it is supposed that this impact is negligible. What is not taken into account, however, is the fact that the very brisk consumption of R by the first reaction limits its availability to the second reaction. Further study (Butzow and Stankis 1992; Eichhorn et al. 1994; Butzow et al. 1997) showed that this removal accounted entirely for the supposed specificity of the second reaction to degrade R*.

Threshold processes that go beyond the trivial are not difficult to construct, especially in naive systems, such as classical quantitative genetics, that rely heavily on linearity.

EXAMPLE 3.27. Let us suppose the following set of assumptions that are neither implausible nor inconsistent. There is a simple threshold that relates the fragility of bone to the content of calcium phosphate. In accordance with the Law of mass action, the rate at which calcium phosphate is laid down in bone is proportional to the product of the concentrations of calcium ion and phosphate ion, so that the pairs of values giving any particular ion product plotted against their individual concentrations will follow a hyperbola. Suppose that the levels of these two ions are inherited as simple Galton-Fisher variables, so that the concentrations in any offspring will be the averages of the corresponding quantities in the parents. It is, then, easy to see that although the points for the parents may both fall below the threshold, the expected value in the progeny will be above the threshold. Treated as a black box (q.v.), the pattern of inheritance would be puzzling (Murphy, Berger, et al. 1988).

Competition in thresholds may make for puzzlement in clinical practice as well. We cite one instance that is well known to physicians but nonetheless apt for our purposes.

EXAMPLE 3.28. A patient with vascular disease in one leg has the typical signs of intermittent claudication; that is, during exercise of that leg there is lameness due to pain (with certain distinctive characteristics that need not concern us here) that gradually increases until further exercise becomes prohibitive. If the exercise is stopped, the pain will gradually subside. It arises, just as angina pectoris does in coronary disease, because the flow through the diseased artery does not meet the actual demands of the exercising muscle. The patient now undergoes an operation in which the diseased artery is replaced, and the intermittent claudication disappears. However, after full recuperation, the patient taking brisk exercise develops angina pectoris. It might easily be supposed that the latter is a complication of the operation. However, commonly it can be shown that the coronary artery disease was present, though silent, long before the intermittent claudication; but it has now become manifest because the bottleneck imposed by the claudication has been removed, and the least healthy part of the remaining cardiovascular system, the coronary arteries, now constitute the bottleneck. If the coronary artery disease could in turn be dealt with by operation, the next bottleneck might be in the heart valves and the new symptom be shortness of breath.

This illustration paves the way for the next section.

SUBSTANTIAL AND NEGLIGIBLE OVERLAP

If there are millions of strawberry bushes and two gatherers, there need never be any clash, and it is hard to excuse possessive squabbles between them. If there are three bushes and fifty gatherers, competition becomes an overwhelming issue. In Probabilistic terms, in the first case the proportions are such that independent harvesting by the gleaners may be treated as virtually disjoint, and the union is simply the sum, a linear relationship; in the second case this approximation (of ignoring the overlap) is too inaccurate, and the union falls progressively shorter of the sum.

It is simple to extend these arguments. At the level of bedside Medicine the competition is weak and largely limited by cost; but for heart transplants the bottleneck is not so much cost as the supply of skilled surgeons or the number of hearts donated.

Without proposing any concrete Ethical decision, it seems to us clear that a principle that is tolerable, even highly desirable, in certain contexts may not be sound for all situations. This relationship, coherent but in historical Ethics fragmented, leads naturally to our next topic.

THE TEMPORAL AND LOGICAL ORDER OF KNOWLEDGE

The truth or falsity of what purports to be an eternal or permanent principle has nothing to do with when it was first stated. Tautologously, eternal statements are outside of time. But one must here distinguish between the content of a statement and how far it is appropriate to believe or accept it; that is the distinction between ontology and epistemology. To the doctrinaire conservative an old principle is worthy of respect, and conversely to the radical mind. But to the nondoctrinaire, the conflict is largely spurious. The fact that the principle is both old and in active use will mean (among other things) that it has probably survived extensive testing; and the more tests, the more momentum it plausibly acquires, and the harder it is to replace or modify it. The loyalty of the conservative often comes from a confusion between age and experience, like supposing that the wise are to be found among the elderly rather than among the experienced. A decision based on current knowledge is in a fair way to become a precedent, that is, a principle to be "in possession" of our respect. The onus of proof, by serious evidence or by putting forward a better decision, lies on those who would demolish it. The conservative mind attaches much weight to the momentum; the radical mind, as C. S. Lewis (1955) has pointed out, tends to the error of supposing that it is in the nature of knowledge to decay over time and that, if old, it is by that fact alone in a fair way to being dismissed.

There remains the liberal view that the case should be judged and repeatedly rejudged on its *manifest* merits. Indeed, a principle that has been often challenged without failing should be respected; but if, though old, it has gone a long time without being asserted or challenged, it is apt to fall into disuse. The lack of recent challenges of the phlogiston theory of combustion means that it is not above criticism but beneath it; and the opposite is true of the principle that for a human to remain alive requires a steady supply of water.

Nevertheless, in argument from precedent there is a confusion of two clear issues. The most obvious truths and sound decisions based on them are apt to be formulated early in the history of a culture, when their evidential merit lies not in their antiquity but in their obviousness or plausibility. However, there is another merit competing with obviousness, namely, experience; but experience takes time. Thus, early decisions capitalize on obviousness whereas late ones capitalize on experience. Furthermore, the merits of formalized experience are within the domain of fact, not feeling. Among the common reactions to Darwinism (a conjecture poorly articulated by scientific standards, and difficult to document satisfactorily) was the early criticism that nobody had witnessed evolution occurring: we do not see monkeys turning into human beings. This argument supposes that a few thousand years of documented history are sufficient experience on which to make a judgment of what the theory had surmised may happen in millions of years.

It is only too easy to miss slight and slow trends, an oversight that may lead to petrification of either a belief or a system of behavior. In most systems there are or have previously been irregular devices for patching up incongruities (in law, equity; in biology, ad hoc hypostasis; in astrophysics, epicycles). But it seems that they are mostly devices for saving the appearances. The flaws would be better dealt with by recognizing that any formulation based on finite reasoning and limited experience is a more or less sophisticated approximation; and that there is much value in an openness to reformulation, not endlessly discarding one theory for another but seeking further refinement.

PUBLIC ETHICS AND PRIVATE ETHICS

There is a common, informal, attitude that the individual should be at liberty to do anything that does no harm to others. It embodies a protest against gratuitous interference by society in the private life of the individual. The protester is not necessarily more lax than the legalist; but perhaps finds impertinent the substitution of puritanism (legislated morality for all) for asceticism (freely chosen in private morality). As we saw in a previous section, judgment about whether or not any putatively private Act is independent of others is difficult; and legalistic ethicists complain that the proponents of this principle seldom try to make it conscientiously.

Leaving aside the merits of this claim, the question arises how far privacy may be seen to extend. Arguably a public assassination is more to be deplored than a secret murder, because it is apt to cause more civic disruption. Sexual activity that on any scale of strictness is proper in private may be considered grossly unethical in public. Inflammatory political opinions legitimate in dinner conversation create quite different Ethical problems from what may, without change, become incitement to riot in public. It is not our goal to discuss these general topics or to propose Legal policy. We merely cite them as agreed examples where distinctions are legitimately made according to the degree of privacy.

One of the key dimensions of an Ethical analysis must, then, always be *how many persons are involved in the Act.*

EXAMPLE 3.29. The decision by the Supreme Court of the United States in Roe *v* Wade (1973), while in no sense Ethically binding, draws a line that can be the basis of Ethical discussion. It states that before a certain stage of pregnancy the issue of abortion is a private matter between the mother and her physician. Now, clearly (to put firm though wide limits on the discussion), on the one hand, no modern court would sustain the principle that whether or not parents kill their newborn child is a private matter for them—although Roman law and the custom of Sparta gave that power to the *paterfamilias.* On the other hand, the court would argue that (with certain safeguards for the immature and the mentally retarded, and with constraints on incest) it is no business of the court to decree with whom a woman may have sexual intercourse. That is not to deny that in some societies fornication is a crime. We are not concerned here with making Ethical judgments. We simply point out that however much they may vary as to where the line is drawn, societies distinguish between what is lawful in private and what in public. Even the strictest religions at their most oppressive draw a distinction between private sins that call for private rebuke and public sins that incur public censure, excommunication, and banishment. In general we agree that publicness is a dimension of Ethics, even of the Ethics of personal Acts.

EXAMPLE 3.30. Use of some revolutionary new treatment of a serious disease raises certain questions, which we shall not attempt to address here. However, we may distinguish two kinds of Ethical issues involved:

1. *Private Ethics:* There are issues to be weighed of short-term and long-term risk; consent of the subjects; delegated consent from parent or guardian; the use of volunteers, of convicts, of the mentally retarded; the qualifications of the experimenter; the soundness of the scientific underpinning; and much more. The previously sluggish public conscience has been alerted in recent years, and there is little informed complaint about either the need for Ethical review or the requirement that the research be done in accordance with current knowledge and understanding.

2. *Public Ethics:* While it is one matter to do such studies in private,

it is an entirely different matter to make public claims about successes. On the one hand there is the issue of the information being made available to the public; informing the political support for policies of the granting agencies; the priority of those making the discovery. On the other hand there are Ethical issues over false hopes; the forming of false Ethical attitudes among physicians not schooled in the techniques of avoiding pitfalls of scientific inference; precocious constraints on controlled trials needed to establish sound information. One must wonder how well this Ethical aspect of therapeutics (as distinct from fulfilling Legal requirements) is addressed.

TRIVIAL ETHICS

There is a Legal principle of convenience that the law does not deal with trifles. Unless an action either has some gravity in itself or is a test case of an important guiding principle in Legal judgments, it should not distract from the more serious business of the court. There is a tendency, to our minds a dangerous one, to intrude this principle into Ethics where there are no rival litigators demanding rapid relief for their problems. No doubt the more weighty Ethical issues give the most emphatic proof that Ethics has serious matters to confront. But we see their major and too often emotional issues as interfering with the cultivation, both personal and scholarly, of balanced and rational judgment. The big and dramatic issues—abortion, cardiac transplants, test-tube babies, brainwashing, human experimentation, the brain-dead, sexual seduction of the mentally retarded, and the like—mobilize much emotion.

There is another, more insidious, difficulty in preserving Ethical detachment.[4] There is a generalization, hard to document but attributable in substance to Norbert Wiener, that the closer a study comes to addressing human beings, the less it is amenable to disinterested rigor. The ideal of scientific rigor is physics; biology at large is much less rigorous, and human biology less rigorous still. Studies of human behavior are perhaps the least rigorous of all. Indeed, wisdom has decreed that much of the education of psychiatrists be directed to making them aware of personal differences and distortions in anybody's approach (including their own) in matters in which the person would be a party at interest. No doubt the problem is due in part to emotion and sentiment, and in another large part to the difficulties of maintaining rigor in complex systems, but the deepest problem

---

4. Current cant denotes what we are addressing as *objectivity,* a word that no doubt was once useful but as a result of overuse as an emotive term of self-approbation has to our minds become virtually meaningless for purposes of serious discussion.

is the reflexive character of studying human behavior. An ancient principle of symmetry is being violated: those doing the analysis are themselves part of what is being analyzed, and it is not at all obvious that they can ever do the analysis impartially. "No man shall be judge in his own cause." We have more to say about this matter in Chapters 4, 14, and 15.

Nevertheless, there seems little hope of escaping the need for optimal Ethical analysis. The best hope seems to lie in cultivating simultaneously the qualities of sensitivity, dispassion, and thoroughness. Now, there are better and worse ways of seeking them. The fledgling tightrope walker is advised to practice a foot above a mattress rather than two hundred feet above Niagara Falls; pianists should cut their teeth on *Tunes for Tiny Tots* rather than Liszt's *Transcendental Studies*. So it seems prudent to develop and sound out Ethics by many preliminary analyses of small problems, although the impatient are apt to dismiss them as trivial because they generate no deep emotion.

EXAMPLE 3.31. One seldom sees in textbooks of Medical Ethics analysis of such topics as circumcision in infancy. Yet it is a model topic that illustrates many issues—for instance, the limits of the arrogation of consent; the claims of preventive Medicine and their relationship to urgency (or lack of it); what mutilation consists of, and when it may be justified; as to ritual circumcision, the issue of the individual's freedom to choose a religion, and the broader question of what limits there are on anyone (including parents) presuming to prescribe the education and irreversible formation, physical or psychological, of children. Yet the common reaction would be that all this fuss is being lavished on the removal of a few grams of tissue. By this, as it were, Ethical disdain we repeatedly miss the chance to develop a spirit of cool Ethical analysis and instead let what is called Medical Ethics degenerate into a heated exercise in little more than common politics.

EXAMPLE 3.32. To judge by the tone of nonacademic Medical Ethics, there are big differences among attitudes to a blood transfusion, a marrow transplant, and a kidney transplant. The clinical differences—risk to donor and recipient, permanency of the impact on the donor, assurance of success, and much more—are easy enough to identify. But if Medical Ethics has anything to say about the one and not about the other, it would be interesting to have an explicit statement of where *in principle* the intrinsic differences lie. Arguably, Ethical *isolation* of the three cases, one from another, is an infringement of the principle of conterminality. Yet apart from objections in conscience, Medical Ethics would regard technically competent blood transfusion as of no importance (except, perhaps, for the danger that it will spread infections). Our implied demand for ontological cohesion (a matter taken up in Chapter 5) is not at all to deny that cardiac transplantation raises radically new issues in epistemology (at various levels including scientific proof of efficacy), in the ontology of life, human life, and personhood, as well as in the Ethical analysis.

We believe that indulging what we might call scale-dependent Ethics in any field inspires no confidence in the probity of the Ethics. There is probably as much importance, if not more (in terms of lives threatened, if nothing else), to exploring the Ethics of whether office workers with the common cold should be required to stay at home until recovered, as there is to the Ethics of research on recombinant DNA. But we might foresee a deplorable attitude that to talk about the Ethics of the management of the common cold is a macabre parody. Insisting on scale-dependence is like supposing that the aim of piano playing is to interpret concertos, and that therefore the pianist should never practice five-finger exercises. We suggest the following principle:

• No Ethical problems are important or trivial purely on grounds of scale.

COMMENT. When we say that there are no Ethical problems that are trivial by reason of scale, we do not mean that there are no trivial Ethical problems at all. There is some danger in the other extreme: to see radical Ethical problems in every possible activity—making telephone calls, putting stamps on letters, cleaning the office. Medical practice would rapidly become unwieldy if every action had to be analyzed in this fashion. Nor are we proposing that slippery-slope Ethics (q.v.) be assiduously cultivated. What we urge is the distinction between Ethical problems that are easily solved (e.g., the operation for acute appendicitis) and in that sense are trivial; and Ethical problems that are intricate and full of interest, but trivial only in the vulgar sense that they would not make the newspaper headlines. In the same way, a mathematical problem may be trivial because it is solved and the answer is well known. *But no unsolved mathematical problem is trivial in the mathematical sense.* It is the goal of mathematics to have available an answer, or at least the apparatus for finding the answer, for any problem that can be cast in mathematical terms. Just so, we suggest that an unsolved Ethical problem is never trivial, however small its impact on the world of concrete experience.

4 Philosophical Interfaces

The principal purpose of this book is not to prescribe how Ethics is to be developed or applied, or what the qualities and merits of various solutions to Ethical problems may be and how we might judge them. Rather, it is to identify and declare the need for vigilance over a special task that may be stated in the following terms. Consider a methodical attempt to amalgamate, or at least to appose or put in contact, aspects of Ethics and of Medicine.

• Then the terms in which the Medical contribution is cast must be safeguarded.

They must be authentic and experiential, not casual and ill-informed inventions of those expert in other fields but not in Medicine. Our goal is to foster the best and most faithful formulations of both Medicine and Ethics with a view to integrating them. The challenge is not to make an exhaustive listing of particular instances, but rather to inspect the methods to be used for doing so.

It is fitting that we should be diffident about the niceties of Philosophy just as it is that the Philosopher be diffident about Medicine or science. Every dog barks in his own yard. But barking dogs are better employed when they are hunting together than when they are disputing bones and territory. However, both groups of experts suffer from the fact that there is not (and, indeed, perhaps could not be) a broker competent to assume responsibility for establishing the union. Clinicians and the scientists of health and disease are therefore obliged to do the best they can to clarify the biological and Medical issues; and then—the major task—to try to identify the appropriate points of contact in Philosophy and Ethics and open up negotiations on these terms. However, if the latter are to be anything more than bland expressions of goodwill, some risks will be involved. Moreover, one cannot communicate in any technical detail without technical words and (what is much more important) technical content. Hence the need for this chapter and the one that follows. Of course, it is not intended as the last word on the terms of the negotiation; it is much more like the first. We shall be surprised, indeed disappointed, if there are no amendments and corrections to their opening formulation forthcoming from the Philosophers and especially the ethicists. Even then, much iteration will no doubt prove necessary. This chapter is inevitably fragmented since, by implication at least, it covers a wide area. We group the topics as best we can, even sacrificing some technical detail to coherence.

THREE DISCIPLINES OF SPECULATION

We have so far rather informally used two technical Philosophical terms, *epistemology* and *ontology*, that we have borrowed, giving them something of our own special meanings. Somewhat belatedly, perhaps, we shall attempt to explore how they are to be defined. To align in parallel the structures of Medicine and Philosophy, we shall introduce a third term, *provenience*, the standing of which is less conventional but which is nonetheless important to safeguard Medical representations. By way of an introduction we may set up a simple familiar relationship, which we intend not as an exposition but as an analogy.

A Talking Point

Suppose that an unknown quantity has to be estimated empirically. (We say nothing further at this stage about the quantity or about the domain of the inquiry.) The process involves three considerations:

1. The quantity must exist, or be believed to exist, or (at the very least) be surmised to exist.
2. There must be available evidence bearing on the value of the quantity.
3. There must be a method of analysis with the aid of which the answer is to be inferred.

EXAMPLE 4.1. Thus, in the scientific domain, demographers may wish to find the size of the population of Baltimore. First, with some care they define exactly what they mean by the various terms (*Baltimore, size, population,* etc.). They peremptorily dismiss, as absurd, the idea that the quantity should not exist, even in principle. (Whether or not it is feasible to find the answer exactly is a quite different issue that makes no difference to that assumption.) Second, they construct a sampling strategy and collect the data. Third, they employ some Statistical procedure of estimation, the relevance and properties of which should be well known from Statistical theory. They are then ready to publish an estimate and an accompanying statement of assurance about it (e.g., a standard error or confidence limits). At that stage the task is finished and the answer is, by nature, stochastic; that is, it is not a statement of unconditionally guaranteed truth (as the solution to an equation might be) but one that is claimed to be more or less close to the truth.

The structure of this task may be discerned in many other kinds of problems undertaken by different kinds of investigators using perhaps quite different methods: mathematicians, historians, particle physicists, literary critics, social anthropologists, cognitive psychologists, and whatnot. Each of the three components may, when necessary, be expanded to any degree of elaborateness. Instead of a simple statement of the number of inhabitants of Baltimore, or of the value of a physical constant, or of whether a painting is an authentic Vermeer, the first component may be a matter of a highly sophisticated physical theory, or a conjecture about a lost civilization. The second component may involve an intricate experiment by an exclusive device such as a cyclotron or the Hubble space telescope; it may mean an exhaustive search for evidence, the nature of which cannot even be guessed at in advance and may emerge only in the light of subsequent findings. The third component may demand during the analysis an ingenious exploration of code-breaking invented expressly for that purpose, which can be recorded only after the fact but cannot be prescribed.

In principle, the three components may be quite distinct and different undertakings. In practice, there will at times be fuzzy boundaries. But also the fact that we have numbered them does not mean that they have to be carried out once for all and in any particular order. There may be endless iteration, "backing and filling," between the data and the attempts at code-breaking, for instance. As the evidence is more thoroughly scrutinized, the formulation of the first component may need to be revised, perhaps radically revised.

Example 4.2. Cosmologists seeking how the various biological species originated, for instance, were persuaded by the evidence to consider possibilities other than special creation or some other teleology including Wallace-Darwin evolution among the candidates. But that broadening of outlook did not at all mean that the *search for an explanation* was in any way being compromised.

Example 4.3. Rutherford's attempts to split the atom by bombarding it with small particles compelled him to abandon the idea that an atom is a compact and physically indecomposable solid, and to conclude that it is a porous structure the vast majority of which is empty space. However disconcerting, research is always apt to disrupt; only the shallow suppose that its only purpose is to confirm preconceived ideas. Nevertheless, Rutherford did not abandon the idea that the atom has *some* structure, not to be invented but certainly something yet to be discovered. The first component was preserved despite the radical change.

Later theoretical physicists were compelled to give up some time-honored paraphernalia: such cardinal demands as that there has to be a mechanically faithful model, that the model must be not only conceivable but imaginable, that the theory have a commonsense referent, and all the rest. Indeed, they were prepared to settle for naked statements in mathematical symbols that can be manipulated by arcane rules subsequently developed from quaternions, tensor calculus, theory of strings, and the like. The apparatus of inference (the third consideration) from Random variables unexpectedly became a literal representation of the reality being sought: the distribution of a particle became the particle itself. Yet with all these unsettling disruptions, the same structures, however distorted, survive.

Heartened by this cosmic robustness, we may, at least by analogy, attempt to identify counterparts of the components of Philosophy to which we might turn and attempt communication (subject, of course, to the ratification of the Philosophers themselves).

Ontology

Identified as a branch of metaphysics, *ontology* is variously, and in some ways not very helpfully, defined as "the study of the nature and relations of being or of a theory about the same" (*Webster's* 1988). Other definitions found in texts by distinguished Philosophers (chosen casually rather than in any systematic survey) are in many cases agreeably informal and sometimes include incisive contrasts that anticipate our concerns with the next topic. Flew (1989: 51) gives us this definition: "Ontology is concerned with what there is, whereas epistemology is the study of how we know, if we know and what we know." Searle (1992: 18) puts it thus: "There is a distinction between answers to the questions, What is it? (ontology), How do we find out about it? (epistemology), and What does it do? (causation)." Cantore (1977: 11) is more decorous but more daunting: ontology is "the reflective study of the objective intelligibility of reality made accessible to man through his own knowledge."

Most scientists would agree that in some sense there is a quarry to their pursuits: an entity, to be discovered, not invented, having some quality of invariance that allows meaning to the statement that such and such a theory is an accurate portrayal of that quarry. Even those such as Wittgenstein and Russell, who in their early writings abandoned metaphysics, and Ayer (1946), who vehemently denounced even the idea of metaphysics, seem to have found it necessary to conserve the notion of ontology. Russell (1940:

22) explicitly repudiated the most extreme interpretation of this view later: "I conclude that 'truth' is the fundamental concept, and that 'knowledge' must be defined in terms of 'truth', not vice versa." The only serious writers who seem to be trying (somewhat ambiguously) to demolish even ontology are the most positivistic of the subjective Probabilist-Statisticians (see Kyburg and Smokler 1964); but their treatment is so formalistic as to leave it unclear whether their studies ever have any point of contact with ontology.

Epistemology

Traditionally termed Major Logic, epistemology deals with "the study or a theory of the nature and grounds of knowledge especially with reference to its limits and validity" (*Webster's* 1988). The rather less austere definitions of Flew and of Searle have been quoted above. Popper (1959: 15) writes, "The central problem of epistemology has always been and still is the problem of the growth of knowledge," a definition that we find rather too all-embracing to be helpful in distinguishing epistemology from ontology. (We do not find it at all easy to think of what in the domain of Philosophical inquiry would be excluded by Popper's definition.) Cantore (1977: 11) designates epistemology as "the study of knowledge as an activity of the subject."

Authors seem to use the adjectives *epistemic* and *epistemological* as interchangeable, and we shall follow suit.

COMMENT. Insofar as epistemology may be cast as the ombudsman of Philosophy, to keep speculation sound, and charged with the task of laying down the rules and method for doing so, it clearly has vast scope. However (to appeal to an old dictum), who is to guard the guards themselves? Not only must ontology respect epistemic standards, but epistemology must itself be subject to ontological analysis. If it were to be asserted (for instance) that, in mathematics, Logic is a self-sufficient, self-governing, self-correcting discipline, then that would itself be an ontological statement and (we hasten to add) not at all a self-evident one. Indeed, however incompletely, epistemology must help to police epistemology itself, as ontology should (as it were) ontologize itself; that is, its explorations and speculations should include, among other objects, itself.[1] We are led to suspect that these two terms *epistemology* and *ontology* are best seen as describing *attitudes* and *disciplines* rather than boundaries drawn about some constricted domains of application, much as, in coordinate systems, the various coordinates (or axes) represent incommensurable directions rather

1. Here again we encounter the Chinese-box phenomenon of Chapter 3.

than specific finite quantities. Just so, genetics, biochemistry, and cardiology are in no useful sense competing for territory but are three separate attitudes often addressed to the very same data.

These definitions leave these subjects broad enough to allow the greatest comfort of debate. Epistemology seems to cover at least two major topics that prompt us to propose a third term.

Provenience

Medicine, like all fields with both a scholarly and a professional perspective, has a complicated structure and operates under the moral weight of its own imminence. Medical scholarship involves both the collecting of evidence and the formal analysis of it. These two matters in science, and especially in the complexities of Medicine, are viewed as operations radically differing in method, field of expertise, and the nature and quality of the statements made. A very large part of the collection of data operates under the protection, but also the discipline, of epidemiology, or population genetics, or Psychology and psychopathology, or pathology and other clinical sciences. The strictly formalistic analysis (the second consideration) of the data is the special domain of the Statisticians and the mathematical Statisticians, who (a lively interest in the issues involved notwithstanding) have professionally, for the most part, been scrupulously careful to keep away from any issue of the *biological meaning of the data* as distinct from the *formal meaning of the mathematics*.[2]

We may, then, choose to regard these various kinds of activities as subdivisions of epistemology. However, we prefer to confine the term *epistemology* to the task of interpreting and disputing the meaning of the evidence, and to accommodate the collecting of evidence in a third division that we designate *provenience* (which, having its own adjective ready-made,

2. For instance, when Statisticians test hypotheses about genetic data, what is tested is not, strictly, whether "the inheritance of a trait is autosomal recessive" but whether "the value of the segregation ratio in the progeny of two carrier parents is 1 in 4" and corresponding ratios for other mating patterns. Failure to grasp that Statistical hypotheses deal with *values of parameters,* not with *actual biological entities,* may lead to absurdities (Murphy 1981c). Again, a test—based on a specified size of sample and a specified size of test (significance level)— of the number of loci controlling a trait might propose the value 2 under the null hypothesis against the value 5.3 under the alternative hypothesis dictated by the conditions of the experiment. This might be required despite the fact that "5.3 loci" has no genetic meaning. If duly warned that the answers under both hypotheses must be integer, Statisticians, with some loss in the tidiness of the answer, could readily meet this requirement. But most mathematical Statisticians would probably consider it not their responsibility to inquire after that constraint, which they see as a matter for the scientist to declare beforehand and not as a pentheric protest. Authentic *bio*statisticians or *bio*mathematicians would regard it as a major responsibility to inquire about such details, and to make sure that they understand the biological nature of the experiment sufficiently to make a sound judgment on their own.

seems to us a better term in this context than the more familiar word *provenance*). We define it thus:

DEFINITION. *Provenience* is that domain of scientific inquiry concerned with the identification, specification, and safeguarding of the standards of procurement of empirical evidence. It covers both the soundness and properties of the scientific methods used and the formal concerns of sampling.

We propose the corresponding adjective *provenient*.

We cannot undertake here any detailed account of the contents of provenience. Much of it is the stock-in-trade of the wise and experienced epidemiologist and is discussed in textbooks of epidemiology. Specially Medical features of it (e.g., the nature of gray-box modeling, which we address in Chapter 5) are the subjects of a former publication (Murphy 1997). Chemical, physical, and kindred technical methods are ordinarily policed by the parent discipline, but certain aspects (e.g., reproducibility in aliquots, common confounding of effects, etc.) may call for epidemiological attention.

The neglect of provenience in the broad domain of Ethics and Philosophy of science we consider deplorable. It has deep roots. Traditional Philosophy (which we do not presume to judge) treated scholarly inquiry as a matter of coherent argumentation (epistemology) about the inner nature of things (ontology). But the empirical data were seen as patent, obvious, deserving no more special and coherent concern than an adequate supply of oxygen so that Philosophers could speak to one another. It would be difficult, for instance, to imagine any Philosopher up to and including Hume ever seeing fit to address formal sampling theory; and the concerns of the founders of that field (notably Bayes and Bernoulli) were treated as minor technical matters, no doubt so readily resolvable that the epistemologist could deal with them in a footnote to sound speculation. That attitude is still rife among physicists and chemists, to whom the notion of "representative sampling" still seems trivial. If a sample is heterogeneous, why, it can be purified by various techniques (filtering, recrystallization, and whatnot), the "impurities" discarded, and the purified compound then examined at leisure. That may be all very well in high-resolution fields of the study of phenomena, the ontology of which is assured. It is emphatically not all very well in biology and Medicine, where there is no a priori agreement as to which is the compound of interest and which the contaminant, where epistemology will make little progress so long as they are divorced from provenient methods.

It is interesting to note how physical cosmology in the twentieth century has rather shamefacedly embraced the matter of *abundance* of the various elements; and to note the absurd analytical refinement of the chemistry of samples taken from the surface of the moon and treated as (in some useful sense) "typical samples," although selected by methods that an epidemiologist or a Statistician could only regard as ludicrous, from a sample space that cannot even be defined. These niceties might make no difference to Aristotle or Galileo or Francis Bacon, but they would make an enormous difference to Bayes or Fisher or Kolmogorov. There is, of course, no reason why epistemologists should not undertake the responsibilities of provenience; all we can say is that they have not done so. It is remarkable, for instance, that Popper (1959, 1963) either totally overlooked or systematically ignored the relationship or, at the very least, the analogy between his principle of deductive testing and the Neyman-Pearson theory of power (Murphy 1982). Other than Hacking (1965), we would be hard put to name a professional Philosopher exhibiting any interest in provenience and stochastic inference. Carnap's interest was in probability (1966). Von Mises, despite his ontological interests (1939), would be reckoned a mathematician. As it is, the load of the fundamental theory of Statistical inference has fallen on the mathematical Statisticians; and we regard that as right and proper.

COMMENT. This third division, provenience, is only too easily brushed aside as a mere ornament. The seasoned scholar does not need to be reminded of the perils of abstraction, which facilitates coherent argument by weeding out much distracting detail from the fine flowers of thought. Enchanting as that metaphor may be, however, it presupposes the skill to tell a weed from a flower. That is no easy matter in so convoluted a field as Medicine. And it is made no easier by the often quite erroneous perceptions of Medicine that are contained in either the lighthearted incursions of the outside expert or the sententious statements of the Medical textbooks themselves.

EXAMPLE 4.4. A notoriously difficult topic, and (as we see in Chapter 10) one that is in the very thick of Medical Ethics, is the nature of Diagnosis (the diagnostic process). In the last fifty years there has been a massive increase in the number and scope of methods and tests available (which make for more reliable and precise Diagnosis), and in the extent of their use in practice. The price of this enrichment is that it has made the process of arriving at a correct diagnosis no easier. The great majority of such tests are of little general help and contribute most when the possible diagnoses have been reduced to a reasonably small working list. Together with the many snags of such tests (risks, expenses, delays, multiplicity of false positives, and all the rest), that elaborate change has raised major Ethical problems in its own right, some of which we address in later chapters. But the concrete task of the clinician in actual practice — sitting down with pen and paper and a few traditional clinical instruments to record some clues, and to plot the diagnostic strategy by talking for a limited time with the patient—is as difficult as ever, and perhaps more so. The simplicities of well-meant computer models of Bayes's theory, or of branching processes, do not touch the real issues at all. Histories are taken from patients; and patients may be confused or inarticulate, are often anxious, and are seldom trained semanticists or linguistic Philosophers. At their best, the Medical textbooks give accounts of how one might take an ideal history from an ideal, completely truthful and coherent, patient, and with such people computer methods might conceivably work. But we suspect that putting them forward as working models of Diagnosis as a process is the product of unalloyed thought rather than analysis of empirical data on how good clinicians actually operate. For instance, as we have pointed out (Murphy 1988), the alert clinician is always suspicious of the patient whose history is too orderly, too exact, too perfectly typical. The possibility that the patient is a neurotic or a malingerer and has studied the subject in a textbook should never be wholly out of the clinician's consciousness. But it is difficult to imagine how (without a great deal more precise and subtle information) a computer program could be written to take care of the telltale warning signs. How could a momentary hesitation in filling out a questionnaire be recovered by the computer? And if these are the problems in general internal Medicine, the difficulties would be far greater in psychiatric Diagnosis. When such an ill-conceived model of a wealth of thoroughly unambiguous, truthful, and reliable data in binary or measurable form is converted into the kind of stick figure that an abstraction extracts, it is scarcely to be wondered at if the conclusions reached by theory are so often rejected out of hand by the clinician.

SUBVERSION OF TERMS

From the ambiguities in the way in which areas of inquiry are so commonly formulated and the insights that painfully emerge from confronting them, there grew up early in the twentieth century the custom of beginning the reply to any formal inquiry, however innocent, with the formula "It depends what you mean by. . . ." Indeed, at one period some Philosophers were seduced into thinking of the entire corpus of Philosophy as the art of uncovering meanings (Ayer 1946; Wittgenstein 1969). Certainly, neglecting the precision of the meanings conduces to bad Philosophy and especially treacherous Logic. Studied neglect and obscuration of meaning are relentlessly exploited in the more disreputable rhetoric.

Malapropism

Technical terms are often misused by those moved by poetry rather than meaning.

EXAMPLE 4.5. The word *allergy* has a technical meaning, expressly invented to describe an intricate, wholly unconscious, type of body reaction that occurs upon exposure to certain foreign antigens. Occasional forays beyond that meaning have done nothing for the advancement of the study of allergy as a reputable clinical science. In journalese and soapbox oratory *allergy* has come to denote repugnance, a perception of something to be avoided (*Webster's* 1988: sense 4). It would be comforting to think that this misuse is never any more harmful than an unhappy but frank metaphor.

EXAMPLE 4.6. The word *inferno,* which means "the nether regions," Hell, is more and more used to connote great heat, the "blazing inferno" of the large burning building. The term, and nothing more, is borrowed from Dante's *Divine Comedy* (1300) and scarcely attains the dignity of being even a metaphor.[3]

One could instance any number of malapropisms that patients use, which need not concern us here. But there are many examples in which any scholarly analysis might more safely be applied to the data (which the clinician must hunt down) rather than the inferences from them (which is commonly what the patient offers).

The malapropism is by no means confined to the outsider but is embarrassingly often perpetrated by the professional who hears a term but never takes the trouble to find out what it means, even approximately. Examples are *inferiority complex, stress syndrome, epileptic equivalent,* and *adiadokokinesis.* We briefly address one such term that has some importance later, notably in Chapter 11.

EXAMPLE 4.7. Many probability distributions are symmetrical about some central point, notably the Gaussian ("normal") distribution. The notion "central point" is somewhat vague, but to the eye it is commonly seen as the location of the highest point, or the *mode,* and there is much talk of the significance of having more than one mode. In other cases (the lognormal and the gamma distributions being of particular import and familiar in Medicine) the pattern is not symmetrical but has a long tail "to the right" (i.e., toward the higher values of the variable). This pattern is called *positive skewness.* Sometimes, as we shall see in Chapter 11, in the empirical survivorship and, theoretically, in the *bingo* model, the opposite asymmetry occurs and there is said to be *negative skewness.* Unfortunately, there is a widespread misuse of the term *skewness* to mean *bias* or a systematic shift of the distribution. Then the statement "survivorship is negatively skewed" is taken erroneously to be an assertion that survivorship may be

---

3. Outside of a few lines in Canto IX, and a few more casual references in Canto XV, Dante's description of Hell scarcely mentions fire. The depths of Hell are freezing cold.

negative, which (all are agreed) makes no sense whatsoever. All the innocent statement is saying is that if the mode for survival is, say, 60 years, the chances of dying before age 10 are greater than the chances of living beyond age 110. (For the word *bias* to have any meaning in this context, one would have to define what the parameters of the distribution are and what the mean of the estimators are, which are totally different issues.)

EXAMPLE 4.8. It is a common mistake for a patient to complain of blindness in one eye (which, taken as a trustworthy statement, suggests a disorder located in that eye) and the clinician to record that without comment. Closer attention to detail may make it clear that the patient has blindness *in one visual field,* a homonymous field defect (which suggests a disorder posterior to the chiasma). The correct interpretation of what the patient is trying to communicate is likely to make an enormous difference to prognosis and management.

Such cases could be endlessly (but rather pointlessly) listed.

Unidentified Associations

A much more subtle and intractable contamination of words is the set of almost unidentified associations—flavors, commonly but not exclusively emotional—with which they become permeated. It is easy to compile a list of words such as *nice, silly, cretin, egregious, random,* and *gas* in which the associations have taken over entirely, so that even in the best writing we have divorced them from what the original meanings of these words were: *fastidious, blessed, Christian, outstanding, impulsive,* and *chaos,* respectively. This kind of drift may be unfortunate, but it is probably inevitable, and students of language have long since made their peace with it.[4]

The real danger lies elsewhere, however, and may be unappreciated, sometimes even after direct challenge.

EXAMPLE 4.9. The word *abolish* is widely used and understood. But consulting dictionaries may do little to define the correct context. A German visitor used the phrase "I used to have a dog; but he became sick and I had to have him abolished." In vain might he search *Webster's* (1988) for clues as to what makes that sentence ridiculous: that the word *abolish* has connotations of grandeur, abstraction, solemnity.

---

4. An interesting word is *leech.* It is commonly but erroneously thought to be a facetious transfer from the bloodsucking worm *Hirudo medicinalis* to the physicians, implying that the latter are bloodsuckers. In fact the original meaning of the word *leech* was *physician;* it is the attribution to the bloodsucker that is the facetious usage.

EXAMPLE 4.10. An instance rather nearer to Ethical concerns is the difference between *small* and *little* as applied to, say, a baby, a child, a school, a town. *Webster's* (1988), in one of the occasional sections on synonyms, says nothing of the overtone of appeal to chivalry in the word *little*. A small baby is one with low birth dimensions. A little baby is something helpless and appealing. "There is a small boy at the door" as like as not hints at mischief and nuisance; "There is a little boy at the door" conjures up a vision of his timidity, vulnerability, and other needs that we must be prepared to meet.

We may note that the wherewithal to discover these nuances of meaning short of prolonged total immersion in the culture is better provided in some languages than in others; see, for example, the distinctions for French given by Genouvrier, Desirat, and Horde (1977). Deliberately manipulating these niceties is the stock-in-trade of the more disreputable rhetoric. What is more, images are used in the same fashion.

There is a growing practice with the immediacy of the modern media for deliberate, often highly autocratic, trifling with the overtones of words. Even as we write there is being debated a deplorably artificial code of what is called the "politically correct," the kind of fad that would set itself up to compete with diplomacy without making any investment in either cultivating the perception or acquiring the experience to do it constructively. We regard it as a dangerous type of abuse. Even to cite examples is a touchy matter. To be wholly opposed to changes in the meanings of words would not only be foolish, it would be ineffectual. If total disruption of communication is to be avoided, however, the shifts of usage and evaluation must occur gradually and not be, like spring fashions, artificially changed every year by a privileged, but not for that reason endowed, class that have access to radio and television.

EXAMPLE 4.11. It now seems doubtful that the word *race* (in the anthropological sense) is so sharply focused or has such decisive characteristics as have been imputed in the past. Nevertheless, it still has a rough utility to investigators of population movements and such matters as the frequency of certain genes and genetic diseases. In his fourth edition McKusick (1975: table 53) gave a listing of many such disorders. Such a listing may actually help in Diagnosis in a disorder that may be commonplace to clinicians habitually working in one community and extremely obscure to those elsewhere. (A notable example is the prevalence of the bizarre and protean disorder familial Mediterranean fever in patients of Armenian descent). But we have all met those, even a few academic colleagues, who have decided to regard the words *race, racial,* and *racism* as all equally obscene. Since these words certainly retain some minor scientific relevance (despite the abundant genetic evidence of widespread miscegenation), banishing them means that more or less elaborate Greek or Latin vocabulary *(deme, ethnic group, reproductive isolate)* has to be imported to fulfill the very same function (indifferent resolving power and all) from which the word *race* has been outlawed.

There seems to be an active campaign against the use of the word *tribe,* which some regard as offensive. If successful, it will presumably create problems for the biological taxonomist, who will perhaps have to study Basque to find a suitably strange (and for the time being inoffensive) word to denote that level of taxonomic split immediately below that of the suborder.

COMMENT. This discussion may appear to be laboring minor points. We are convinced, however, that the wholesale imputing of connotations by fiat and the hawking of more and more arcane euphemisms—*draconian* for *cruel,* or *conflict of interest* for *jobbery,* or *disinformation* for *lies,* or *lobbying* for *bribery*—present almost insurmountable barriers to Ethical discussion unless terms are defined and preserved with the most excruciating care. Nevertheless, this recourse has its own perils, as we shall now try to expound.

SPURIOUS DEFINITENESS

Our task calls for much dissection of words, for in the main we communicate with words and all the perils attached to them. But words are only words. In nontrivial cases the principal difficulty commonly lies deeper. The main goal is not to play ducks and drakes with what words to use but to consider what notions purport to underlie them with which we have to deal. How far is the use of any word at all to be taken as a metaphysical endorsement of an idea? We deliberately choose an old example in which passions no longer run high.

EXAMPLE 4.12. Eddington (1928), in an informal account of microphysics written for the intelligent laity, discussed the fine structure of the floor and the furniture of a house as an assembly of subatomic particles filling only a minute fraction of the space they occupied, holding him up by constantly bombarding him like a swarm of bees. The solidity perceived in these gross structures, floor and furniture, is in fact illusory. The Philosopher L. Susan Stebbing (1944: 43), a contemporary of his, in criticizing his text on Philosophical grounds asks, "What can be meant by saying that 'the plank has no solidity of substance'? If a plank is not solid, then what is the meaning of the word solidity?" Stebbing flatly asserts, "Stepping on a plank is not in the least like stepping on a swarm of flies." Well, that was a typical challenge of the period (and one now sadly dated). We infer that

Stebbing was raising the objection that Eddington's use of the word *solid,* even in a pure negation, clearly implies that there are other things that are indeed solid, and that for some reason the authentic property of solidity is denied to his furniture. We shall have nothing to say about the soundness of this or any other assertion of hers.

It seems to us, however, that Eddington's point was that the word *solidity* and whatever its mental associations may be are fictive, and that it is certainly not a term to be employed or deployed in ultimate authentic questions in physics. Eddington, after all, is appealing to a respectable body of scientific theory and experiment. It is not at all clear what Stebbing would accept as an alternative interpretation, and we cannot undertake to argue her undeclared brief. On the other hand, in ordinary conversation there is a word *solidity* that presumably has some meaning even if it is only a crude one with little utility. Then it must be that the attribute of solidity, beyond a certain level of resolution, is not observable as a distinctive phenomenon at all and can serve no useful purpose, even as a fiction. It might be a proper and useful term, even a most fundamental one, in jurisprudence, orthopedics, or architecture, none of which addresses questions at the subatomic level. If so, then these three fields would have to assume the responsibility for defining the term. But it is useless issuing a subpoena or a set of building codes to a theoretical particle physicist and expecting, in any context whatsoever, an expert opinion on solidity, which, to such experts, is a nonquality. In the same way, "The sky is blue" is no doubt a statement of great comfort to writers of love songs and to painters and chambers of commerce, and it is perhaps pointless to tell them that the sky is not any color at all (as they could easily see in a flight on the Concorde). Dante, for instance, knew that on a brilliantly sunny, cloudless Italian day, predominantly the sky is white.

· At the outset of any discussion among experts of different persuasions, then, it is vital for serious purpose or useful outcome to address, examine, and if necessary define the terms exchanged in an appropriate analysis.

It is wise, however, to beware of the risks of implying, seeking, or in any way invoking the vaguely imputed phenomenology of such terms. The ethicists may discuss (say) *normality* to their hearts' content, with all the rights and privileges pertaining thereto. (We devote Chapter 8 to discussing it.) They are given due notice, however, that *there is no guarantee that any counterpart to their notion of that term exists in Medicine or that, in particular, in attempting to apply their speculations to Medicine, they will be able to find competent and pliant Medical experts to back them up.* Moreover, they may claim no right to demand one, and there is no onus on the part of Medicine to identify, provide, or seek any such counterpart to which the pronouncements of the ethicist may apply. This warning is not mere truculence. It is a necessary precaution to safeguard the authenticity of the Medical input into Ethics.

The matter of ontological and technical definiteness is sufficiently important in Medicine and Medical science to warrant the special discussion on ontological coherence in Chapter 5. We defer further discussion until then.

VOCABULARY AND DISPUTED IDENTITIES

The intricate topic of disputed identities represents the intersection between the last two sections. It can be only briefly sketched and sparsely illustrated. The problems of imprecision in vocabulary can hardly need more emphasis at this stage. The use of any purely lay vocabulary will no doubt always alert the thoughtful to the risks of imprecision and ambiguity. Medicine, science, and Philosophy all have rich technical vocabularies that, even with the most austere and economical policies, continue to grow; and as they do, ideally they endow scholarly discussion with incisive new tools.

The most treacherous kind of words are those that lie in between, that may or may not be regarded as lay words *(sick, tired, weak, dizzy)*; lay words artificially endowed with highly technical meanings *(likelihood, linkage, probability, strangeness, chaos)*; unabashed technicalities *(neurovegetative dystonia, variable expressivity, anticipation, Banti's syndrome, the Hayflick phenomenon)* that were introduced for good reason but, being obscure or frequently misused, must be kept under careful scrutiny. Reluctance on the part of either the scientist or the Philosopher in challenging the meaning, the metaphysical support, and the rhetorical overtones of any word used is to be deplored where there is any shadow of doubt on these points.

EXAMPLE 4.13. An outstanding specimen of the technical term that exhibits something of these perils, and is itself of serious importance to Ethics, is the word *fitness*. In the first place it is a lay word that is riddled with ambiguity. It has a great many meanings related to physical state and performance, appositeness, moral worth, decorum. It is sometimes a term of approbation, sometimes a nonprejudicial descriptor. Under the pressure of attempts to popularize Darwinism and the cult of progress at the hands of Thomas Huxley and Herbert Spencer under the motto "survival of the fittest," it has tended to be used mainly as a term of approval and aspiration. That motto itself was soon shown to be tautologous ("the survival of the survivors") and naturally to be neither verified nor falsified nor authenticated. It remained a vibrant slogan awash with emotion and desperately in search of a meaning. There have been a number of attempts after the fact to try to construct for it some useful scientific signification. Population geneticists have made two attempts (genetic fitness, or effective fertility; and evolutionary fitness, or the probability that a line will not become extinct either by selection or drift); there have been countless clinical and athletic uses; there have been cultural and social uses. It is scarcely surprising that there have occasionally been confusions among them, notably in the star-crossed historical eugenics movement.

Often, ludicrous conclusions are reached by sylleptic Logic (Murphy 1972) ("equivocation"), in which diverse senses are used in the premises and the conclusion. We take the matter up in dealing with normality in Chapter 8. The Philosopher is duly warned. Any vestige of meaning *normality* retains is apt to be swamped by the noise.

We note and commend, as a *façon de parler*, the guiding standard of whether or not (setting aside anachronisms) a proposition can be translated into Latin (Waugh 1964: 139). It has been extended in Russell's perceptive criterion admirably summarized by Copleston (1967: 224): "The significance of a sentence is that which is common to a sentence in one language and its translation into another language." It is, of course, useless as a *practical* criterion. The translation would have to be a faithful one, and to ensure that, we should have to know what the precise meanings were in the two languages. We should also be in some difficulties about how distinct the two languages would have to be. (Would Czech and Slovak be too close? Or Flemish and Dutch? Or British and American English?) And again, who is to be the arbiter of disputes over what the two languages have in common? Moreover, the best we could ask of this criterion is that it should be sufficient to establish a meaning. We cannot expect it to be a necessary condition, since there is no guarantee that there exists an adequate translation (and not merely an elaborate paraphrase) into any particular language. Nevertheless, Russell's criterion is an ontologically admirable statement of meaning. If a sentence cannot be translated into any other language, there must be a strong suspicion that it conveys no meaning and is merely an artifact of the flaws in the language of its origin (see Example 7.14). This notion is akin to the principle of conterminality. A serious effort in trying to translate faithfully the principle "the survival of the fittest" into a foreign language (or even to paraphrase it coherently in English) will convince the reader that it is empty.

Lexical Demolition

The introduction and elimination of terms (formally by deletions in Medical dictionaries, or informally by the actual use or nonuse of a word) has an incalculable impact on the repertoire of ideas. One could only wish that there were less caprice involved. Sometimes this is done to good purpose. The term *abiotrophy* has come slowly to signify nothing more than the unhelpful quality that a genetic condition comes, for no clearly specified reason, to be manifested later in life. The word is slowly dying out, and since it is a completely black-box term with no heuristic value, it will not be missed.

In contrast, it is remarkable how many technical words that do serve a useful purpose die out. The word *hypotrophy*, now to be found in only a few Medical dictionaries in English, seems to be an accurate term to describe only partial wasting away. *Atrophy*, which (it seems) should indicate total loss, has come to be used instead. It is sometimes clumsily qualified to give the unhappy form *slight atrophy*. On the other hand, the word *dysphonia* (impairment but not total loss of the ability to phonate) seems to have been wholly replaced by *aphonia* (again meaning a total loss) in Spanish. Cardiac *arrhythmia* and *dysrhythmia* are now almost interchangeable terms.

Sabotage by Association

Short of full demolition, words may be colored, restricted, or made more or less useless in coherent discussion by the accumulation of subtle distorting factors that may be perceptible when the words themselves are explicitly examined. It seems extraordinary that there is no English word that is the antonym of *exceed,* and some tedious paraphrase must be used. What is the opposite of "the prescribed amount of wine put in the stew should not be exceeded"? The simple answer, that the opposite is simply to delete the word *not,* misleads, for the word *exceed* (like its cognate *excessive*) has a hidden connotation of disapproval. There is a minimal effective dose of an antibiotic; but centuries of entrenched practice keep us from writing on the medicine bottle, "This dose must be exceeded."

EXAMPLE 4.14. Consider the verb *warm. Webster's* (1988) defines it as "to make warm"; the *Oxford English Dictionary* (1976) gives much the same definition. Both are clearly wrong, for they ignore the fact of polarization of temperature change. *To warm* means to increase the temperature of something until it is warm. To decrease something to that same temperature is not to warm but to cool it. To raise the temperature to the level of vaporization is not to warm but to boil it. The nicety arises because *warm* in English, unlike *chaud* in French or *caliente* in Spanish, describes a state with moderate lower and upper limits. The German cognates of *warm* and *hot*, namely *warm* and *heiß,* are not clearly distinguished. (It is interesting that there is no Spanish word for *simmer;* and the French verb, *mijoter,* contains the prefix *mi-* with its overtones of moderation.)

EXAMPLE 4.15. The clinician may be concerned should a patient's temperature be too high or two low; in cholera, for example, both states occur and are causes for alarm. But how do we describe the state when both have been avoided? The common expression is that the patient's temperature is "stabilized." But that is little more than slang, as a glance at *Webster's* (1988) would make clear. Those who are by any reasonable standard healthy will show variation in temperature, some of it regular circadian changes, and some of it accidental from an assortment of environmental causes. There is little in Medical criteriology that has either ideas or words to address these details of variation; and competent clinical practice is largely a matter of unarticulated judgment. The characteristic waxing and waning of Cheyne-Stokes respiration in depression of the respiratory center, fluctuation of alertness in subdural hematoma, and the contrast in affect between schizophrenia and bipolar mood disorder are notorious pitfalls for the unwary. But at least they tend to be periodic. Too little is perhaps known about the significance of nonperiodic variation in Medicine.

The habit of exaggeration, so vital in the vulgar world of commerce, imparts similar half-hidden polarizations to many laicized words, and a faithful analysis of the ontological issues must be alert to this trend.

EXAMPLE 4.16. A common malapropism that has infested even the majestic aura of the law is the word *average*. It has a technical meaning in Probability and Statistics, originally imported from the vocabulary of the actuaries and the insurers. The average is a property of distributions, not of persons or other individual components of realizations of Random variables. The expression "average man" is meaningless, and it is doubtful that even the law could rescue it as anything more than a vague rhetorical term. Nevertheless, this malapropism flourishes and has acquired a wholly unwarranted connotation of belittlement. To describe a patient as average may not be slanderous, but certainly it is insulting; and there is a widespread implicit feeling that all are entitled to be rated "above average."

5 Ontological Cohesion

Underlying much contemporary discussion of Medical Ethics is the assumption that the terms addressed—*patients, diseases, organs, diagnostic tests, treatments, outcomes*—are as definite as need be and make for precise communication. That is not at all self-evident to us. It is the purpose of this chapter to examine this assumption and to explore what is needed to assure adequate definitions, which will allow Medical Ethics to operate as an autonomous unity.

This book, though aiming for a wider union, starts from the standpoint of the Medical scientist. Even on this narrow footing, however, for some topic of interest to be constructively analyzed from the standpoints of a variety of specialists, there is need to communicate clearly what that topic is. But we are constrained by two commonsense principles. The first is that neologisms should be avoided wherever possible, and when they cannot be avoided they should be defined as clearly as may be. It is a widespread but perilous practice to use common words to which an artificial technical meaning is then attached. The second principle, inevitably somewhat in conflict with the first, is that wherever we use a term in one of its several possible senses, we should qualify it if there is any ambiguity. This caution is all the more needed in compound disciplines such as Medical Ethics.

EXAMPLE 5.1. In any discussion of the theory, science, or Philosophy of law, we are apt to meet the term *jurisprudence*. Now, in one regard Medicine is the practice of a professional field just as academic law is; and the theoretical underpinning of Medicine (i.e., the counterpart of jurisprudence) is denoted by the same word, *Medicine,* a regrettable source of confusion. There is a Logical intersection between Medicine and academic law containing all matters touching both, designated (according to viewpoint) *Medical jurisprudence* or *forensic Medicine,* two terms well established and hallowed by tradition. Nevertheless, a compound discipline such as that intersection is a set in its own right and disjoint from the parent sets. The fully accoutered experts in this compound discipline, whether trained Medically or Legally (or both), would respect precisely the same knowledge and skills. That is not to say that all practitioners, regardless of professional formation, would be equally adept at all details. That is not a reasonable requirement for any practitioner (as, indeed, it would not be even inside one of the component disciplines). But the expert in forensic Medicine may not dismiss any part of it. In contrast, the expert in fine arts might declare mathematics foreign to that discipline (or conversely).[1]

It can be further argued that in the best of all possible worlds, such compound disciplines are autonomous and not to be tampered with by experts from either simple discipline, especially where they are in conflict. For example, in the practice of law and in Medicine the respective notions of tactical proof have very different technical meanings, for the law is ordinarily adversarial and Medicine is not. But in forensic Medicine both senses might be unacceptable and a new one required. Now, there is an age-old argument as to the scope of Philosophy. There have been extreme views. Some make the widest arrogations: Philosophy is the overseer of all natural scholarship (so that there are still university chairs of "Natural Philosophy," meaning in fact chairs of science, and often not even theory of science at that). Others preach extreme nihilism: "The problem of philosophy is to prove that there are no philosophic problems" (Wittgenstein 1969). True, the autonomous discipline science—in its usual, unqualified, modern connotation as the investigation of natural phenomena by structured analysis and interpretation of systematically collected, empirical, data—is an invention of the nineteenth century, but of course as an activity it goes back to at least Roger Bacon and Albertus Magnus, to the Arabs and the Greeks, especially Archimedes, and in some sense indefinitely far back in history. Science and Philosophy stem from a common origin, just as the English and American languages do. They share a common heritage and vocabulary. Nothing is to be gained by partisan arguments about which is the older, the more deeply rooted, or the more correct. Philosophy and science have diverged by specialization and have been in some measure estranged; and as with British and American English, there are disputed matters where we keep painfully rediscovering a true, well-nigh forgotten, communality. At such encounters, scientists have no authority to decide what Philosophers should be studying. On the other hand, Philosophers, especially those who studiously avoid involvement in the science concerned, have no self-evident mandate to constrain scientists from drawing on the common heritage.

For historic reasons and because of the complexity of the topic, Medicine has its own position. It is not historically a branch of ordinary science, and Medicine-as-science is the result of a rather modern treaty that has been immensely important to the welfare of both. Nor has Medicine any

1. An individual painter such as Escher might make extensive use of imported mathematics. But that does not impose the reasonable expectation that an expert in fine arts should even be prepared to discuss mathematics, let alone be competent in it. On the other hand, it is reasonable to expect all such experts to understand the Laws of perspective.

right to dictate the content of science, nor may science set itself up as the last court of appeal for Medicine. When there is an overlap between the fields, it is better treated as an authentic intersection in which both topics may on their own terms appeal to an expanding common heritage. Flawed as they are, the terms *Medical science* and *scientific Medicine* do not denote the same topic, as one might have hoped. It is well to remember that Medicine has made fundamental and lasting contributions to science, of which the most conspicuous in the twentieth century lie perhaps in certain special topics of immunology and genetics.

These comments are not intended as a declaration of sovereignty or as a drawing up of frontiers. Neither stance would serve any purpose and might imperil much-needed, but tenuous, interactions among Philosophy, science, and Medicine. Rather, the message is a much deeper one. The analysis by the Medical theorist and that by the professional Philosopher may be widely different, although at a yet more profound level the differences may be fully reconcilable. Meanwhile, there may be only modest hopes for useful exchange. Yet we have found from our own experience that analysis of Medical problems leads us, often unwittingly, to hark back to a more primitive, anaplastic stage of scholarship, such as animated the endeavors of Leibniz, Descartes, and Pascal, to name but three ancestral scholars each having irreproachable credentials as an authentic Philosopher, mathematician, and scientist.

SOME EXOTERIC ASPECTS OF MEDICINE

Medical theorists are called on to grapple with a certain set of conspicuous and obtrusive problems that confront investigators, such as pathogenetics; epidemiology; nosology (the classification of disease); the optimization of Diagnosis; the basis of Probability theory and its concepts of Randomness, independence, and sample space; Statistics and its concepts of Randomness, independence, and sample space; the nature of disease and defect; normality; and modeling (in several different senses). Of their very nature these problems are not to be solved by simply collecting data, by leafing through the standard Medical textbooks, or by devising new tests or reporting fresh sources of diversity. For reasons that are hard to state but are apparent to all who have grappled with them, these topics must sooner or later be accountable to criteria (e.g., parsimony, consistency, falsifiability) that lie outside the domain of empirical science. This forum has plenty of vital content and at least some rudimentary theory, much of it buried in the past—in Galen, Sydenham, and Descartes, for instance—and some of it engaging many contemporary Medical scholars. It is a minor matter whether it is properly cast as part of Philosophy or part of a fundamental theory of Medicine. Its reality, which is at least as compelling as forensic Medicine, will not be greatly changed by what name it is given, or even if it has none. But there seems little doubt to us that it would be very much the better for a healthy dialogue with Philosophical ontologists.

BLACK AND WHITE BOXES

If the scheme explored in Chapter 2 is to have some pertinence, then an Ethical system seems to represent an encounter and an exchange among three topics (axioms, consequences, and practice; *A, C,* and *P*). To facilitate these aims, their subject matters must in some sense enjoy a commensurability: they must address the same kinds of things, even though they may be cast in different terms, dimensions, and moods. What are these things? How are they to be converted into useful negotiable forms? It is scarcely surprising that the various elements—empirical, esthetic, Moral, Logical— are in one way or another represented in all, no one of which in isolation encompasses a complete Ethics.

The depths, the penetration, of the Ethics may be graded in many ways. Our concern in this chapter is what we may call the black-box/white-box scale. The notion is borrowed from the physical theorists.[2] The behavior of a structure with output (discernible behavior) may be investigated under the assumption-of-convenience that it either has no intelligible inner workings or that they are inaccessible to direct study. The investigation then consists solely of observing how the structure's behavior (output) is changed by exposing it to changes in stimuli (the input). This strategy is said to treat the structure as a *black box.* At the other extreme, all the inner workings of the structure may be fully known, understood, and made available in the analysis. The investigation then treats the structure as a *white box.* (This course may, however, have to be compromised because of the technical demands that the white-box analysis makes, and other methods such as Monte Carlo simulation may have to be used instead.)

Most empirical realities lie between these two extremes and may be said to be boxes of a variable degree of grayness. The input into the black box may itself be gray. It seems clear that by analogy Ethics might be treated as operating on its natural materials, where structure, input, and output are somewhere on the black-to-white scale.

EXAMPLE 5.2. In Ethical discussion the issue may arise of how much freedom should be given to mentally retarded adults. A black-box analysis would take all the issues at highly intuitive levels: everybody knows what

---

2. It also has a more macabre connotation. The Chernobyl disaster was a result of mistaken action in the face of a system that was both complex and inadequately understood, the very type of our topic. *Chernobyl* means *black and white* in Ukrainian.

freedom, given, mentally retarded, adults, and *should* mean, or else it is impossible to analyze them and fruitless to try. The decision is then to be made by the use of common sense and wise judgment, both of which tools are the blackest of the black. A fully white-box treatment would explore these terms in exhaustive detail, teasing out all the (perhaps very complicated) ramifications of the terms used in the analysis.

The progress of science, and of physics in particular, is a steady pursuit of whiter and whiter boxes. But not all the scholarly interests are quite so relentlessly reductionistic. Indeed, one concern of inferential science (typically in Statistics) is to devise *robust* methods, that is, methods (such as nonparametric analysis) that aim at a maximum degree of utility for any given degree of grayness.[3] It is understandable that in practical situations we must usually make do with intermediate shades of gray. (Withering's introduction of digitalis in the treatment of heart failure without any controlled trial is a classic example.) But in important issues, at least, even the most hardened user of black-box analysis must have misgivings about settling for criteria on a gratuitously dark scale and with a dubious or perhaps quite unknown robustness.

SOME ONTOLOGICAL ASPECTS OF COHERENCE

We have said that Ethics and its gray-box rating permeate all three of the components *(A, C,* and *P)* addressed in Chapter 2. In this book we repeatedly use terms that are traditionally regarded as exclusively scientific or exclusively Philosophical. We intend no violence to them; to the contrary, we try to use them in what seems to be proper form. But it is not entirely within our control if they involve some minor distortions, for the very process of annealing, say, theoretical Philosophy to theoretical Medicine may expose certain problems over compatibility for sundry reasons, not the least being the indeterminacies of the Medical viewpoint.

EXAMPLE 5.3. Where there is doubt, the question is whether the substance of the doubt is the shortcomings of our method and analysis (epistemic doubt) or is an intrinsic part of the process itself, as appears to be true of quantum mechanics[4] (ontological doubt). This question has usually not been wholly resolved, and indeed, according to theory (e.g., of Chaotic

3. A familiar example is regression analysis by least-squares analysis in which the *scientific ideas* involved enjoy the robustness of crass measures of relatedness without any explicit model of the mechanism; and the *Statistics* capitalizes on the robustness of the Gauss-Markov theorem.

4. It is only fair to note that there are articulate dissident opinions about quantum indeterminacy (Bohm 1957).

processes), no resolution may ever be possible. Perhaps that lack of resolution is not disturbing to the Philosopher or to the scientist, but for motives and reasons that are not readily analyzed, it seems to be important both to the clinician and to the patient. It is, for instance, a major issue in genetic counseling how far the doubt is epistemic (and in principle remediable by better phenotyping and intrauterine diagnosis) and how far it is ontological and only to be remedied by as yet undeveloped methods such as choice of the inseminating sperm.

We hope that this anticipatory disclaimer sounds neither too ominous nor too sinister a note. Nevertheless, it must be made, for without it there may be much misunderstanding. For purposes of Ethics, our preferred position would be to identify a particular discipline designated Medical ontology, for preference one that is not a botching of two highly specialized fields but a true untampered, rather primitive, intersection between them. It might be wondered what there is so special about the need for such a discipline as Medical ontology. All that we shall say here is that our study group, starting out in an attempt to contribute to the field of Medical Ethics, encountered many gaps in the coherence and understanding of Medicine, and (what is much more serious) a general failure of Medicine and Medical practitioners to recognize that the gaps even exist. Needless to say, there results a serious lack of apparatus for addressing these gaps even wholly inside Medicine. Until some serious improvement is achieved, it seems vain to try even to identify the issues necessary for any kind of practical deontology.

The issues of editing, analyzing, manipulating, and Logically applying empirical evidence (what we conceive to be the responsibilities of epistemology) are necessary preliminaries to Ethical analysis. At first the shortcomings in Medical theory seem to be epistemic, but it soon becomes apparent that the real gap is a much deeper and more disturbing one. However, all these activities are vain if it is not clear *what it is that the data deal with*. There seems to be little point in trying to explore the Ethical aspects of the management of *pus* and *ichor* in relationship to health by collecting data, however extensively or systematically, when it is not at all clear what, if anything, the two terms mean and how, if at all, they differ. That dispute loomed large in the writings of the German pathologists in the nineteenth century; but the term *ichor* seems to have disappeared for the worst of reasons and in the worst possible way. Medical scientists simply stopped writing about it, and the notion fell out of fashion. We identify this as "the worst possible way" because even after a long and arid struggle, nothing whatsoever has been learned, not even some consoling scintilla of wisdom bought at a great price about how such an inquiry should, and should not, have been conducted.

It will be clear from what follows that the basic matters of the inner nature of Medical issues together with the canons of their coherence (i.e., what we denote as *Medical ontology*) are more important than the methods of inquiring into those issues *(Medical epistemology)*. Without a commensurate attention to ontology, in the long run Medicine will become a myopic grappling with received but unexamined goals.

EXAMPLE 5.4. Much has been written on population dynamics as a means of describing and understanding, say, hypertension or diabetes, by analyzing the frequencies in the population and the selective processes that sustain them. Now, that approach has been successfully applied to, for instance, Mendelian inborn errors of metabolism, where the trait is defined in a specific enzyme that may be studied chemically quite independently of the population frequencies. However, it is useless, even at the level of technical analysis, if the terms *hypertension* and *diabetes* cannot even be defined. It is tedious enough looking for a needle in a haystack. It is a hopeless quest if there is no agreement as to the difference between a needle and a wisp of hay. Defining hypertension by choosing some arbitrary cutoff point separating "normal blood pressure" from "high blood pressure" may play havoc with the population genetics, for even a small change to another (also arbitrary) blood pressure level may make all the difference between quantitatively sustaining and refuting a hypothesis about the inheritance. That makeshift, gray-box method is not robust.

However, the entire ontology of Medicine is a much wider subject. Examples of the general topics have been listed above. We cannot hope to address or even review them here. They must be left to publications elsewhere, although some will be cited from time to time. Our interests here will be narrowed to some of the major issues that arise in Medical ontology in connection with Medical Ethics. The object is not at all to deal with defining broad Ethical principles *(Major Ethics),* with applying these principles to particular classes of issues *(Minor Ethics),* and least of all with resolving particular cases *(Medical casuistry).* Our aim is to explore the implications of assumptions, often wholly implicit, that have emerged in makeshift attempts to bridge the gap between Ethical theory and Medical Ethics.

ONTOLOGY AND IDENTITY

The ease with which we may identify terms of discussion varies widely. Consider first a rather extreme case.

EXAMPLE 5.5. A perfect diamond is a crystal of pure carbon. It is one of the hardest physical bodies known. In consequence, it has physical limits that are sharp, unambiguous, and precisely defined by its atomic organization and not merely by its chemical composition. Because of its remarkable optical properties it has great esthetic purity. It has disproportionate commercial value, which is not to be improved by coating it with noncrystalline carbon, however pure. *Diamond* is as precise a term as a lawyer might hope for. Economically, diamond, like gold and other precious metals and stones, is a classic hedge against inflation, with the added virtue that it is not abraded by handling.

Consider now an intermediate case.

EXAMPLE 5.6. Human beings fall into two classes, male and female. Sexuality is probably the most important natural factor in the preservation of the human race. Every society has to some degree and by some measures been concerned to intervene to protect, regulate, and police it. It is widely perceived by very diverse religions to be a cornerstone, or at least a test case, of Morality. The major topic in Legal concerns with obscenity is behavior between the two sexes; to a lesser degree, the focus is behavior of persons of the same sex; and only to a minute degree is it violence, drugs, or crime. Gender is the object of much concern in the provision of public lavatories, athletic competition, clothing design. In another perspective, there have been constant upheavals over the last hundred years or so about inequity in the Legal and social treatment of the sexes, and in the general working of common justice. Clearly, gender and sexuality are very important issues in several spheres. The definition of gender—a key issue if political and social reform are to have any bite—is reasonably sound, provided it is not examined too closely. Anatomical appearance, histology of germinal tissue, cytology, psychology, chromosomal analysis, reproductive capacity, hormone assay, behavior, mystical appraisals, and surely many more criteria have been put forward at various times to define or delimit gender. No one of them is foolproof; and while all the criteria will tend to agree, discrepancies can nevertheless be found for each, singly or in combinations. Nor is that surprising. There seem to be a small number of persons of a genuine intermediate gender, having, for instance, testicular tissue on one side and ovarian tissue on the other. To those who can tolerate some measure of conceptual untidiness, the notion of gender works well as a whole, and the occasional exceptions may be dismissed as distractions.

However, there are two issues other than tidiness of identification that go deeper and are not nearly so easily brushed aside. For one thing, there are practical matters, like the exigencies of the law.

EXAMPLE 5.7. For definiteness, let us suppose that a person has the condition known as testicular feminization, which seems without reasonable doubt to be an X-linked recessive Mendelian condition (McKusick 1994: entry *313680). Unsuspectingly, and on commonplace anatomical criteria, he is judged to be female and brought up as such. Eventually he marries a male by due legal process. The union will be judged heterosexual if gender is interpreted by overt anatomical phenotype, but homosexual if appeal is made to biopsy of germinal cells. Homosexual unions are illegal in many countries and are considered by certain religions grossly immoral. Again, the father of this patient of mistaken gender may have a title to be inherited only by a male, or he may have made a will leaving more money to his sons than to his daughters. In both matters it may be argued that a gross miscarriage of justice may result from continuing to treat the geno-typically male person as female. No doubt these issues may be disposed of by juridical contrivances, but they will give little satisfaction to the geneti-cist or the Moral Philosopher.

The other issue is deeper still and much the more difficult. If there is a satisfactory definition (of gender), then the problems we have discussed in Examples 5.6 and 5.7 so far are to be seen as epistemic. That is, there is an undisputed goal, compliance with the law; the Medical problem is in dis-cerning the implications of the data; and the Ethical problem is applying them in making judgments about action. Now, the various sources for judg-ing gender are more or less reliable diagnostic tests. But what is the thing of which each of these tests makes a reliable (but not necessarily foolproof) statement? How can we define what is to be meant by *reliability?* Is there something else that is the point of the point, the gold standard, the *essence* of gender, that is being tested for? There lies at the heart of this ontological question the supposition that out of a set of diverse and conflicting empiri-cal data, some one datum, or perhaps some perfectly concordant subset of them, is to be put in a preferred position ontologically; and all discrepan-cies between this preferred set and the rest of the data will be identified as errors in the rest and never identified as errors in the preferred criterion. The only alternative seems to be to treat all the data with parity and devise some sound and self-evidently respectable method, the form of which has yet to be clarified, for negotiating a consensus (a consensus, not a com-promise) among the experts. There is precedent. The atomic number, an empirically discovered fact, has come to be the definition of each particu-lar element. (However, that criterion was not available in 1850.) To define the essence of something in terms of its properties leaves it at the mercy of new properties that must be included with the rest, and will lead to differ-ent estimates of misclassification and change the importances (weights) of the other criteria relative to one another. To propose as final any particular principle of identification is a bold commitment.

Consider a third level of definiteness.

EXAMPLE 5.8. The care of an abused child is a matter of concern to the law courts. A new law prescribes that the appropriate social services coun-cil (or some such body) shall arrange the placement of the abused child in a home that will be removed from the sphere of influence of the abusive parents. No doubt but that the ruling is a compassionate and constructive embodiment of something very important. On these grounds alone the law has serious merit. But unless it goes into explicit detail, to the Medical scientist it will be Ethically useless. It is not at all easy to see what *sphere of influence* means; it is even more difficult to define the criteria that may be used, for instance, as a gauge of compliance of the placement with the spirit of the law. Finally, under the consistential principle, in the event, it is likely to prove impossible to assess whether the remedy was effective. The epistemic problems are difficult; the ontological problems seem to be insuperable.

POSSIBLE STANDARDS FOR IDENTITY

Now, what emerges from these last three examples? The ideal kind of trait to deal with in Medicine is one in which three standards are met:

1. The trait should correspond to an actual and accessible test (i.e., a state or criterion) in quite unambiguous terms, and that test should tolerate no other trait. In brief, ontologically the test is to be both a sufficient and a necessary condition for defining the trait.
2. The trait should have an identity in some natural sense that is distinct from the means of examining it. That is, under the peril of the charge of triviality, the definition of the trait and the criterion may not be conterminous.

EXAMPLE 5.9. To define the term *giant* arbitrarily to denote any human being over seven feet tall is to intend the term to be applied to all over seven feet and none under that height. The criterion, then, is both necessary and sufficient for the designation. But that involves us in certain beliefs that may be unpalatable to us. For instance, that there are more men giants than women giants; that there are no child giants; that a giant who has both legs amputated is no longer a giant; that osteoporosis may cure gigantism; and so forth.

These absurdities are aggravated for more labile criteria, for example, that a patient has hypertension before breakfast but not after, or on some days but not others, and so on. The clinician may have a pentheric demand that a chronic disease does not behave in such a labile capricious fashion. In Medical practice, the criterion of the natural identity of a state is in most instances a total concordance in the results of many Logically distinct tests.

3. There should exist no other tests that show those persons exhibiting the trait to be heterogeneous.

EXAMPLE 5.10. Genetics, to cite one source of examples, has in many cases shown that what appeared to be a homogeneous Mendelian (unilocal) condition may be due to genes at quite different genetic loci, a fact that is taken to demonstrate heterogeneity. But that criterion would be difficult to extend to that vastly more important group of traits that are under the control of many loci.[5] However, clinicians might pentherically refuse to be overawed by that fact. They may think that the main point of defining a particular disease is to represent implications, treatment, and prognosis; and the actual root cause may be of little or no relevance to any.

ONTOLOGY AND IDENTITY (CONTINUED)

Let us now apply these standards to the three cases discussed above. The perfect diamond (Example 5.5) fulfills the first by its physical definition in space: it is by definition confined to its hull, which comprises nothing but the diamond (the hypothetically perfect diamond does not contain impurities or air bubbles). It also fulfills the second standard: the natural identity is one single continuous crystal of carbon. As we saw in Example 5.4, it certainly fulfills the third standard, since the findings of several other tests confirm, and none disproves, the claim of homogeneity. Note that this example is somewhat artificial, since we specified that the diamond be pure and perfectly cut. In any practical example we might be less assured. The carbon may contain some radioactive ^{14}C that will eventually decay, with some loss of material that will have an ambiguous relationship to the non-decaying carbon; there will be minute impurities; and so on. But at least we are highly confident about its overall nature. We have very little misgiving about what "the diamond" denotes: whether any particular point in space is inside the diamond or outside it, or whether there is any reasonable doubt about its entity, or whether the entity so defined serves a useful purpose.

Gender (Examples 5.6–5.7) is a much less satisfactory trait. We may define ourselves out of the problem, arbitrarily identifying the male gender by the presence of Y antigen, for instance. But it would remain an artificial definition that would lead to messy complications in particular cases. For instance, hermaphrodites who do not coincidentally lack Y antigen would be declared male. Taking the evidence as a whole, the diversity of the tests, the imperfect agreement among them, the overt existence of exceptions (hermaphrodites), and the disputed practical criteria of gender, it seems appropriate to conclude that gender is an imperfect idea with at least some

5. Such so-called Galton-Fisher traits are typically expressed in a single measurement (e.g., height, weight, blood pressure, blood glucose level) the value of which in any particular person is due to the combined effect of genes at many loci. It is clear, however, that within a single system the same effect may be produced by different combinations of contributions. What does that imply about the meaning of *homogeneity*?

ontological fuzziness and certainly epistemic doubt. There seem to be no good grounds for singling out any one criterion for special treatment as the essence of gender against which other tests have to be validated.[6]

The notion of the sphere of influence (Example 5.8) simply does not lead to a ghost of an analysis. In a spirit of compassion, we would hope that whoever has the task of interpreting the Legal decisions will exhibit some common sense. For the child to go on living with the abusive parents would clearly be noncompliant. To prevent all communication whatsoever between the parents and the child, even of the most indirect kind, would be compliant but might be judged too harsh. But any kind of cogent formal analysis is a hopeless undertaking.

ONTOLOGICAL DENSITY

We shall now try to introduce a little more precision into these ideas (Murphy 1981b). For simplicity, we first suppose that the test (criterion) is a measurement on a continuous scale. The measurements from a population that possesses the state of interest occur only between two values, A and B (we shall call it literally or by analogy the *diagnostic range*), and none of the population without the state have measurements that fall between A and B. The grouping of the trait is compact and pure. There is no epistemic doubt. These properties ensure sharp definition of the trait, and we shall say that it shows *high ontological density with respect to that measurement (or test)*. If an entity has high ontological density with respect to two or more independent traits (as the diamond does), then the overall ontological density is correspondingly higher. The scope of the idea of ontological density is in no way restricted to measurement. What we call physical life is ontologically very dense with respect to the presence of DNA. (However, DNA may be only an impurity, as a bloodstain on a window would be, and as to origin, the DNA might be synthetic; so the identification of DNA with life is not foolproof.) Physical life is nothing like so dense with respect to another test, namely, the ability to solve more or less complicated problems by formal means. Many living systems have little or no discernible skill at it, whereas computers may perform very successfully.

The density may concern some very abstract test. We do not wish to provide a delimiting principle that would constrain the possible scope. *Ontological density* is, more than anything else, a relative term and a precise but elastic one. It is intended to avoid repeated use of long circumlocu-

6. There is a curious anomaly of identification. The 46XY karyotype is male, the 46XX karyotype female. In the Turner syndrome the karyotype 45X is commonly called the "incomplete female" state. But since no second sex chromosome (X or Y) is present, there is just as good a warrant for calling the phenotype the "incomplete male" state.

tions. It may be quantitated; but that is not the only form it can take, nor should undue importance be attached to that fact.

EXAMPLE 5.11. A cooking pot may be chemically pure iron. But not all pieces of iron are cooking pots, nor are all cooking pots pure iron. We might decide that *cooking pot* is a broad term: roughly, it denotes something that is little damaged by heat and can be stably balanced so as to leave at least one region on its surface that is continuous, nonporous, and concave below some contour. The challenge is not only or mainly that it may be difficult to identify whether any particular object is a cooking pot (that is an epistemic issue). An archaeologist might find it difficult to cope with the ontological question of what the essence of a cooking pot is. Moreover, a cooking pot may have poorly defined limits.

An example may help to illustrate these realities in human biology.

EXAMPLE 5.12. Geneticists pursuing Mendel's primordial observations found it necessary to suppose the existence of a genetic "atom," that is, a fundamental unit of minimal size that could not be subdivided without total disruption of its genetic function. Later it was arbitrarily called the gene. So far so good. But what is this function? What are the characteristic qualities of a gene? Geneticists, thinking of the phenomena of breeding systems, found themselves addressing four properties all of which were supposed conterminous:

1. The gene is the unit transmitted entire from one generation to the next: unlike genetic material in general, it does not recombine. Hence we have the definition that the gene is the limit of possible (nondestructive) recombination, or *recon*.
2. The gene is the target of discontinuous change that results from outside forces. Hence, the gene is the unit of mutation, or *muton*.
3. The gene is the segment of genetic material that must exist entire in at least one chromosome for normal functioning to occur. Thus, even for recessive characters, two minor defects in different parts of the two members of the pair of genes do not compensate for ("complement") each other. The gene in this aspect is known as the *cistron*.
4. The gene is the segment of genetic material that contains the information necessary for the elaboration of one polypeptide chain, the subunit of protein. This segment has been informally called the *peptidon* (though this usage was never widespread).

Until the modern era of biochemical and microbial genetics, these four concepts of the word *gene* could be, and were, used interchangeably. Indeed, there was little evidence for supposing them to be in conflict, and the words *recon, muton, cistron,* and *peptidon* did not even exist because there was no need to invent them. So long as the resolution of the system under examination was sufficiently low, no inconsistency was apparent. But the development from the mid-1950s onward made it necessary to discard the monolithic gene model used fruitfully for nearly half a century. Various specialists made a choice, and each kind made a distinct image. The linkage analyst worked in recons and pieced together *linkage groups* and eventually a *genetic map.* The cytogeneticist dealt with the chromosomes and devised a *karyotypic map.* Somatic cell geneticists used heterokaryons to make *cell assignments* and in collaboration with the linkage analysts and the cytogeneticists undertook the perplexing problem of setting up a correspondence between the microanatomy of the chromosomes and the behavior of the genes in genetic segregation. The biochemical geneticist by various ingenious devices explored the mechanics of how the genetic code was translated to produce phenotypes; and, especially with the introduction of restriction fragment analysis, complemented at a higher level of resolution the endeavors of the linkage analyst and the oddities of disequilibrium studies by the population geneticist. As a concerted approach to rationalizing genetics, it has been admirable.

It would be a long story to relate what these splendid and exciting advances have done to the ontology of the gene. Not, of course, that sound and pertinent knowledge can in the long run impede or tarnish the ontological analysis: there is nothing to be said for living in a fool's paradise. But it looks very much at the present time as if what may emerge in due course will be an elaborate set of answers to a totally different set of questions from those that were being asked in the 1930s. For one thing, the working gene, the structure that actually executes the message transmitted in the genome, is now seen as something that is edited in an elaborate way by peeling off packing material (exons and introns) that takes no intrinsic part in the genetic process. But that last statement is at once suspect. Regardless of evolution altogether, the facts must meet a question cast in strictly genetic terms: Why is the packing material conserved in the face of the constant attrition by new mutation? (Moreover, there is the added complication that the packing material often seems to contain genes of its own arranged in a bizarre fashion.)

It is not an idle question to ask whether the idea of a gene is still useful for any purpose other than a kind of crude shorthand to provide rough answers to practical but often crude questions. That such a doubt arises is itself rather dismaying. Even twenty years ago it would have been dismissed as idle and mischievous sniping at genetics, clearly the great and confident hope of understanding the inner nature of biology. It probably still is that hope; but the terms of the understanding to which it may ultimately lead may not include the gene but be something that at this stage is too elusive even to be guessed at.

A purist, then, will insist that in the final analysis, to identify the essence of certain classes of disease as nothing other than the inevitable and unassisted operation of a single gene may be yet another (although vastly more refined) level of ontological approximation. We still have not attained our metaphysical ideal of the perfectly defined trait. On top of these concerns at (as it were) the high-resolution mapping, the microcosmos of the trait, there are shaping up enormous clouds in our understanding of the macrocosmos of the disease. We may merely mention the problems of property emergence (an old will-o'-the-wisp of the Philosophers (Lonergan 1957; Passmire 1966; J. Cohen and Stewart 1994)) now evident in the theory of complex systems with special importance in ontogeny (Waddington 1957; Grüneberg 1963; Murphy and Pyeritz 1986; Edelman 1988, 1992); the developments in the theory of dynamic systems (Hirsch and Smale 1974), theory of Chaos (Devaney 1989), and fractals (Mandelbrot 1977); the rapid advances in modeling how the brain functions; and many other topics. From the standpoint of fruitful scientific inquiry, biology is at a peak of unprecedented richness. Nor should this feast be grounds for dismay to the ontologist. At the least, however, it should make for some mistrust about glib and precociously smooth answers in science or in Ethics.

THE INNER IDENTITY

The standards of the ideal trait given earlier will do very well as a bridge to deeper insight, but they seem cumbersome and do not quite ring true. The third standard supposes that we know what we mean by *homogeneity*, and in practice we mostly identify the lack of heterogeneity by default. The first standard really begs the question, because criteria of nontrivial *necessity* and *sufficiency* can be applied only after the essence of the trait is defined. The second standard is a hedge against precisely the risk of triviality; but it raises questions that need further exploration.

Two perennial questions lie at the bottom of this analysis: the ontology of Randomness, and the nature of empirical redundancy.

Randomness

Consider a trait that is specifiable by the outcome of a test on a continuous scale. If there exists a class of subjects homogeneous with respect to that trait, why are the data from the members of that class not all identical? Yet in fact it is overwhelmingly difficult to think of any precise trait in biology that behaves in this perfectly homogeneous way. There are a number of conventional answers:

1. If they are not all the same, then tautologously the class is not homogeneous. This nominalistic answer saves the purity at the expense of demolishing virtually all empirical candidates.
2. The results are all the same, but that fact is obscured by irrelevant but real technical error. To support this explanation requires inquiry into the nature and properties of this putative error.
3. The homogeneity resides in the cause (e.g., in the gene), not in the outcome (the phenotype). There may be modifying factors in the environment, or in other factors (such as other genetic loci) that are unknown or only dimly identified. In effect we have a mixture of a white box and a black box. No progress will be made with the claim for a candidate without identifying those factors more fully. If this explanation is true, the necessary-and-sufficient claim is at least quantitatively in peril.
4. There is a genuine but irreducible Random component in the execution of the process. Here the term *Random* denotes a phenomenon that can in principle be formally described (by a distribution function or a set of literal or fictive axioms). Although it may be generated by a *randomizing device,* its output has no prescribed cause and therefore must be irrelevant to the phenotype except in that it undermines its precision. It is not to be a euphemism for ignorance. This Randomness may have selective value (Murphy 1981c). After all the systematic components subsumed under it have been carefully identified and removed, ontologically it is a perfect and unassailable black box.

Redundancy

Redundancy may be purely Logical: the same entity is masquerading under two disguises.

EXAMPLE 5.13. The pulse pressure *(P)* is by definition the systolic pressure *(S)* minus the diastolic pressure *(D).* Given any two of these three quantities, one may readily find the third. To be given all three is clearly a Logical redundancy, even if all are measured separately.

Of course, the theory of the Statistical estimation of parameters thrives on Logical redundancy, namely, the use of replicate readings of the same quantity. In typical, more ambitious, problems, there will be multiple parameters to be estimated under a parametric model. Finding the true values of the parameters is the preoccupation, what we may call the veridical concern, of Statistics. The aptness of the model is the veridical concern of Statistical tests of *goodness-of-fit.* But the terms and structure of the model (except in that they may make the Statistical estimation more or less complicated) are the veridical concern not of Statistics (which treats them as an ontological black box) but of the parent discipline that generated them (physics, biology, psychometry, economics, etc.). Wherever there is a formal redundancy in the model (as in Example 5.13) so that the Statistician is trying to estimate S, D, or P by ignoring the fact that estimating P is the same as estimating $(S - D)$, then either there will be intractable problems[7] or what is being estimated is largely epistemic noise.

Here, however, we are concerned with empirical redundancy; and wherever it is exact, or nearly so, the scientist always has misgivings that there is a Logical redundancy.

EXAMPLE 5.14. In physics, the weight of a body and its inertia give individual estimates of its mass that agree as perfectly as the resolving power allows. Einstein's suspicion that this agreement was an artifact due to a Logical redundancy led him to reformulate physics in the theory of general relativity in such a way as to eliminate gravitation and dispose of the redundancy.

Is the set of perfectly agreeing attributes of the diamond just such a redundancy? Very likely it is. The optical properties and the hardness account for many of the attributes and are common results of the crystalline structure, which itself is a subject of physical chemistry. This outcome may appear to undermine the claim that the diamond is a near-ideal trait. Indeed. But it has also furnished a unifying explanation that by its very explicitness provides all the physical coherence we could hope for, in the same way that general relativity theory unified weight and inertia and much more besides. We seem to have reverted to a monolithic theory, an ontology with a single generative structure. But no doubt all would agree that it is much more satisfying, more reassuring.

EXAMPLE 5.15. Clinicians and especially clinical geneticists may notice that a number of superficially disparate characters tend to *run together* (to put it in plain English), to be found in a cluster more often than might be expected if they were unrelated. With sound Probabilistic assessment of properly collected data and repeated failure to explain this association, they celebrate by translating this *concurrence*, a Latin word, into Greek and call it a *syndrome*. In time, as experience increases and the scientific method is refined, all features turn out to be traceable to one clear cause, often a genetic one. The word *syndrome* is then dropped out, the name of the condition is appropriately modified to something more illuminating, and the path of connection is replaced by a "pedigree of causes" from a unified principle. As before, the key to the inquiry (the multiplicity of concordances) is the final causality.

7. For example, because of singularity or ill-conditioning of the information matrix.

The Authenticity of Covariance

One source of confusion in exploring ontological coherence is to suppose that what is a perfectly well defined event in one theoretical discipline may have no counterpart in another. This is a matter of real concern in Probability (as a branch of mathematics) and Statistics (as a branch of science). We cite one instance.

EXAMPLE 5.16. In Probability theory there is a well-defined quality for a wide class of bivariate distributions, called the *covariance*. The technical details do not concern us here; but broadly it is used as an index of relatedness of two Random variables (or *variates*). Now, in some cases, at least, much of that relatedness is due to a straightforward deterministic so-called structural relationship. For instance, if we plot temperatures measured by the Fahrenheit and centigrade thermometers (both of which are dealing with the linear expansion of mercury by heat), then there should be a perfect linear correspondence. In other cases, it is claimed that some of the relationship in covariance may lie in the fact that the Random parts of the measurements vary together (i.e., *covary*). However, deep within this formulation there are two assumptions that seem to be in conflict. First, covariance by definition can exist only between two variables both of which are at least in part Random. Second, the strictly Random component cannot be accounted for by any cause, or else it would be perfectly predictable from the state of that cause, in which case it could not be Random. Yet the idea of *co*variance seems to make no physical sense unless there is some message that is influencing the two variables to behave in a related fashion. But how can two causeless effects be sharing a common cause? Surely there must be serious doubt that (on these terms) covariance can ever exist in empirical phenomena. What does this misgiving do to the standing of the syndrome-as-concurrence?

CONCLUDING COMMENT

Perhaps the elaborateness of this examination has dismayed many. Two notes of general caution seem worthy of mention.

The first is that the wealth of undiscovered detail does not of itself warrant an attitude of incontinent nihilism. The matters that we believe in are, generally, much more robust than the terms in which we try to understand them. A middle-aged man with an acute attack of gout, whatever his intellectual equipment—be he a philosophical materialist, idealist, or transcendentalist, whether a population geneticist, an orthopedist, a hermit in the wilderness, a journalist, or a poet—has an inalienable pain in his toe that distresses and is likely to get him to seek relief; and no elegance of speculation will alter the uncompromising quiddity of that fact. It will be evident that we see ontology as important in setting out on Ethical inquiry; but it is not so important that defects in it should totally paralyze or invalidate the Ethics. No doubt but that the flaws introduced by imminent demands will call for refinement and amendment, but not in general for an eradication, root and branch, of everything that has ever been said, thought, or done. If we have not found the 24-karat golden truth, we may not in fact be very far from it.

The other, more earthy caution is that Ethics, like Medicine, or the practice of law, or engineering, is an imminent topic. There are problems here and now that need its attention; and if on the grounds of incomplete understanding, Ethics refuses to offer anything at all, why, nature abhors a vacuum, and a makeshift decision will be made by one means or another. Like as not, the makeshift decision will be called Ethics to the embarrassment of all. We fear that that is what has happened to so-called Medical Ethics and that it accounts for the incoherent terms in which it is so commonly cast. It is far better to formulate imminent Medical Ethics as a dynamic field that is being actively explored, exactly as science is and exactly as Philosophical Ethics is. The answers of casuistry or even Minor Ethics, then, are represented as incomplete and approximate, apt to change, even to change radically; nevertheless, at any moment of challenge the current best judgment can be stated with some confidence. But it is pernicious to think that any such Ethical opinion is forever exempt from reconsideration in the light of deeper and better understanding.

II Some Important Structures

In this second section of the book we propose to examine in some detail the nature of the terms met in the usual discourse of Medical Ethics. The task is that of the matchmaker rather than of the lover. It is a concern with communication between the ethicist and the clinician rather than with either specialty in its own right. We do well to recall Dickens's satire (1837: chap. 51) of the editor of the *Eatanswill Gazette* who, having read in the encyclopedia two articles, one on China and one on Philosophy, felt himself equipped to write a "copious review" on Chinese Philosophy. It is saner to recall Russell's principle (Copleston 1967) that the meaning of a sentence is what it has in common with its translation into a foreign language. In the vocabulary of theory of sets, Medical Ethics is the *intersection* of Medicine and Ethics, not the *union* of them. It is not a body of Ethical theory developed by other people at another time and in some other place with a few savory fragments of fashionable Medicine inserted into it like anchovies in an olive, and ornamented with a few fashionably content-free buzzwords. Nor is it Medicine with a smattering of Ethical garnish. Unless Medical Ethics has the same meaning in both Medicine and Ethics, it might as well not exist at all.

But the matchmaker must at least be prepared to listen to multiple, perhaps frankly conflicting, demands; without being a lawyer or a pastoral theologian, sociologist, psychiatrist, or banking economist, yet know something of each topic; and not be afraid to use this knowledge or to seek more as needed. Obviously we are at times goaded into making sorties over the border into the territory of other experts, sometimes to make frankly brutal smash-and-grab raids. But these excursions imply no disloyalty to our main purpose.

We start in Chapter 6 with an analysis of the traditional issues of Ethics, namely, Things and Acts. Chapter 7 takes on the problem of whether there are means of establishing a rate of exchange among facts, goals, and strategies. The proposed solution is an authentic understanding of Law as an expression of relationship and law as juridical.

Chapters 8 and 9 are concerned with more pragmatic issues. Chapter 8 addresses the entrenched notions of normality and disease about which Medical activities revolve. In Chapter 9 we deal with the pressing, if necessarily abstract, topic of assessing the reliability and precision of Medical evidence as raw material for Ethical practice.

Finally in Chapter 10 we give an outline of the anatomy of what the applied Statistician would call relevant decision theory. This activity is to be seen as a restricted device for optimizing certain arbitrarily defined goals (whether material, Moral, or esthetic) rather than establishing a preemptive criterion that is to dominate actual Ethical decisions.

6 Thing and Act

A t the outset we recognize that there is a large technical literature on the Philosophy of Thing and Act. We may instance the monograph on Thing by Heidegger (1967), which draws on a rich tradition from Kant. Much of the literature falls under what has come to be called the Philosophy of mind (Shaffer 1993), of great theoretical interest but as much concerned with thinking about things as about the things themselves, and unlikely to be helpful to a scientist trying to address the elements of discourse. The review by Lonergan (1957), though old, is still an authoritative starting point. We cannot wholly escape this tradition or ignore it altogether. The more we know of it, however, the more we see it as indeed a technical literature of Philosophers, and the less germane it seems to our authentic purpose. Just as the physicists do, we consider that the safeguarding of our fundamental ideas is our own internal responsibility, and that while we gratefully accept all helpful contributions, we should not look to Philosophy or the Philosopher to do our routine job for us, any more than we look to the mathematician to supervise and analyze physiology or the Greek scholar to tell us the difference between *paranoia* and *metanoia;* seeking enlightenment on the latter topic in, say, Liddell (1889) would in fact lead the practicing modern psychiatrist grossly astray.

The conception of the gene as the fundamental unit of genetic inheritance is a problem of Philosophy, just as the spelling of *pityriasis* is a lexicographical one; but from their sheer involvement in these entities and ideas about them, physicians must ordinarily learn to be their own experts. It is only when physicians aspire to interdisciplinary exchange and consultation that they have to be made aware that *artifact* has one meaning in Medicine and an entirely different one in archaeology, or that *elastic* has exactly opposite meanings in dermatology and physics. The same ambiguity, but greatly aggravated, haunts communication of notions, ideas, mechanisms, and models, conceptualizations that are used glibly enough in ordinary daily exchanges.

However, the real problems lie even deeper. One might reasonably suppose that Ethics, being traditionally a branch of Philosophy, would use the word *thing* in the same way that (say) Kant, Husserl, Heidegger, Brentano, and Wittgenstein do. But not only do we doubt that that is true, we

also doubt that the several meanings of the various groups of metaphysicians themselves have much in common; and presumably Ayer, and in their
early writings Russell and Wittgenstein (who at that stage expressly repudiated metaphysics), must have had some entirely different way of treating it. Meanwhile, the conscientious clinician has to have dealings with
the ethicist about what meanings (if any) they have for terms like *suffering,*
melancholia, drunk, energy, and *well-being* that perceived as words will be
familiar to both groups, but that used as terms of discourse may swamp
any interchange with impenetrable ambiguity.

We shall do our best. But the reader has been duly warned of the difficulties we foresee. We have no delusion that what we have to say will please
all parties. The saving grace is that our goal is much narrower than a full-
blooded analysis would demand.

THE FUNDAMENTAL SETTING

We start by supposing that authentic Medical problems are to be translated into terms that Ethics might address, and that any Ethical conclusions
that result are to be translated back into the verbal currency of Medicine.
This criterion of what we may call *analytical fidelity* has a simple analogy
in elementary mathematics.

EXAMPLE 6.1. Complicated calculation of some pragmatic problem
involving, say, multiplication of negative fractional powers of irrational
numbers may be made practical by using the logarithms of the quantities
concerned. But at the end of the calculations the answer must be expressed
in the original terms; that is, an intermediate answer as a logarithm must
be converted into its antilogarithm.

Just so, the Ethics of a clinical problem is no doubt best handled inside
the apparatus of Ethics. But to be useful to the clinician, it must eventually be interpretable as a clinical statement. And it is our perceived duty to
safeguard both of the translations. That may seem obvious to the point of
triteness. Perhaps we shall convince readers that, however trite, it has received so little attention that in many, perhaps almost all, cases the Ethical
consultation has met with little authentic success.

The traditional machinery seems to have relied heavily on the notions
of Thing and Act. Now, they are two robust terms: it may not be at all
easy to devise an entity that (without doing violence to its nature) can be
called neither "a thing" nor "an act." In the terms of Example 5.9, the idea
of a giant may be of low ontological density; but if all endeavors to discern
useful groupings of heights should fail, one may by the process of abstraction to a higher level call height a thing and growth an act. As we might ex-

pect, however, for practically nothing one gets practically nothing. We have (so to speak) made Things safe for ethicists but in so doing have robbed the term of much of its ontology. There is a useful distinction between what can be measured and what can be only categorized. By decree, categories can be treated as measures (e.g., as the number of successes, X, in a binomial process of order N becomes a measure). But as Abraham Lincoln so earthily put it, calling the tail of a dog a leg does not make it a leg (Bartlett 1962: 542). Thimblerigging of terms does not change the properties of the term rigged. By the time the specificity has been bled out of the ultimate terms of discourse, no useful statements may survive the generalization.

Now, a billiard ball, judged by its crass physical properties, would have high ontological density: it has a sharply defined exterior that is reinforced by its necessarily spherical shape; it is stout, not easily broken, homogeneous, and highly elastic (in the technical physical sense that it resists stretching, squeezing, and deformation); in its appropriate use it behaves virtually as one mass. In a world of upholstery and rice pudding and fluffy toys, it appears to enjoy something of the adamantine quality of the atom. It is a useful image of the decisive type of Thing.

•   Note that we are not using its physical properties to define the being of the billiard ball. They serve merely as a rough indication that the billiard ball is sufficiently defined to be an object of useful discourse. No matter what licensing boards may prescribe, one does not, by analogy, define a physician as one who has acquired a certificate or memorized a certain number of facts. But at least these qualities are some kind of screening test, however crass, that might help us in trying to discern what we mean by "a physician." It is not at all evident that the essence of a physician can ever be adequate defined.

One way of assessing Things is to consider how far they share characteristics. One billiard ball may impart its momentum to another and be stopped dead in the impact. Just so, a Thing called a cause may set in motion another Thing called an effect and spend itself in the process.

Now, this *billiard-ball theory* of Ethics,[1] though a reasonable first approximation, seems usually to be quite inadequate for analysis of many refined problems.

Criminal Insanity

EXAMPLE 6.2. In the administration of law, the interpretation of the facts implied in the *McNaughton* rules (see Lindeman and Mcintyre 1961:

---

1. We use the term as a brief phrase to summarize "atomic" Ethics, but not derisively, although we disagree profoundly with it. Moreover, this scheme is not related to the common ascription to the theories of Hobbes.

332), for adjudication in a defense against a criminal charge on grounds of insanity, is that in its daily operation the mind behaves as a complex of components of high ontological density. It is as if the "faculty" of understanding were one unit of a computer that had failed and might, in principle, be fully restored by replacing it. The gist of *McNaughton* was whether the man accused of an assassination and claimed to be laboring under some delusion or misunderstanding had behaved as a sane person would have done if the content of the delusion had been true. In a word, it countenanced insanity as a *pure defect of cognition.* For a century this vision dominated the psychiatric defense on grounds of insanity. Since then a succession of Legal rulings, authoritative statements by forensic psychiatrists, and the promulgations of responsible and learned bodies have progressively eroded the reputability of *McNaughton.* In 1929 "irresistible impulse" was admitted as a defense, while nevertheless distinguishing and excluding impulses that were not irresistible, simply unresisted (Smith *v* United States 1929). In the celebrated *Durham* decision in 1954, Bazelon greatly widened the scope of the defense of insanity (Durham *v* United States 1954). The scope of the new ruling was so wide that later judgments recognized that *Durham* was being abused, and they redressed it. A judgment by Leventhal sought a more temperate course, which nonetheless included disturbed emotion as a reasonable substance for a defense (United States *v* Brawner 1972). Thus, the defense on grounds of insanity now extended beyond cognition, to the other two main features of conation and affect.[2] The thoughtful review by Capron (1972) is interesting reading. Robitscher, both a physician and a lawyer, gives an account (1966: chap. 9) that is both Medical and Legal, with historical details.

COMMENT.   The ethicist must surely be disturbed by the fact that *McNaughton* was held in high repute for so long. Regardless of the merits of the judgment in *McNaughton,* it seems to be a flagrant example of attempting to canonize axiomatic judgments stemming from what purported to be common sense with no regard for empirical fact. We cannot fault it for a lack of scientific fact that was not available a century and a half ago. Even so, it must surely be rated as an impenetrably aprioristic standpoint both to believe that an insane mind operates in the same way as a sane one except for a few errors of briefing, and to have no phronetic concern over whether the decisions arrived at were at all incongruous. The *McNaughton* rule would rate as *A- -* on the scale described in Chapter 2. Moreover, it was allowed no scrutiny as fact and thus seems to have been awarded a higher standing and protection against reform. However, that is something

2. These three aspects of attention are implicitly Kantian in spirit and represent a vestige of the old tradition in which Psychology was a branch of Philosophy. We encounter them in somewhat greater detail in Chapter 15.

of a diversion from our concerns here. The more disturbing ontological fact is that so intricate and subtle a phenomenon as the human mind has undergone a facile dissection into constructive components that, without a scintilla of evidence, have been endowed with high ontological density. But, of course, understanding the mind is not the only kind of problem that has suffered this fate.

Complex Action

In Medical Ethics, the notion that a medical procedure, even a surgical operation, is a single indecomposable Act simply will not suffice. To motivate this discussion further, let us consider the Ethical criterion known as the *principle of double effect*. We would like to make it clear at this stage that we are not concerned with the *fairness,* the *truth,* or the *usefulness* (or otherwise) of this principle or even whether it is totally out of fashion; we discuss it merely to show a commonplace attitude that is posited in arguments of this kind.[3]

Say that an Act *A* has two consequences: *B*, which is proximate (most immediate) and intended, and *C*, which is remote and unintended. It is argued that (given certain premises, which are irrelevant to the discussion) if *B* (the proximate consequence) is good and *C* (the remote consequence) is bad, then the Act *A* is ethical; but if *B* is bad, then *A* is not ethical, even if *C* is good. (*Good, bad,* and *ethical* are here undefined terms. Those who think of this argument at a purely Logical level will not be distracted by them. Also, there are problems concerned in the word *intended,* which we discuss in Chapter 13.)

EXAMPLE 6.3. A surgeon diagnoses a cancer of the prostate in a patient, a disorder curable but life-threatening. He performs an operation *(A)* to remove the cancer, which eliminates the danger or most of it, a good effect *(B)*, but which may also sterilize the patient, a bad effect *(C)*. Since *B* is a proximate (direct) effect and *C* a remote (indirect) one, then *A* is ethical.

Leaving to one side the question of whether the Ethics is sound or the conclusions warranted, let us analyze more closely the ontology of the terms of this argument. This principle of double effect is addressed here because it puts a heavy strain on the billiard-ball properties of Thing and Act. (If *A, B,* and *C* are not discrete, sharply defined, and cleanly separable, the utility of the whole principle is in ruins.) On these terms, the principle declares that there shall be no "package deals." We may not arbitrarily decide to lump *A* and one of its effects together as one Act just because it suits us to do so; nor may we lump *B* and *C* together as one effect. Furthermore,

3. For detailed discussion of the principle of double effect, see McCormick 1977.

B and *C* must both be ontologically dense; if the argument were to concede that there is overlap, we have no natural way of resolving ambiguities about which is proximate and which remote, particularly if they cannot be distinguished ontologically. *A* is treated as one Act; it has no parts, it does not have stages. If, as is common practice, the first step in prostatectomy is to prevent infection by tying off the vasa deferentia (which itself sterilizes), this is to be subsumed under an Act, "prostatectomy."

Second, what is being attacked is a cancer. But who is to say what a cancer is, or what its limits are? Prostatic cancer, probably more than any other cancer we know, is intimately related to the hormonal milieu, so much so that castration is a common ancillary treatment for it. Also, extensive surveys (Whitmore 1956; Sheldon, Williams, and Fraley 1980) have shown that elderly men nearly all have prostatic tissue that, by standard and well-established histological criteria, is cancerous. Is it thus to be argued that these cancerous changes are in some sense "normal" concomitants of aging? (The thorny problem of defining normality is discussed in some detail in Chapter 8.) If so, is it good or bad to remove the prostate and interfere with the "normal" state? Consequentialist ethicists will ask whether this operation improves the prognosis. The evidence is in dispute (Chodak et al. 1994; Lu-Yao et al. 1994; Fleming et al. 1993; Whitmore 1994).

Instances of profound ontological ambiguity such as arise in Example 6.3 could be multiplied, but that would be to paint the lily. We have perhaps made it sufficiently clear that there is need to discuss our fundamental terms, *Things, Acts, normality, disease,* and so forth, in considerable detail.

THING

A fundamental problem in the discussion of Things is to emancipate the mind from notions that are not necessities of thought but mere clutter. To put our analysis on a less fragile basis, we propose to deal only in ideas to which we believe no rational mind will take exception. Rational scientists, for instance, in pursuing their inquiries into the nature of the universe, do not believe that they are elaborating some invention of their own minds, as Shakespeare in writing *Hamlet* might have wondered how he was going to arrange the details of his hero's death. The universal scientific stance is that the inquiring mind is not inventing a world but discovering it. There are bases for discovery that exist apart from the perceivers and their often garbled imagery. Such bases we shall call *existents*.

But clearly (and indeed tautologously) one has no reason to believe that the set of phenomena that human beings have so far observed, directly or indirectly, exhausts the entire set of existents. It seems utterly unreasonable to suppose that before Röntgen's work in 1896 there were no X-rays, and therefore they should not have been considered existents. Nevertheless, there is at least practical utility in distinguishing what has been experienced and what has not. A Thing is an existent that has an impact on the human mind, directly or indirectly, through the organs of sense, through imagination, or through rational speculation, tempered by cogent use of indirect evidence.

THE FORMAL STRUCTURE OF THING

Some classes of existents may not be knowable directly but come to be perceived as an aggregate of existents. Thus, the naked eye cannot see the atoms in a brick, but it can see the aggregate of atoms that make up the brick. The complete set of existents is some enormous but (we will suppose) finite number. There is, then, an even larger number of subsets (i.e., individual selections) that may be made from among the existents. For instance, each existent is a subset. So is the entire set of existents. The total set of subsets is known as the *power set,* and enumerating its contents is an enormously tedious exercise in elementary combinatorics.

Some of these subsets will have a coherent impact on the human mind as Things. Some will be so incoherent that the mind will not see them as in any way related. And also, the coherence of some of them will be evident only at certain times. For instance, there may well be emergent properties perceived only when a certain configuration is attained. Manifestly, the set of existents that to a particular person constitutes Things, even intermittently, corresponds to only a minute proportion of the components of the power set. Some existents, singly or in groups, may have no impact on the mind, because, for example, there is neither a corresponding sensory modality (e.g., one cannot see infrared light) nor an intellectual endowment through which they may be constructed or reconstructed (the temperature of invisible light or infrared-sensitive photographs).

Objectivity and Subjectivity

What we call a Thing has two aspects. First, it corresponds in some way to external actualities or existents. It therefore has *objectivity* in the strict sense. But second, it must have some kind of impact (however remote) on the human mind, or we would have no occasion to consider it. Hence, a Thing also has a component of *subjectivity.* A Thing is thus an interfacing between the existent and the subject perceiving it.[4] This conclusion does

4. Reality is considered by some to be limited to the correspondence between existents and the subjective counterpart. But in our view reality is more than this, for in addition there are existents that have not yet been perceived, as with X-rays before Röntgen or repressed material in the unconscious. On the other hand, there are subjective experiences that occur without there being direct external correspondence to them, such as rainbows, hallucinations,

not commit us to any sensationalistic epistemology. The relationship between existents and the mind is a reciprocal one.

EXAMPLE 6.4. In the *Timaeus*, Plato surmised that sight is something emitted by the eye, somewhat perhaps like a radar beam (Bury 1929). Physics dismisses that surmise: there is no dispute that the light comes from the needle to the eye and not conversely. However, we do well to note that Plato is discussing sight *(horan)*, which he treats as quite separate from light *(phos)*. A burst of electromagnetic energy is not a percept, still less a concept. Diverse objects may bombard the senses with stimuli: the noise of traffic and the flashing of neon signs in Times Square. But the human mind is not obliged to make a Thing out of this aggregate. There are a great many bursts of energy that the senses receive from the exterior of which the mind makes nothing (i.e., no-Thing). To suppose that what we call Things is a simple matter of physical stimuli is perilous reductionism.

Thingness

The mind imposes Thingness on reality at least as much as the converse. Plato's view seems to us correct if we suppose that what the eye is emitting is not a physical process; rather, it is imposing a principle of arbitrary order. In this sense we regard a Thing as an interaction, a reciprocal and complementary relationship between perceiver and existents. This interpretation calls for caution on two points.

First, we cannot look exclusively to the external world of physical phenomena, of measurement and the like, as our basis for the notion of Thingness. The temptation to do so is great, not merely because the *Zeitgeist* is scientific and urges interpretation in terms of a theory of cause, but because within its own domain physics has an epistemology of unrivaled brilliance and resolution.

Second, Thingness is in large degree a product of the mind. The readiness with which the mind will accord to any collection of existents the status of being a Thing depends on the particular preparation of the thoughts. The existent may not mean the same Thing, or even any Thing at all, to every person. The commonsense view of Thing may be sensed differently by different minds.

EXAMPLE 6.5. To the painter, perhaps, a cloud is a Thing, a coherent entity that may be used to convey some artistically unified idea. An air-traffic controller keeping track of six planes inside the same cloud may

---

dreams, or ideals. Since they are actually experienced, they are experiential existents. Reality, to us, includes all the existents.

perceive it as, perhaps, a complex set of quite distinct physical entities among which clear separation (but not, in general, independence) is to be preserved.

Likewise, a stonemason may see stones as Things and an architect may see cathedrals as Things, even though the one may be made from large numbers of the other. Or a tire, a car, and a fleet of cars may all be thought of as Things by different kinds of people concerned with different kinds of speculation.

Consequently, Thingness is subjective, even idiosyncratic to a point that to a physicist such as Feynman (1989: 30 ff.) is foreign—nay, repellent. Complete unanimity about such personal viewpoints is not a reasonable objective. Nor can we reasonably expect complete consistency from the individual thinker, however coherent and articulate. Thus, arguments about Things may appear unambiguous up to a certain level of resolution only. Furthermore, an appeal to particular Things, or even to the idea of Things as subjects of discourse, as if they were immutable Philosophical bedrock on which one might base rigid principles suitable for universal and perpetual arguments (in Ethics, for instance), seems to us to court peril. Things may be invaluable parochial structures, like the facts in a particular domain of application. But we have learned from empirical Psychology how we may be betrayed by our inconsistencies not only of sensation but of perception; and the experiences of twentieth-century physics in particular have taught caution about conceptualizations also, and the dangers of appealing to the obvious, the commonsense, or, more formally, our tenuous epistemological criteria of consistency.

DEFINITION.   A *Thing* is an abstract, arbitrary grouping of interfacings between the human mind and a collection of existents, recognized in the course of action or discourse.

It is in view of the caveats we raised above that we refer to a Thing as abstract and arbitrary. These two points merit further discussion.

A Thing as an Abstract Grouping

That Things are abstract groupings does not deny that a Thing may be completely concrete. A gallstone is a Thing. So is homeostasis (i.e., the set of compensating mechanisms in the body that tend to restore a previous state that has been perturbed). Obviously one can handle, break, throw, or discard a gallstone; one cannot do the same with homeostasis. Nevertheless, it seems to us that homeostasis is at least as worthy a topic for Ethical argument as a gallstone is.

There is no need for any universal quality about a Thing, and indeed there is no uniformity in the kind of criteria of Thingness. We may cite several different criteria.

First, the components of a Thing may have in common physical contiguity. Thus, a brick is an aggregate of atoms that cohere physically and resist considerable efforts used to sunder them. Physical contiguity may at times be much weaker so that the ontological cohesion from this source is more suspect.

EXAMPLE 6.6. The brain contains many so-called nuclei, that is, clusters of cells that are close together but not held together by any strong force. The warrant for ascribing Thingness in that case is communality of function. For instance, one cranial nerve (such as the trochlear) may arise from one nucleus and be distributed to a single muscle (the superior oblique) and nothing else. However, in the trigeminal nerve, for instance, the unity is undermined by the fact that centrally the nerve arises from at least three nuclei, and peripherally it is distributed as a sensory nerve in three major regional branches (whence the name) supplying also motor nerves to the third division of them. In fact, the trigeminal nerve has only a brief coherence. Note also that a single horseshoe-shaped structure, continuous throughout, may appear on the plane of section to comprise two unattached parts.

Second, the components of a Thing may be held together by continuity in time.

EXAMPLE 6.7. The statement "In the last ten years Mr. Jones's liver has developed cirrhosis" seems—at an everyday level of resolution, at least—a clear and reasonably defined statement. Now, in those ten years many, perhaps most, of the atoms in that liver have been replaced; so the Thing of which the cirrhosis is predicated cannot be the atoms, but an identity that has been preserved in its continuity of anatomy and function over time. This phenomenon is expressly discussed by Lonergan (1957).

Third, the Thingness may reside in a very subtle functional coherence that only a skilled mind may perceive.

EXAMPLE 6.8. The early anatomist examining gross structures saw perhaps the adrenal glands as paired organs, and the sympathetic nervous system also as an organ but a quite distinct one. For a great many purposes this delineation of Things may still be useful, as in operative surgery. Endocrinologists, concerned with biochemical activities, would see the matter quite differently. To them the two parts of the adrenal gland are merely accidental neighbors (see Koizumi and Brooks 1980; Yates, Marsh, and Maran 1980). Its medulla produces the hormone epinephrine, a function that it shares with the sympathetic nerve endings, and these two sources of the hormone work together in certain situations, typically involving alarm, pursuit of prey, and the expression of anger. The endocrinologists might see this combination of the adrenal medulla and the sympathetic nerve endings as a single Thing in our sense. The cortex of the adrenal gland produces two quite different hormones with functions most closely related to the endocrine functions of the gonads; the endocrinologist would therefore see the cortex as a second Thing. To Selye, the proponent of the stress syndrome (1936, 1956), however, the juxtaposition of the two components of the adrenal gland is not in any sense accidental. Both components are concerned with adaptation to stressful challenges: the medulla provides the means for immediate but transient response, the cortex the means for more delayed but also more sustained response. In Selye's grand perception, the two parts of the adrenal gland are united by a single purpose: to confront stress. Both medulla and cortex raise the blood sugar and the blood pressure, concomitants of purposeful physical action.

Here, then, even among three kinds of physicians (and there are surely others) we have three viewpoints of the organization (i.e., in the literal sense of "converting into an organ"), a choice of structures each reflecting a distinct set of abstractions, which implies no lack of concreteness, no want of pertinence to practical problems—yet abstractions for all that.

The foregoing three criteria—space, time, and function—are, of course, not intended to exhaust the possible grounds for defining a Thing. They merely illustrate how the notion of a Thing as an abstraction is not necessarily inconsistent with unwavering practicality of purpose.

A Thing as an Arbitrary Grouping

Again we use the term *arbitrary* in its strict, aboriginal meaning. The fashion has developed of using the word in almost a disparaging sense. An "arbitrary decision" is one that is highhanded, capricious, unreasoned, even irresponsible. We intend it not in this way but rather in the sense that has not been entirely lost from the word *arbitration:* a selection is arbitrary if made after serious thought about its nature and consequences, although it does not correspond to any inalienably natural grouping.

EXAMPLE 6.9. The age at which a person is allowed to vote is arbitrary. Obviously, there is no instantaneous change in personality at the age of eighteen (or whatever critical age is chosen) that warrants the use of this age as a watershed for political maturity. Equally obviously, a baby one week old has no political views and is therefore unfitted to vote. Thus, under the democratic principle "one person, one vote," there must be some point at which the dividing line is drawn. The boundary is not drawn to correspond to any well-defined phenomenon (unless it be fusion of the last major epiphyses of the bones); on the other hand, it is not left to caprice. It is determined after mature reflection with the recognition that it has no other intrinsic basis, no principle to which appeal may be made. It is hence necessarily always tentative and for good reason may be modified, radically changed, or totally abandoned.

Nevertheless, an arbitration, however circumspect or punctilious, is not to be seen as an inalienable truth. Water can rise no higher than its source. We cannot accept the notion that what is the result of an arbitrary selection or decision can be made the basis for an argument *in principle*. For instance, the age at which the drinking of alcohol is permitted, and the level of blood alcohol at which driving is to be prohibited, cannot be formulated in any authentic principle. Billiard-ball ethics, which treats of Things, some of which are in fact decreed as if they existed in principle— that is, a priori and not by arbitration—seems to us a dangerous falsification of the subject matter of Medical Ethics.

We may have to modify this disclaimer in particular cases. It may be argued that the *person* is an intrinsic, and not an arbitrary, grouping. But no number of such counterexamples can sustain any general supposition that all, or even most, phenomena called Things correspond to inviolably intrinsic groupings.

The idea that a Thing is arbitrary in the strictest sense connotes ideally that it is defined by consensus.[5] To say that a Thing is arbitrary might be misinterpreted to mean that it is devised by someone for personal, even idiosyncratic, purposes; but in useful discourse a Thing should be seen as the result of free agreement among reasonable persons.

EXAMPLE 6.10. Suppose that in a primitive society most members see a piece of wood as fuel but somebody else perceives it as a weapon. There

5. Like so many words used not on their merits but as "elegant variation," *consensus* has lost much of its savor. It is a "cohesion of thought and belief." It is not a compromise. It is not a majoritarian decision, however large the plurality. Those with any sense of history know that wherever there is dispute, painfully often it is a minority, sometimes only one or two people, who turn out in the long run to be correct, to the humiliation of the majority of experts and their many supporters. Small wonder that this should happen. Truth is not a democratic matter to be decided by vote. So long as there is one sound disputant who sees a flaw in the general belief and articulates it, and so long as that complaint is not adequately answered, then there is no consensus. Of course, we do not claim that even with consensus there is any guarantee against error. But the two best natural steps to truth are complete integrity in the Logic and scholarship, and assurance that error is given a wide margin. Consensus is a fair demonstration of both. By analogy, a pharmacologist trying to find the lethal dose of a drug by administering it to a thousand mice will reach vastly different conclusions if no mice are killed and if only one mouse dies.

is likely to be little progress made in negotiations between them about disarmament. It takes consensus to ensure peace, but only one dissident to imperil it. (It would be laboring the point to remark that even as we write, this seemingly fatuous dispute is exactly analogous to what is going on over the uses, but also perhaps the threat of abuse, of fissionable nuclear material in such countries as North Korea and Iraq.)

Furthermore, the agreement about what is to be called a Thing must not be limited to drawing up some fiction "for purposes of argument." Rational argumentation is not only a matter of axioms and terms but also a search for a fully authentic and rational answer. Shallow statements using the term *disease* (see Chapter 8) or a contrived grouping of medical procedures under the fictive label *operation* (see Example 6.11) are not a sound basis for lasting policy.

The Stability of Things

A consensus is not necessarily permanent. It may have to be modified in time as the existents become more clearly perceived or as radically new knowledge accrues from unexpected sources. Further empirical knowledge may call for a new consensus about a particular Thing, which will have an impact on Ethical argumentation. We refer the reader to the problem of defining human gender in Example 5.6. It is idle to treat systematic doubts on the point as a minute flaw, a wrinkle in the fabric of Medical ontology. Much of the ambiguity is the result of high-resolution science, largely dating from the last thirty years.

We also remind readers of the principle stated at the end of Chapter 3 that no unresolved problem in Ethics is trivial.

We do not expect Things of all kinds to be equally susceptible to change; we expect the definition of gender to be more stable than that of rheumatoid arthritis. In an Ethical system, we find that there is a hierarchy of stability: those Things playing a part in the theoretical underpinning (e.g., personhood) are required to be the most stable; those involved in the construction of working definitions and rules are to be intermediate; and those ordinary Things that are the subject of particular cases are to be the least stable.

ACT

From our definition, Acts are special cases of Things, and all that we have discussed about a Thing applies also to an Act. Nevertheless, because of their central, even essential, role in Ethics, it seems worthwhile to treat

Acts separately. An Act too is abstract and arbitrary. An Act, however, has two distinctive features that must be carefully considered.

A Thing is an object of knowledge, and commonly a passive type of knowledge, whereas an Act is also an object of will — it commonly involves deliberation, value judgment, and execution. The Act of one person may impinge on the consciousness of another just as much as a brick can; but in addition, an Act involves responsibility, which a Thing does not. Accordingly, Acts by their nature fall within the domain of behavior; and if there were no human activity, there would be no need for Ethics. However, it is only in the ontology of Ethics that Things are of importance.

The other distinctive feature is that an Act is dynamic. To be sure, we have considered, by implication at least, that the life history of a Thing is an aspect of it: that a full description of a Thing, such as Mr. Jones's liver, is not merely a matter of spatial features but a spatially three-dimensional entity in time, four dimensions in all. There is, however, a sense in which a Thing exists in an instant of time, that is, time of no duration. But of its very substance an Act involves duration and progression in time. A painting as such is a Thing; a piece of music of its essence has order and duration, and its deployment has the dynamic quality of an Act. Of course, the viewing of the painting is an Act, while an unplayed score or an unreproduced and unheard recording of the music remains a Thing.

We have noted before how the arbitrary limits of a Thing may be changed by expanding or curtailing its extension in space. In a subsidiary degree it may be curtailed or expanded in time. The same arbitrary manipulation of limits may be made on Acts, except that here their loci are interchanged. An Act may be viewed by its narrow spatial repercussions; but the greatest scope for arbitrary extension or contraction of Acts is in time. In this way the billiard-ball Ethics becomes entirely unworkable: what is a remote Act and what a proximate one is no longer necessarily determined by natural boundaries. That occasional counterexamples occur does not really help to solve the ontological problem in general. The important concept is that an Act is not necessarily, or even usually, so clear, concise, and delimited an entity as is commonly supposed, and it does not fall so easily in place in an Ethical consideration.

The Temporal Aspect of an Act

The difficulties posed for a Medical Ethics when an Act is supposed of its nature to be ontologically dense with respect to time can be well illustrated by trying to apply a type of general Ethical principle to a surgical example. In this discussion, of course, we are not concerned with the truth of any judgments expressed by this principle. To make this detachment clear, for the Moral term *good* we substitute *transparent;* for *bad,* we use the word *opaque;* for *indifferent,* the word *translucent;* and for *ethical,* the word *luminous.*[6]

Then suppose we are given the Ethical principle "To perform a bad Act to attain a good result is not ethical." To try to divorce the Logic from the distracting effect of putting in values, let us translate that into the Logically equivalent statement "To perform an opaque Act to attain a transparent result is not luminous."

First, what are the implications of the general principle? They are that we may not make a "package deal" for kinds of Acts. We may not lump together an opaque Act and a transparent Act to get an overall transparent Act, and therefore a luminous result. The combination is not even a translucent Act, which would also be a luminous one. The opaque Act is a deliberate one, and this determines that the whole procedure is opaque and therefore nonluminous. Let us try to apply this to a particular surgical problem.

EXAMPLE 6.11. Suppose that the removal of cancer is transparent, but that injury to healthy bodily tissue is opaque. What, then, are we to make of the operation of nephrectomy for cancer of the kidney? Removal-of-a-healthy-kidney from a living person seems to be an Act of pure mutilation with no redeeming features and therefore opaque. Now, we might simply insist that removal-of-a-cancerous-kidney from a living person is a single transparent Act. That would treat removal-of-a-cancerous-kidney and removal-of-a-healthy-kidney as two different and ontologically indecomposable processes. Then we at once see that in transplant of a kidney, removal-of-a-healthy-kidney from a healthy person is an opaque Act even if the transplantation is transparent. One is performing an opaque Act to attain a transparent result, which is impossible.

However, even where one person only is concerned, it is quite unrealistic to treat nephrectomy as if it were one indecomposable Act. To the contrary, a senior surgeon will quite commonly delegate parts of the operative procedure to juniors, such as making the incision or sewing the wound up afterward. Thus, the first step will be making an incision in the abdominal wall. Is the incision a transparent or translucent Act? Evidently not. Nobody would so regard such an incision made in a healthy person for no good reason. To the contrary, it would be a mutilation and therefore opaque. But the Ethical principle specifically demands that *we may not make a package deal of Acts.* An Act of mutilation is opaque and cannot be made transparent, or even translucent, however transparent the Acts mixed with it. But further, a later step, tying the renal pedicle, is also an opaque

6. The particular substitutions also give an interesting physical analogy that aids in illustrating the questions raised. The model indicates that the decision is good if the model allows light to pass through it.

Act. A surgeon in the abdomen for some other purpose would not tie the pedicle off simply to allow junior assistants to get some surgical experience. So this Act too is incurably opaque.

Yet again, much, perhaps most, of the tissue removed will be noncancerous, and this too is wanton mutilation, and therefore opaque. Furthermore, even the cancerous cells are not abnormal *in toto*. And even the process of sewing up the wound after the operation is a mutilation. Introducing foreign material into the tissues will be met with an inflammatory reaction and perhaps rejection.

It is thus evident that however much of the operation is transparent, several major parts of it, *taken in isolation,* are opaque. And the opaque parts are not in any sense incidental, or indirect, or by-products of something else. They are all deliberate and indispensable Acts or episodes in a continuum of activity. Thus, it seems that removing a kidney (cancerous or not) consists in a sequence of distinguishable steps: except for the *unity of a general purpose,* it is not, like a cue stroke in billiards, readily seen to have any intrinsic unity. Therefore, no such operation—indeed, practically no medical procedure whatever—could be defended under an Ethical principle that treats an Act as if it were indecomposable, unless there were some means of at least establishing some principle of the unity of the Act. That it is not all an inexorable, unitary, process is shown by the fact that virtually the same starting incision may be used in many quite different operations dealing with different diseases in quite different organs. We are unimpressed with the idea that because a procedure is given one name ("nephrectomy"), that decrees it to be a single, indecomposable Act.

The problem is that the limits of an Act are arbitrary, just as are the limits of a Thing. But a course of action occurs in time; thus, when it is analyzed we find that an arbitrary selection of limits in time is made. An adequate Ethical analysis will have to take this into account.

COMMENT.　The reader must not mistake the intent of this example. It must look like beating a dead horse. Whatever the argument says, there are no serious proponents of the view that all operations that involve mutilating normal tissue are unethical. However, it is clear that the Ethical principle as stated—that no package deals involving heterogeneous Acts are admissible—is totally inadequate. It fails the existential test: it does not bear any relationship to how anybody actually behaves or to what anybody recommends. By Flew's reversal principle (1989: 22–24), the unacceptability of the conclusion allows us (in this broad context, at least) to demolish the Ethical principle that the end never justifies the means. Phronesis would not tolerate all this shilly-shallying for an instant.

This discussion of an Act leads naturally to a discussion of continuity and discreteness in human behavior. We shall return to that discussion shortly; but we must first pay some attention to the voluntary aspect of an Act.

The Voluntary Aspect of an Act

In accordance with standard Medical usage, we make a distinction between *Act* and *action*. The two correspond, respectively, to the operation of the so-called voluntary nervous system and somatic musculature in Act; and to the operation of the autonomic nervous system and splanchnic musculature in action or physiologic activity. There are movements that partake of both: the muscles of the upper eyelid, the bladder, and the genitalia.

We have previously noted that an Act is an object of will. The latter property distinguishes an Act from Things in general, and from an action. Tying off the renal pedicle is an Act (or a composite Act). The beating of the surgeon's heart is an action, a physiologic activity.

EXAMPLE 6.12. The respiration of the surgeon is a peculiar and important case; it is neither a pure Act, since it is automatic, for instance, in sleep or in coma; nor is it a pure action, since to some extent it can be modified voluntarily. It is predominantly an action. Breathing in professional singing or in flute playing is primarily an Act. The surgeon losing consciousness from a massive cerebral hemorrhage will continue to breathe, and evidently the breathing is then a pure action of the respiratory center and not an Act. As a further demonstration of the distinctness of the two components, we point to the disorder known as Ondine's curse (sleep apnea): during sleep the automatic action of the respiratory center is lost, and the patient does not have the attention necessary to keep breathing.

Although an Act may be voluntary, there is some difficulty in relating will to Act. Responsibility (which we discuss in some depth in Chapters 14 and 15) implies deliberation and some degree of choice. Reflex activity is strictly a physiologic response to a stimulus. The familiar knee jerk is a reflex; as such, it does not involve deliberation, and indeed the whole process need involve nothing other than certain intact pathways in the spinal cord in a patient paralyzed from the waist down. Nevertheless, besides being mediated through somatic (voluntary) muscle, the knee jerk may be (and often is) stimulated by a voluntary Act. Even when simulated or elicited by a voluntary component, the reflex as such is trivial from an Ethical standpoint.

We note in passing that Philosophers professing so-called eliminative materialism, for example, when writing on the mind-brain problem, would flatly deny that volition has any meaning. Paul Churchland (1984) has expressed that view quite explicitly. Without becoming engaged in controversy on this difficult topic, we would confidently propose to appeal

(minimalistically) to the empirical stance of Searle's "biological natural-
ism" (Searle 1992) that in fact the basic level of operation of the brain is
neurological and not physical; and its clear implication that the basis of
analysis is how the brain in fact works, not how physical reductionism says
it ought to work.

The Cultivation of Fast Responses

There is a common, though malapropian, usage of the term *reflexes* to
refer to those immediate actions that occur in response to unheralded situations. A sportswriter will say of a shortstop that his "reflexes are quick."
Here the response reflects no present deliberation, although in its initial
execution during practice it did. In many cases it would be misleading to
suppose that for that reason no volition is involved. It is clear that volition
may be remote as well as proximate. The apparently involuntary nature
of the Act results from cultivation by practice of a set of responses. It is
in fact a deliberate Act that is by now habitual and thus somewhat like a
conditioned reflex. It may even in some cases become a conditioned reflex,
and no longer an Act. An experienced skater, for instance, will respond
unreflectingly to an irregularity on the surface of the ice; so will the beginner. But the expert responds with cultivated purposive maneuvers that
(like those of the violinist developing the right fingering for a complicated
musical passage) go beyond mere instinctive coordination.

Appreciation of the voluntary character of an Act remains incomplete
if only the conscious level of functioning is considered. The consensus of
psychiatrists from Janet and Charcot onward (and perhaps even earlier)
is that the parliament of the mind is not all conscious, that (to extend the
metaphor) the silent majority of the unconscious mind has a large share of
the Act (see Appendix 1). The motives are often disguised and sometimes
inscrutable. The conscious mind may assign to its decisions its own interpretations, couched in palatable terms, if need be with the help of rationalization. The deliberative aspects of an Act have a variable impact on a decision and what is finally done. How far the unconscious mind may influence
a decision is an open question. It is a complicated problem to determine
how much deliberation may be modified and understood by analysis of the
psyche.

The Continuity or Discreteness of an Act

We denote by the term *continuity* whatever is capable of being infinitely subdivided, and by the term *discreteness* whatever does not exhibit
continuity even in part. As we noted in Chapter 3, current theoretical
physics requires that both activity and matter comprise elements that are

ultimately discrete (quanta of energy and fundamental particles of matter). Human activity is more coarse-grained, and there are no practical difficulties in regarding both Things and Acts as continuous. Nevertheless, both for analysis and for communication, many ethicists prefer to treat comparatively large segments of activity as "acts" and large segments of matter as "things." Without some further warrant, such a view is at best loose and at worst grossly misleading. Several objections may be raised:

1. It is not clear that such groupings are necessary.
2. There seems to be no rigorous basis put forward for the delimitations.
3. Agreement among observers ordinarily is superficial, and a little probing will expose fundamental dispute.
4. Such groupings do not lend themselves to widely applicable principles, and every particular case is then required to be judged on its merits.
5. Things and Acts in this quasi-discrete sense enjoy no invariance. A brick may be viewed as a collection of Things (particles of mud), a Thing-in-itself (a building unit), or part of a Thing (a building). Likewise, tying an artery may be viewed as a set of Acts, an Act-in-itself, or part of an Act (an entire operation).

In the face of these criticisms, and perhaps others, two major questions arise. Is an Ethics based on Acts and Things a necessity of thought, or is it merely one way of looking at the world—a purely cultural pattern, perhaps? Is it possible to construct a consistent, coherent Ethics by abandoning these conventions and substituting continua of activity and matter? Perhaps we have need of both viewpoints. Any answers will be empty if they do not lead to rigorous structures with internal consistency. To delimit an Act as discrete and then go on to examine its parts is absurd. Discreteness implies that the entity has no parts; if it did, it would be not a unit but an aggregate of units. It is illogical and (in Moral issues dishonest) to try to have it both ways.

EXAMPLE 6.13. A man may descend from a mountaintop by jumping off a cliff, by walking down, or by sliding down on skis. We are prepared to concede that jumping may be viewed as an Act in the discrete sense: unaided, he cannot change his course halfway down. In Medicine, analogous cases are so rare and so little to the point that we cannot consider them a sound basis for Medical Ethics. The man walking and the man skiing down the mountain are behaving in much the same way, except that walking consists in small, more or less discrete Acts (taking paces) while sliding is one continuous activity. In either case, every instant of the descent may be viewed as a decision point even if the actual decision is nothing more than an implicit one to continue. Clearly neither man is at any stage committed beyond recall to pursue his original plan.

It is false to approach Medical Ethics as if all, or even most, Medical management were like descent by jumping rather than by skiing or walking. Occasionally this representation may be accurate (e.g., in a semi-instinctive but uncompromising decision in an emergency). For the most part the portrayal as massive, discrete, and irrevocable is a gross distortion.

EXAMPLE 6.14. The ontologist might like to wonder whether a series of ten operations for plastic surgery designed to produce one result is one Act or a series of Acts.

EXAMPLE 6.15. To quote an extreme instance, we wonder whether there would be any serious proponents of the claim that psychoanalysis—several sessions weekly for two, three, four years—is a single Act and does not involve countless thousands of discrete decisions along the way. The psychoanalyst may have a very clear objective that imparts coherence and relevance to the whole process. But would a traditionalist, in calling the whole matter a single Act, be content to judge the process as a whole, and either condemn the whole as unethical because some of the side issues offend or accept it holus-bolus because the overall result is good? Yet once we start chopping this long project into parts, it is difficult to see by what judgment we decide when some intrinsically indivisible component sub-Act has been attained. It seems to us unsound, and in all likelihood unnecessary, to build a system of Ethics on so contrived a foundation.

The most reasonable way seems to us to recognize that—some rare and most atypical cases excepted—the ontology of an Act depends on its arbitrary delineation within a continuum of human activity. Many ethicists, however, do not see it in that light. We are thus led to a definition of the term *Act* as we conceive it in our approach to Ethics:

DEFINITION.   An *Act* is an abstract formulation of a segment in a continuum of activity arbitrarily chosen for analysis of voluntary behavior.

The terms *abstract* and *arbitrary* here have the same force as when applied to define a Thing.

We recognize that, for an Act as for a Thing, there may exist some properties external to the observer, either real or figmented, that lead to a sound arbitrary judgment being made; nevertheless, even if the judgment proves both useful and apt in many cases, it must not be confused with a rigorous demonstration, and the Act or Thing does not of itself necessarily have any intrinsic qualities. In the discussion of Thing we have already commented at length on the contribution of objective and subjective components in this kind of judgment. In addition, if any Ethical system could not accommodate originality and departure from established custom in dealing with Medical problems, there would be no prospect of change, and hence no improvement. The correspondence between an Act as dissected by observers and the Act as the actor personally sees it is an intricate (and perhaps elusive) undertaking that we address in Chapters 14 and 15.

Finally, whether we take as an Act a "small" division, such as making an incision during a nephrectomy, or a "large" one, such as long-term psychiatric treatment, we are on safe ground only so long as we recognize that the Act is a construct, and as such it may have to undergo further modifications. As soon as these crude and artificial structures start to impede our insight or to misrepresent the truth, they should be discarded. The warrant for this course of action is unabashed phronesis. But that does not deny that crude structures may have heuristic value. An air pilot finds the airport by radar but lands the plane by sight. Acts and Things may help in the broad development of Ethics; but that is no reason for believing they will have any permanent place in Medical Ethics.

CONCLUSION

The analysis in this chapter leads to the inferences that a Thing is whatever is perceived and agreed upon as a Thing; and that an Act is whatever portion of voluntary activity is perceived and agreed upon as an Act. The directness of these statements may perhaps seem surprising, but it is fully in accord with the rigor and parsimony we believe should be exercised in the formulation of Medical Ethics. Nor should these conclusions, which fall strictly within the domain of Ethics, be taken as representing the whole of our opinions.

We summarize.

First, many assertions are in dispute. But staunch Ethics has to be founded on premises about which there is general agreement. So to the extent that such notions as Thing and Act can be communicated cogently from one reasonable person to another, they are fertile components in a viable Ethical system.

Second, both Thing and Act we recognize as abstractions arbitrarily fashioned from the spatiotemporal continuum.

Third, it will be objected by some that we have dehumanized Ethics by our analysis—that we might as well be discussing geological events on some remote uninhabited planet. We who have ourselves been through countless experiences from human patients are not unsympathetic. However, we give the following reply:

1. An analysis requires abstraction, and abstraction always dehumanizes somewhat. For our part, we are unimpressed with the attention that traditional ethicists have devoted to the particular human confronted with a problem, as distinct from an abstract person confronting an abstract problem or a fictional person confronting a fictional problem. If we cannot improve on this treatment, at least we can plead that, as suppliers from the clinical front, we have not further encumbered the professional burdens of ethicists with false phenomenology.

2. If there are constraints on activity that arise from human nature, they should certainly be incorporated into Ethics. But a distinction is to be made between what ethicists believe they have discerned to be human nature and what ethicists (being members of that species) have misread into the data of science. If, for instance, it were discovered that all of human behavior is cultural and has no genetic component, this discovery would surely have quite profound implications for Ethics. It would be intolerable, however, to let a system of Ethics be based on a misinterpretation of such scientific evidence. It seems to us, moreover, that it is insufficient to propose a system of Ethics the sole virtue of which is internal consistency. This too easily degenerates into the purely axiomatic Ethics that stood up so poorly to scrutiny in Chapter 2.

3. Human beings contemplating the external world may be engaged in a much more trivial activity than contemplating each other; but undoubtedly they are in a more secure position scientifically, Psychologically, metamathematically, and epistemologically. We confront the problems arising from the essentially reflexive analysis of human nature in Chapter 15. The task is not easy, and the conclusions are likely to be controversial and unacceptable to many. Perhaps we may be forgiven for postponing the issue at this stage and concentrating our attention on a smaller body of relatively noncontroversial topics.

Finally, in Chapter 1 we characterized the purpose of Medical Ethics: it is to help in the making of decisions in concrete cases. Our analysis of Thing and Act has been directed with this goal in mind. One way of stating the minimum goal is that Ethics is to define and identify the connection between possible outcomes and the courses of action necessary to attain them (as is explored in Chapter 10). Thus, for example, where a patient's blood sugar is dangerously low (hypoglycemia), then, on the broad assumption that it is desirable to live, glucose must be administered. Strictly speaking, the connection between the objective of keeping the patient alive and the need to administer sugar is independent of (1) whether hypoglycemia exists as a discrete condition (a Thing) or whether it shades noncritically and imperceptibly into "normal" levels of blood glucose (a continuum); and (2) whether a glass of sugared water drunk rapidly is regarded as one bolus (an Act) or a continuous activity with finite duration.

We would point out, however—and it is a matter often overlooked by those espousing a strongly personalistic Ethics—that more practical good is done in Medicine by those who take the correct course (even in contempt or cynicism or with the grossest of personal intentions) than by those who act incompetently or inappropriately with the noblest of personal sentiments. There seems to be at least some value in distinguishing a code of Ethics from any actual Agent, in exactly the same way that one distinguishes between the theory of accountancy and a particular accountant who does or does not cheat when filling out his own income tax form; or between the rules of football and a referee who honestly or dishonestly applies them in a particular game.

7 Facts, Goals, and Strategies

In this chapter we address how Medical science may contribute material for Ethical reasoning. It covers interlocking topics that require some preliminary individual discussion. It draws on material already discussed, notably cardinality and dimensionality (from Chapter 3).

Readers will perhaps be prepared to put up with the somewhat fragmentary character of these preliminaries, the mutual pertinence of which should become clear in the latter part of the chapter. As an inducement we may give a brief sketch of where we are going.

THE FUNDAMENTAL TASK

Medical Ethics is concerned with co-adapting two major features: the facts from the empirical world of Medicine; and the behavior of the parties concerned—the physician, the patient, the relatives, and the representatives of society—in relation to the facts. The next steps are Moral and deontological, that is, directed to translating the propositions of Ethics into obligations. Taken as a whole, the endeavor seems to be doomed to failure. It is often said that one cannot deduce a conclusion of obligation from propositions of fact. C. S. Lewis (1947) cast it in grammatical terms: statements of fact are in the indicative mood; the Moral proposition, a command to act, is in the imperative; and the two are *incommensurable*.

EXAMPLE 7.1. Suppose that an examiner asks a candidate to identify the inventor of sonata form, adding, "I will give you a hint. The battle of Tagliacozzo took place in 1268." The candidate will be perplexed. How could these two facts, apparently so disparate, bear any relationship to each other? Could one even imagine a theory that would connect them nontrivially? It is not that the two matters are incompatible, that they clash in any way, for a clash involves, so to speak, a confrontation within a single arena. The difficulty is the exact opposite of a clash: they are so disparate that they share no *point d'appui*.

————

This lack of engagement between the facts and obligation is the essence of the quandary of incommensurability. Indeed, G. E. Moore (1903) reached a kind of Ethical nihilism that argues that principles of conduct are not deducible.

The criticism of incommensurability in Moral argument, however commonsensical, depends on assumptions that we shall make explicit. Although Morals and deontology (the study of obligations) do not directly impinge on Ethics (the study of human Acts and their consequences), confusion about the role of Morals has greatly added to confusion about the role of Ethics. The misunderstanding lies in the meaning of *Law*, which is critical for grasp of the structure of both.

SOME LOGICAL POINTS

No doubt readers will be familiar with elementary, Aristotelian, deductive Logic. However, because we want to use it in a rather unorthodox fashion, we shall define a few terms and give some examples.

DEFINITION. *Syllepsis* is a rhetorical figure in which, in juxtaposition, the same word is used in two different senses. Commonly one sense is literal, the other metaphorical.

EXAMPLE 7.2. In the sentence "The thief took a fond farewell and several valuable bracelets," the word *took* is being used of two objects with differing connotations, one metaphorical and abstract, one literal and physical.

DEFINITION. A *syllogism* is a logical method of drawing a conclusion from the juxtaposition of two statements of fact, called premises, one of which (the major premise) makes a predication of a set of which the other (the minor premise) is a subset.

EXAMPLE 7.3

Major premise: To live, all mammals require oxygen.
Minor premise: All bears are mammals.
Conclusion: Therefore, to live, all bears require oxygen.

Textbooks of Logic discuss in detail the rules for reaching *valid* conclusions from premises. If the premises are true, then we are guaranteed that the conclusion of a valid syllogism is also true. Validity is a property of Logic, truth a quality of propositions. So an inference may be valid, or true, or both, or neither. Deplorably, the two terms *truth* and *validity* are commonly confused. At a more practical (and hence more vulnerable) level, the rules are extended to making inferences about fact from data (Murphy, Rosell, and Rosell 1982). Details of these rules will not in general concern us here.

Sometimes a syllogism is formally valid but more or less misleading because of syllepsis in two or more of the components. One has only to think of the many meanings of *good* or *love* to see how readily argument, even by valid syllogisms, may be perverted. We shall discuss this error later; but its obvious perils have suggested the term *sylleptic syllogism* (Murphy 1972). It is known in classical Logic as equivocation; however, the word *equivocation* has so often been used as a euphemism for *lying* that it is now hopelessly debased.

EXAMPLE 7.4

Major premise: It is good for young boys to be normal.
Minor premise: It is normal for young boys to fall out of trees.
Conclusion: Therefore, it is good for young boys to fall out of trees.

Here *normal* is being used in two of its many senses (Murphy 1997). In the major premise it implies something like an ideal—the identification of something to be desired or aspired to. In the minor premise it is descriptive, meaning that it is very common for boys to fall out of trees. The former sense is (if you like) Platonic, the latter empirical. Although the syllogism is again valid, the conclusion is false because the terms are incommensurable. While the term *good* is appropriate to the sense of the word *normal* in the major premise, it is quite incongruous to understand it of the sense in which it is used in the minor. It is no more self-evidently true that something is good because it is common than it is self-evidently good that ^{32}P has a half-life of 14.3 days.

Let us take a more subtle variant.

EXAMPLE 7.5

Major premise: It is malpractice for doctors to give poison to their patients.
Minor premise: Morphine is a poison.
Conclusion: Therefore, it is malpractice for doctors to give morphine to their patients.

Set aside the moral overtones of this syllogism. It is perfectly valid. The word *poison* has the same meaning in the two premises. In the major premise, however, it denotes the giving of some substance in sufficiently large doses to inflict deliberate and unnecessary harm. In the minor premise it is a due warning to be put on certain bottles—not to mean that its contents should not be taken at all, but to mean that the dosage is critically important. Both usages are correct, but for a proper syllogism, in both premises there would have to be a statement about quantity.

DEFINITION.   An *enthymeme* is a syllogism that purports to be valid but is formally incomplete because of suppression of either one premise or the conclusion.

The suppressed term may be a premise.

EXAMPLE 7.6

Major premise: It is immoral to kill innocent people.
Conclusion: Therefore, waging war is immoral.

Here the minor premise "Waging war kills innocent people" is implied but not made explicit.

The conclusion may be implied but not expressed.

EXAMPLE 7.7

Major premise: Failing hearts dilate.
Minor premise: Mrs. Jones's heart is not dilated.

Here the conclusion "Therefore Mrs. Jones's heart is not failing" is suppressed.

There may even be double enthymemes in which two propositions are suppressed.

MEANING

At this stage we need a brief comment on the vast topic of the meaning of *meaning*. The topic is exhaustively examined in the classic text by Ogden and Richards (1960); but for our purposes here, a very little of it will suffice. This episode is prompted by semantic rather than ontological motives, and it aims to make only some simple distinctions.

EXAMPLE 7.8. Consider the meaning of the proposition "Smoking is carcinogenic." We can envisage at least three meanings pertinent to our topic:

1. *Deciphered meaning:* Smoking leads to cancer.
2. *Relational meaning:* Smoking is at least a contributory cause of cancer.
3. *Implicative meaning:* Whoever smokes is more liable to get cancer.

There are aspects of all three that might be discussed at length. Roughly:
The first answer is simply a translation of the technical term *carcinogenic.*[1]

The second answer addresses the meaning as a scientific proposition on which the evidence has a bearing.

The third answer defines a possible consequence of the individual's decision to smoke. It alone has Ethical overtones, for it addresses the personal appropriation of the interpretation of a relational statement, and that ties a free and responsible personal conduct to its consequences. It is also new in that it means a jump from a secure generality to a particular person. As such, it may indeed not be a sound jump, for it may be that increased liability attaches only to a well-defined, or at least definable, group. For instance, some geneticists have furnished evidence that perhaps only those with deficiency of the enzyme aryl hydrocarbon hydroxylase have the increased liability (Kellermann, Shaw, and Luyter-Kellermann 1973; Khouri et al. 1982). When a Statistical statement is being made about the whole population or about some person yet to be picked at random from it, there is an element of chance. Once the person has been picked, there may still be uncertainty because the person's genotype is unknown, but this is a reflection only of our lack of information about the genotype, and there is no Objective uncertainty. If we suppose that the surmise about the enzyme is true, then the uncertainty is epistemic, not ontological. Many individuals have claimed the right to decide (rationally or not) whether they are personally at risk; and certainly the Ethical implications for the individual would, in principle, be quite different from the implications in a public health campaign, for slogans have no room for subordinate clauses. So the zealot often overlooks—unwittingly, one hopes—the radical distinction between the statements "All smokers are at 50% risk of cancer" and "50% of smokers are at 100% risk of cancer." (The two models produce the *same average rate of cancer* among smokers.)[2] The scientific evidence in this case is not good enough to pursue this particular example cogently. But there are well-

1. A more vivid example of deciphered meaning would be to apply it to the dictum "Ontogeny recapitulates phylogeny," an admirably compact evolutionary principle and insight, but one worded with discouraging abstruseness.

2. Suppose that the genotype is unknown and the issue is the total lifetime risk of lung cancer in a sample of unrelated individuals from an infinite population. It is readily shown (e.g., by the use of compound Probability generating functions) that the Random variable follows the same distribution (e.g., the binomial or the Lexis distribution) regardless of whether the uncertainty is ontological or epistemic.

established instances in which dangers attach only to some already well-defined genetic states (such as deficiency of glucose-6-phosphate dehydrogenase, which causes adverse hematological reactions to certain drugs).

A MORE GENERAL FORM OF ARGUMENT

While two propositions may be incommensurable so that one cannot argue from the one to the other, a bridge may be provided by a third proposition that is formally incommensurable with both. A few simple physical illustrations may pave the way for a helpful analogy.

EXAMPLE 7.9. If the distance between two points is 10 inches, then (by international convention) it is also exactly 254 mm. Here there is no problem at all of incommensurability. The comparative distances can be found by multiplication, or read off from markings on the upper and lower sides of a single-dimensioned diagram like a ruler (Figure 7.1A).

EXAMPLE 7.10. The area of a circle may be expressed in a simple formula as a function of its radius; and the relationship may be displayed by a curved line on a planar, or two-dimensioned, diagram (Figure 7.1B).

EXAMPLE 7.11. The volume of a cylinder depends on, and can be calculated from, two *predictor variables*, namely, the length (or height) of the cylinder and the thickness (or diameter) of the circular face; and it may be displayed in a spatial or three-dimensional diagram (Figure 7.1C). The whole relationship can be represented as a curved surface embedded in space. It will be clear that for any fixed diameter, the volume will be strictly proportional to the height, and for any fixed height it increases with the diameter in a curved relationship. We notice, however, that nothing in the diagram reflects any relationship at all between height and diameter. Height and diameter are *independent*. But they are not *incommensurable*; in fact they may be, and usually will be, measured in precisely the same units, say, centimeters.

Now, let us apply these ideas to a familiar problem where the predictor variables are independent but incommensurable.

EXAMPLE 7.12. In the golden age before Einstein, it was evident that distance and time are incommensurable. They do not deal with the same quantity. In the physical sense, they are not expressed in the same dimensions. In contrast, miles and kilometers can be expressed one in terms of the other. The rate of exchange between them is a simple dimensionless ratio, and no combination of circumstances will make the ratio any different. On

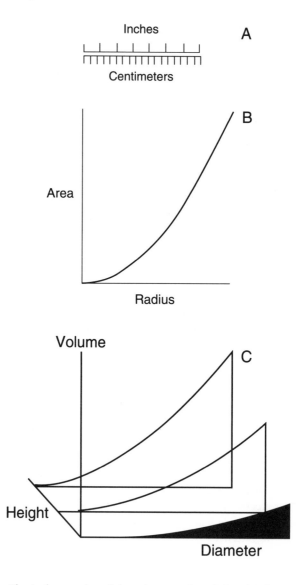

Figure 7.1   Physical examples of the existence of a relationship between measurable quantities. *A:* Two one-dimensional scales. *B:* The area of a circle and its radius. *C:* The volume of a cylinder and its length (or height) and thickness (or diameter).

the other hand, distance and time are in different units. The distance be-tween Baltimore and Toronto is unrelated to time; the ratio between them is not a simple dimensionless quantity but a quantity in compound units (e.g., velocity in miles per hour). We do not get the same result if we deal in miles per minute or kilometers per hour. The structure of the composite quantity, speed, provides the clue to the means by which the quantities can be made to conform. Is there any way in which the statement "It is 480 miles from Baltimore to Toronto" can be made equivalent to the statement "The messenger will take ten hours to go from Baltimore to Toronto"? Obviously yes, if we add the third statement "The messenger travels be-tween Baltimore and Toronto at an average velocity of 48 miles per hour."

Of course, not all sets of compound statements can be made to cohere in this fashion. The rules for how and when they may be created are laid down in the field of dimensional analysis in physics. Briefly, when each term of a proper formula is written out with its correct dimensions, after appropriate cancellations the dimensions of the two sides will be the same. By the criterion of incommensurability we would say, "You cannot deduce a time from a distance." And, as it stands, that would be quite correct. Let us now address that limitation.

THE NATURE OF COMPOUND ETHICAL PROPOSITIONS

The next step is complementary. The argument that we cited asserts that propositions of fact and Moral conclusions are incommensurable. But surely that assertion depends on exactly what is meant by *Moral conclusion*. Is it so obvious that a Moral proposition is incommensurable with propo-sitions of fact—even of simple physical fact?

In order to develop the argument coherently, however, we must discuss some other fundamental notions and define some more terms.

The Optative Mood

To begin with, it will be helpful to extend the grammatical analogy to include the *optative* mood. This mood, encountered in various Indo-European languages, notably Classical Greek, expresses wish, desire, aspi-ration.[3] An optative proposition is not a statement of fact (indicative) or a

3. A colleague has complained bitterly about a dispute with some (nameless) scholars who failed to recognize that the word *might* in a phrase such as "They died that we might live" is an obligatory subjunctive in a subordinate adverbial clause of purpose. His complaint is that they supposed the word *might* to connote an actuarial statement—that it means "They died so as to increase the probability that we shall live." Wherever modern English is spoken and understood in such a fashion, the Greek optative mood (which cannot be unambiguously

command to action (imperative). We shall represent these three moods as a paradigm, with a letter to designate each, as follows:

Optative: Would that (𝕎)
Indicative: Is (𝕁)
Imperative: Must (𝕄)

Strictly, *must* is not an imperative any more than *you are obliged to* is. That is because the politeness of the times has replaced a frank command by a politer form (which, however, is just as exacting).

Two Types of Law

Empirical scientists with a taste for philosophizing (with an emphatically lower-case *p*) make much of the difference between scientific Law and juridical law. They point out that a scientific Law that for centuries has withstood all assaults may yet be destroyed by some simple, well-established counterexample. In contrast, breaking a juridical law does not have this effect. If a person parks a car beside a fire hydrant, the juridical law has not suddenly ceased to exist. To the contrary, the crime gives the police the chance to assert the power of the law. The most feeble laws are those that are never enforced. Thus (the argument goes), the word *law* is used in two senses, scientific or descriptive, and Legal or prescriptive. What is true of it in the one sense is untrue in the other.

We claim that this line of argument is a misrepresentation, which the more juridical of the Moralists have themselves abetted. However, we must first clarify terms carefully.

The Ethical, the Deontological, and the Moral

By *Ethics* we mean the study of the relationships between human Acts and their consequences (insofar as they can be studied in the unaided light of reason) as a source of principles of conduct that will, in some sense, be seen to be optimal.

Appeals that go beyond reason (such as to revelation) do not fall within Ethics unless the (presumably transcendental) relationships and the consequences are capable of being explicated. Ethics implies a concern with three matters: orderliness in the empirical world (we do not live in chaos); fact; and a sense of responsibility.

---

translated even into Latin) does not stand a chance. The translator then has to use artificial constructions such as "Would that the patient may survive the operation!" or "Oh, that the population of the city be spared the cholera!"—literary contrivances that give English translation of Greek poetry a bad name.

Deontology is defined by *Webster's* (1988) as "the theory or study of moral obligation." This meaning is deeper than the confrontational meaning we have given to Ethics, and it might lead to certain conclusions that are not demonstrably optimal. A familiar Medical analogy would be the difference between biochemistry and nutrition, the former being a pure, disengaged, intellectual discipline (analogous to Ethics) and the latter a particular topic of adapting biochemistry to certain defined benefits for society (analogous to deontology). Unlike a nutritionist, a biochemist does not have to address the question of what state of nutrition is desirable and should be promoted. For instance, the drive to truth is hardly to be denied; but it is not at all obvious what the truth is, what the consequence of knowing it may be, or whether there may be multiple, mutually contradictory, claimants to the truth, each of which is internally consistent.

Morals is another topic beyond the scope of this book. We mention it simply for completeness and to avoid confusion both about what we discuss and about what matters we avoid. We mean by this term a code of behavior that proposes to meet the obligations identified by deontology and other pertinent forms of study such as revelation, corporate social values, or political discourse. Morals is much more elaborate, subtle, and personal than we are prepared to address here.[4]

Roughly, we may identify Ethics with the indicative; the deontological with the optative; and the Moral with the imperative. The scene is now set for our main task.

SYLLOGISMS OF MIXED MOOD

Classically, syllogisms deal with matters of assertion. Then by definition the two premises and the conclusion are all in the indicative mood, and the pattern will then be represented as $\mathbf{J} \cdot \mathbf{J} \cdot \mathbf{J}$. Syllogisms are not usually concerned with Moral propositions. Nevertheless, we see no formal reason why they should not be applied to Moral problems. The term *mood*, although taken by analogy from grammar, seems to prove a peculiarly apt pun for the discussion. There is no reason why a Moral proposition cannot be safely *manipulated* as a purely formal statement.

EXAMPLE 7.13. The statement "Colonel Jones gets angry every time bimetallism is mentioned" may tell us that he is seething with moral indignation and outrage at the economic theory; but his anger is just as much a fact as the weather. A political pollster can recognize (or at least infer) the

---

4. The better to ensure that there is no intrusion of our private opinions, we have totally bypassed this topic of Morals. Readers are unwise to make any inferences whatsoever from our silence on this or other topics.

fact of the anger without sharing it or even understanding it and may duly record it in the course of an election.

The reluctance that many would have to apply Logical syllogisms to Moral issues lies more in mood, in attitude of mind to the matter considered, than in the form of the statement. Unconsciously a line is drawn between statements like "All elephants are big" and those like "All hermits are deprived of human company" because unless so endowed, bigness in elephants excites neither approbation nor disapproval. But statements of the form "All monks are cenobitic" is another matter, for the latter word is not commonplace. Few would accept Logical manipulations of it without some suspicion that it is subtly tinged with occult moral values. For that matter, bigness in elephants may in special circumstances be made into a statement of economic, or even of quasi-moral, value.

We are better occupied hunting for occult syllepsis.

EXAMPLE 7.14. An aspirant for office may be a fitting (suitable) candidate; a tailor may be fitting (adjusting) clothes; and an uncontrolled epileptic may be having a fit (attack) now. In a purely verbal sense, we may say, "They are all fitting." But it seems doubtful that that conjunction of ideas has in itself any meaning.

Ethical and Moral Syllogisms

To assert that something is *good* or *Moral* or *indefensible* need not present any Logical (as distinct from veridical) difficulties any more than to assert that it is *transparent* or *opaque* (see Example 6.11). In fact, it will have been noted that in Example 7.6 we deal with the immorality of war, which in content is obviously a Moral assertion. However, there we dealt with the Moral judgments as if they were arbitrary assertions in the indicative mood. Many would not agree with one or the other of the premises and would dispute the truth of the conclusion. Even so, they would not dispute that the (implied) conclusion is the only one that can be validly reached from those premises. To repair the conclusion, they must reform the premises.

In what follows, then, we ask readers for the time being to direct their attention to form rather than to content. They are welcome to make any reservations they please, including flat negation, about the truth or otherwise of any of the premises or the conclusions. It will be our argument that the Moral syllogism may be expressed as two premises, in the optative and the indicative respectively, and a valid conclusion reached in the imperative.

Well, but it will be argued that our concern here is not with Morals but with Ethics, and it is difficult to believe that Moral conclusions can be reached simply by any reasoning that is to have the intellectually coercive force of a purely indicative conclusion. We continue to have the option to smoke tobacco, and plenty of reasonable people continue to smoke despite the undisputed association between smoking and serious disease. Society denies citizens that type of option in certain cases, such as taking certain drugs or not wearing seat belts when driving, and in doing so excites much criticism and protest.

A strictly Ethical approach to behavior (i.e., a confrontation of decisions with their effects and with no deontological component) seems to us to be of the form 𝔍·𝔍·𝔍; that is, all the terms are in the indicative and commensurable as to mood, and the function of the syllogism is to provide a confrontation of terms.

We might summarize this distinction as follows:

	Logical and Ethical Syllogisms	Deontological and Moral Syllogisms
Major premise	𝔍	𝔚
Minor premise	𝔍	𝔍
Conclusion	𝔍	𝔐

The foregoing is a traditional distinction and certainly a grammatical one. Nevertheless, we do not necessarily think that it is Logically real or that the incommensurability as to mood of the terms in the deontological and Moral syllogisms has necessarily any reality at a speculative level, however wide the gap may appear to be in practice.

We believe that the illusion of incommensurability of the terms arises from attempts to confer on the imperative something that is totally other, something that, unlike a scientific Law, refers not to matters of fact but to something that is arbitrary. The suspicion is much greater in the Moral than in the deontological sphere. The imperative can in fact be seen as a conditional statement of putatively objective fact: "*If* you wish . . . , *then* you must. . . ."

EXAMPLE 7.15. Take a fairly straightforward example that, whatever the grammatical forms, will be seen as in the indicative throughout: "One cannot be a vegetarian and eat pork." The auxiliary verb is *can,* which is reassuring. It emerges as merely the statement of a non-Thing. The Logical intersection of vegetarians and pork eaters is zero, the null set, with zero measure. One cannot be a six-legged quadruped. These are not prohibitions at all but simple statements of the meanings of words and the properties of Things. There is no such thing as a four-sided triangle; therefore one *cannot* draw a four-sided triangle. To achieve that power it will be necessary to attach some new meanings to the words, as when (for instance) one may have a regular polygon of six and a half sides or an irrational number of sides, notions that ordinarily seem quite meaningless but nevertheless may be consistently used (Murphy, Berger, et al. 1989).

Now, note that the foregoing treatment involves taking no Ethical stand at all about whether it is desirable to be a vegetarian or whether it is appropriate to act in accordance with any conclusion reached in the indicative proposition. We have in fact taken the extreme confrontational position (see Chapter 2, under "Confrontational Ethics"): here are the facts and the relationships; make of them what you will.

Let us take a more intricate case.

EXAMPLE 7.16. Consider two well-known proverbs: "Who sups with the Devil must have a long spoon" and "You cannot play with pitch and not be defiled." Clearly the meanings are much the same: to consort with evil is corrupting. The reader at this stage is asked to treat the terms *evil* and *corrupting* as undefined matters of external fact, disregarding any moral significance or overtones. Predication of *evil* for the purposes of this argument need have no more moral a quality than the statement "If you sleep in the dew you will wake stiff." [5]

Now, the interesting feature of these two proverbs, which are so similar in meaning, is that they are very different in grammatical form. The former is in the imperative mood (or, to be more exact, contains the equivalent courtesy form *must*). The latter is in the indicative and almost has the form of a scientific Law: in a detached, dispassionate way, it asserts that being defiled is an objective consequence of playing with pitch, without taking any formal stance as to whether or not it is good to be defiled. Clearly the gist of the two proverbs (both enthymemes) could be fully expanded in Ethical terms as described in the first column of Table 7.1. All statements being in the indicative mood, and the syllogism formally valid *modus ponens,* there is no difficulty with the Logic.

Now, as we have repeatedly said, it is not our goal in this book to deal with Ethics as such, and still less with deontology or Morals. It is quite enough to grapple with scientific and Medical issues. But to present the latter in coherent and negotiable form, we are required to make Logical juxtapositions that display the connections between certain courses of action and certain consequences. Any actual Ethical engagement would involve an appeal to the ethicist for certain facts and relationships; and on the

---

5. To refuse to distinguish between the form of an abstract argument and its content would be to act like the accountant who cannot maintain a balance sheet for a business without wondering whether Bill Smith treats his rheumatism with aspirin or butazolidine and whether George Brown will spend his three weeks of vacation in Mallorca or Rio de Janeiro. The accountant may be a personal friend of both, but that has nothing to do with his being or not being a competent accountant.

Table 7.1. Ethical and Moral Syllogisms Compared

	Ethical Syllogism	Moral Syllogism
Major premise	All detriments are avoided by ethical minds (𝔍)	It is good not to be defiled (𝔐)
Minor premise	All hazards are detriments (𝔍)	To consort with evil is to be defiled (𝔍)
Conclusion	All hazards are avoided by ethical minds (𝔍)	A human being must not consort with evil (𝔐)

part of the clinician and the scientist the concern is to supply details that are to the point. The ethicist would certainly want to have this information but may not even be aware that it exists. With the utmost diffidence, we also provide in Table 7.1 something like a ghost of a Moral syllogism, in parallel with a possible set of arbitrary values. But we are expressly not declaring (as scientific and clinical matters) that these values are appropriate or to the point.

The reader is, of course, not asked to subscribe to either set of premises given in the table. The Ethical syllogism could be "saved at any price" by giving any desired meanings to the terms *detriments, hazards,* and *ethical minds*—certainly we have tried our best to define the assertions contained in it.

Skeptical readers may still feel they are being insidiously subverted, although we are not even claiming that the conclusions are true, merely that the syllogisms are valid. Accordingly, we shall continue to stress that Ethical argumentation is not the procession of an imperative; not a recommendation to act; not even the expression of an opinion; but merely a confrontation between a human Act and its consequences. In effect, the proverb "You cannot play with pitch and not be defiled" has the content of the minor premise: it is a double enthymeme, the major premise and the conclusion being suppressed. It implies how the rational person would act (which is a response and hence an occult imperative)—by avoiding certain contacts that might as well be good as evil, for all the validity of the syllogism is concerned—to attain some objective (not to be defiled), which is an optative. The other proverb, "Who sups with the Devil must have a long spoon," is also a double enthymeme: it is a conclusion with a suppression of the optative and the indicative.

COMMENT.   There will be formal criticisms about the structure of the Moral syllogism as a whole: the contents of the propositions deal with different matters. But its validity is in fact explicated in the Ethical syllogism in parallel, which is itself valid. However, the soundness is not determined by the mere correctness of the form. In the same way, in Example 7.12 (quibbles aside) the conclusion is undoubtedly correct; yet the individual statements are not about the same thing, and would not (for instance) be invariant under changes of scale and units. It is no doubt debatable whether the form of that example can be defended as a Logical deduction. But there is certainly a process of deduction, and the conclusion is correct.

The juridical aspect of the Moral syllogism contrasts with the rational aspect of the Ethical syllogism. It happens that Moral arguments are often expressed as enthymemes or double enthymemes (with only the imperative conclusion); Ethical arguments seem typically to be fully explicit. And that contrast is a measure of the dispassion of the two fields. Moral arguments have a (perhaps wholly appropriate) flavor of rhetoric, which is as out of place in Ethics as it is in mathematics.

The Force of the Conclusion

The question now arises as to what we mean by the conclusion of the Ethical syllogism or the imperative component of the Moral syllogism. Evidently neither is very different from a scientific Law. No one is under any physical compulsion to obey the imperative, using the word *obey* in a Moral sense; that is, a free person may refuse to comply with the imperative. The consequence of the imperative is simply that to refuse to comply is inseparable from forgoing an optative. A man is free to jump out a window from the tenth floor of a building; but he is not free to survive if he does so. The notice "Beware of falling rocks" can be viewed as not a command but a piece of advice. It contrasts with "Trespassers will be prosecuted," which is a juridical threat in which the relationship between the Act of trespassing and the response is an extrinsic and arbitrary one.

It transpires, then, that there is indeed a syllepsis in this discussion about Law, but it has been falsely located. The Law in the scientific sense and the Law in the Ethical sense are in essence the same. They are not really in different moods; they are both indicative. In our opinion the Law in the Moral sense and the Law in the scientific sense are also similar. The syllepsis lies in the word *obey*. It is clear that *obey* is used in at least two senses. When we say that chemical reactions "obey the Law of conservation of energy," we mean that they conform to it, that it describes how such reactions behave. It is not a Moral prescription but a pure description from which, strictly, not even causal inferences may be made.

In the domain of human Acts, however, there is an added ambiguity in *obey* that stems from the nature of human freedom. Shipley (1984) identifies the origin of *obey* as the French-Germanic verb *oyer*, meaning "to hear and heed," and its familiar form from the town-crier *oyez*, from the Latin *audire*. It thus seems clear that the primordial sense was a Moral one, and that its use in the Laws of physics is derived and metaphorical. A man jumping to his death out a window may well be said in the primordial sense to be disobeying what some readers will see as Ethical or Moral Law; that is, his Act is not in conformity with the optatives of a man who is (in some as yet undefined sense) good. Nevertheless, in the derived metaphorical sense he is obeying a biological Law about the effects of physical injury on survival every bit as faithfully as a purely physical body may be said to be obeying the Law of gravitation or of the conservation of energy.

We may restate this argument in the interest of clarity. A scientific Law about cause and effect assumes the form "If X, then Y." If a particular set of circumstances X prevail, then a particular outcome Y is to be expected. The system obeys the Law if the Law is true. The force of the Law is its truth, not the arbitrary exercise of some retributive power. We commonly suppose that the soundness of a scientific Law is shown by the predictability of the outcome. However, this relationship is not necessarily so, for prediction is, strictly, an epistemic attribute of the human observer (scientist) and only secondarily (if at all) ontologically related to that which is, to the truth addressed. Prediction, even in a completely deterministic system, may not be possible because not all the circumstances may be known. But this ignorance is no reason for supposing that the outcome does not conform to some Law.

One area of mounting interest is what is known in the theory of dynamic systems analysis as Chaos (Gleick 1987; Devaney 1989). There exist systems in which the outcomes of certain states are inexorably determined; but for the outcome to be known, the state of the system must be known with perfect precision (i.e., measurable quantities must be known correct to an infinite number of decimal places). In practice, because of the coarseness of even our most refined observations, such precision is impossible, and then not even approximate statements may be made about the outcome. In effect, the system behaves as if Random, so that the outcomes from two states that differ only to the most minute extent imaginable are quite contrary. This theory, though latent since the time of Poincaré, was given its first great impetus by Lorenz's attempt (1963) to construct a theory of weather.

OBEDIENCE AS SYLLEPTIC

Now, what about obedience in the Moral sense? In the scientific sense of *obey*, every human being continually obeys the Moral Law.[6] Here the Moral Law would not have the juridical form "Thou shalt not kill" but a

---

6. We note that this discussion involves the implicit assumption that a Moral Law can exist without (for example) leading to self-contradiction.

descriptive form: "If you kill, it will have such-and-such consequences to yourself and others." These consequences may be Legal (killing is a crime), or Psychological (killing blunts compassion), or Moral (killing corrupts), or spiritual (killing is damning) and so forth.

After all, it would be difficult for matters to be otherwise. A scientific Law may have a more or less sound theory underlying it; but it is really descriptive process, ultimately generated by, and ruthlessly tested against, empirical observation. We have no particular reason to suppose that the scientific Law of behavior will be easy to discover. For that matter there is no strong scientific presumption, and no guarantee, that any such Law exists; or if it does, that scientists (who in this context are studying a group of organisms to which they themselves belong) can understand it. But if there is a Law and we discover it, and if the test that it is indeed a *scientific* Law is that the observations of how human beings behave conforms to the Law, then human beings (in that sense) obey the Law in exactly the same sense that they obey the Law of gravity or the conservation of energy. That is not a conclusion, it is a tautology. Whether the scientific Law is ontologically anterior to the behavior observed in the components of the system or vice versa is not a problem we can decide by observation alone, since the two coexist and scientific observation is made in time. We might as well say that the Law obeys the behavior; and certainly this is closer to the order in which we grasp scientific truth. In following that line of reasoning, however, we are in some danger of creating a new syllepsis out of the meaning of the word *behavior*. Of course the moralist (using the term in its original sense) may discuss how human beings *behave in the face of danger*. However, the physicist will discuss how such and such a system *behaves in a magnetic field,* a sense that (like *obey*) is a metaphorical borrowing to which has been attached what is not evidently the same meaning. Whether these meanings are truly the same, or whether the behavior of the human being has an added dimension of freedom, is a matter that may be endlessly discussed. It has no doubt loomed large in the councils of the behaviorists, metaphysical, methodological, and Logical (Flew 1989: 296). But once we concede any added freedom, then we are obliged to distinguish between two senses of the word *behavior*. In any case, law in the forensic sense conceived as a juridical enactment is clearly anterior to any behavior.

DEFINITION.   A *scientific Law* is a statement of the outcome of a set of circumstances, states, and properties that includes Acts done in response to the circumstances themselves.

Note that while the content of the Law will very likely differ according to the types of entities concerned—inanimate objects, vegetables, animals of various degrees of complexity, unreflecting animals, and deliberating human beings—the epistemology of the definition remains the same.

On the other hand, law (in the juridical sense) is commonly treated as a kind of coercion, social, political, Legal, or Moral, to act in a certain way in certain circumstances. It may not escape from all Philosophical constraints, since jurisprudence looks for at least minimal requirements from a coherent theory of what is right. Political law is something enacted for the putative good of society as a whole and not, except perhaps accidentally, to protect the individual from himself or herself. In the political sphere, there is perhaps no other course. Moral Law, however, is another matter and one worthy of deeper consideration.

If we revert to the syllogistical formulation of Moral Law, we see that the optative deals with the broad policy about the objectives, the indicative with the means to the objectives, and the imperative with the course of action in the particular instance. By analogy we may say that the optative is the plan of campaign, the indicative is strategy, and the imperative is the tactics. What we call *legalism* is the exclusive preoccupation with the imperative: the frame of mind of the soldier who exercises no discretion and does exactly whatever his battle orders may indicate, no more, no less. It is, to a degree, a safe policy. He may argue that he has neither the facts nor the training to warrant overriding his orders in the face of some unexpected event. In military Ethics, in particular, there is commonly such a concern with the secrecy and confidentiality of the plans that the soldier on the firing line is required to behave as part of a system that is mystifying to all but the inner circle of the general staff. This detached attitude has two obvious weaknesses. First, at times such obedience is no defense against charges of misconduct. Soldiers cannot plead that they were "only carrying out orders" if these orders include the wanton killing of little children. This Moral prohibition overrides battle orders, however arcane. In the second place, faithfulness to orders based on unreasoning conformity to prescription demands extraordinary, heroic, self-abnegation. Such discipline is apt to be brittle. The consequences of an awakening critical sense in the totally unprepared mind may be disastrous. A field officer may have never previously thought at all about what underlies his battle orders, may have been cut off from fundamental information and strongly discouraged from trying to acquire it. If he decides in an emergency to abandon the orders, he is apt to act unadvisedly.

A Note on a Radical Ambiguity

We may interject at this stage a radical ambiguity, previously hinted at, over the attempts by the soldier or the field officer (or their clinical counterparts in the chain of command in, say, a complicated operation or Medical treatment) to consider the ontology of the Ethics in use. Consequences come into the process in two ways that may be confused:

1.   The type of Ethics will exhibit one of two or perhaps more *orientations* in the precedence. The extreme of the strict axiomatic

system $(A--$; see Figure 2.1) will demand that in deciding what is Ethical, the consequences are neither here nor there. The course of action is rigidly dictated by axioms, and the consequences are not under the control of the person acting. This extreme view would be softened somewhat in a system $(Ac-)$ that regards the foreseen consequences themselves as a component of the axiomatics. The price paid by the consequences may be regarded as so disproportionately severe as to veto the course reached by the axiomatics. At the other extreme, the consequences may so dominate the Ethics $(-C-)$ as to override all veto by the axiomatics: the principle that (without any reservations) the end justifies the means. That too might be softened (to $aC-$ or aCp, etc.). The impact of consequences here is Ethical.

2.   However, the consequences come into the Ethical decision in an entirely different way. Take the case of extreme axiomatic, doctrinaire, Ethics. The consequences are given no Ethical weight, but they do bear on the meaning of the Act and are therefore ontological.

EXAMPLE 7.17. As a general principle, the outcome of any therapeutic procedure involves some uncertainty, some of it due to lack of information, but not all of it; and Chaotic systems (q.v.) may behave like Random ones. A surgeon may judge that the risk from an operation, though small, is not altogether negligible, whereas the outlook without the operation, though not totally hopeless, is poor. On balance, certain principles (which we address in Chapter 10) applied by axiomatic Ethics will decide in favor of operation. That is a Probabilistic matter.

However, the scientist will insist that *anything that purports to be a Probabilistic statement or a clinical judgment must be based on something, some evidence or rational argument.*

Appeal to Probabilities has no Ethical standing at all if the so-called Probabilities have no means of subsistence whatsoever; for instance, if the sample space cannot be defined, no sampling procedure is prescribed, there are no data, then no ontological statement can even be made about what the Probability statement means. To push this argument to the extreme, if there is no possible diagnosis at all, however crude, and no judgment even about whether the broadest clinical measures are supportive, then the Ethical analysis has no domain of action. It is on a par with trying to determine what the behavior of a system subject to an impossible combination of circumstances would be. It is not possible to have any Ethical analysis where there is neither information nor understanding.

In the military metaphor, even those who base their battle orders on tactical understanding can too easily fall into the trap of underinformed decision. The tactician does not readily see the connection between two things widely separated in space or time: an immediate effect is readily (sometimes too readily) accepted. A tactician who sees a group of human beings fall ill after eating a certain kind of mushroom more or less easily connects cause and effect and, valuing good health, will avoid these mushrooms. By contrast, there is a long interval between the first contact with leprosy and the first signs of the disease,[7] and a tactical viewpoint may miss the connection. Suppose there is a long incubation period between, say, habitual lying and its consequences. Why there should be this long gap is not clear in either the pathological case or the Moral one; no doubt in some way it reflects the complicated nature of the mechanisms involved. It may, for instance, be a multiple-hit phenomenon (q.v.).

The basing of a system of Morals on a tactical understanding (i.e., as one might say, on working principles rather than on fundamental issues or sound inferences from them) is liable to reproduce the juridical error of the field officer more gradually and on a larger scale, and (such is the accommodating nature of the human mind) a miscarriage of tactics may disturb the conscience less. Far worse crimes have been committed in the deliberate and measured application of principle (such as that left-handedness is a perversion that education must stamp out) than in uncritical obedience to a regulation. An unjust war (which is fought after weighty deliberation) is more evil than the unjust hanging of a man (which is merely a deplorable miscarriage of justice), but it commonly raises less public sense of outrage. However, to decide whether a war is just is much more difficult than to decide whether someone is guilty of a capital crime; and among wars, it is harder to justify wars of principle (e.g., so-styled holy wars) than wars of defense against some supposed aggression. But after all, tactical insight is itself only a limited range of vision. Ultimately, Ethical principles are reached largely in the light of experience. We may formulate them by noting the consequences of certain Acts; or because we deduce what the optimal function of a mechanism might be; or when we consult the common aspirations of society; or some such. It is evident, however, that all depend on experience gained with, and from, the passage of time; little heed would be paid to the Ethical speculations of a mind from outer space, however intelligent, whose sole knowledge of the human species was based on a split second of observation or one detailed photograph. While the ethicity of action with immediate consequences only is easy to work out, the longer the incubation period, the harder the formulation of the principles. The same is true wherever the connection between cause and effect is obscure. The peoples of the Middle East learned early the immediate dangers

---

7. It is tempting to suppose that leprosy is commonly used as an image of evil, not so much because it is disfiguring as because there is a long latent period before its consequences become evident.

of trichinosis from eating pork; but even now we are not altogether sure of the impact of diet on atherosclerosis.

It is to be expected, then, that a law will be received with an enthusiasm in proportion to the readiness with which it is seen to have beneficial consequences. Only young children, the retarded, or the psychotic have to be told not to put their hands in the fire, so no public laws are required on the point; but legislation that would prevent slowly acting causes of cancer forty years later is likely to be grudgingly received.

In the face of the foregoing we make one assertion and one disclaimer.

First, the assertion. Whereas Ethical analyses are rational, and whereas the major source of rational understanding of nature in the scientific sphere is a coherent collection and rigorous analysis of empirical fact, then (Murphy 1981c):

• Deontology demands a commitment to pursue accessible scientific truth.

It would seem very strange to us that those wanting to act in accordance with the interests of society would not wish to equip themselves to promote these interests. We hear much debate about whether or not some critical experiment involving risks for human subjects is ethical—and this is by no means an easy problem to solve in all cases. But surely any experiment, even one that is totally without risk or cost, that is so ill-designed that it will admit of no sound conclusions at all may be summarily condemned as indefensible.

Second, the disclaimer is about the exhaustiveness of the treatment of Law. To extend the previous analogy, battle orders imply lesser insight than tactics, and tactics is less farsighted than strategy; but there is no reason for supposing that the plan of campaign represents the last word on behavior. In the political sphere there may be matters of national policy more important than strategy, as MacArthur had to learn; and national policy may at times have to be subordinated to international policy, as the politicians sometimes have to learn from the statesmen. And some, at least, would admit that there are higher matters still to be weighed. In the analogy, to regard Medical Ethics as something like a war and, like it, to some extent self-sufficient, is not to deny that there may be overriding considerations. But it seems only fair to the physicians to allow them to protest that the decision to which they defer is not a Medical one. This explicit protest places a heavy onus on the overriding authority.

The Law and Freedom

We recognize that here we are in some danger of either treading on territory we have declared out of bounds to us or (what is almost as bad) being suspected of it. Our domain of Medicine and biology nevertheless contains a large component of existential commitment to these precarious topics. That is especially true of psychiatry, clinical genetics, and genetic counseling, in which we can claim some expertise and extensive experience. We proceed, therefore, under these credentials. If, as is more than likely, we are led to much the same verbal forms of questions as other experts (metaphysicians, lawyers, political theorists, Moral Philosophers) address, and our analyses and conclusions are somewhat at variance with theirs, that points up all the more the need for constructive dialogue and the goal of mutual correction, adjustment, and consensus.

It is commonly supposed that laws restrict freedom. Laws are usually defended on the grounds that they are restrictions applied to human beings individually for the good of human beings collectively. This claim may be sound, but it is perhaps worth exploring. Two distinctions are to the point.

First, law in the prescriptive, juridical sense may be an inadequate representation of the ideal Law because of the imperfections of the legislators, or the limits of the feasible, or some such accidental shortcoming. Ethical arguments are best conducted in terms of the ideal Law, and then (where necessity exacts) perhaps adjusted to the realities of existential and experiential law.

Second, whole volumes could be written about the nature of freedom. We shall take the word in the common sense rather than a severely ontological one, rendered somewhat abstractly:

DEFINITION. *Freedom* is that state that promotes, wherever possible, opportunities for making deliberative choices in matters that bear on the future state of the individual.

We recognize a further extension to freedom that represents at least the next element in the Chinese box of choice. The apparatus of freedom includes emancipation from Emerson's "foolish consistency." Freedom must include the wherewithal to rise above conclusions that are inexorable but distasteful consequences of a narrow analysis, namely, by appeal to those qualities that we have earlier identified as illation and phronesis (qq.v.).

There is little doubt that in the sphere of physical Law, knowledge promotes freedom and conversely.

EXAMPLE 7.18. If human beings wish to fly, then some knowledge of the Laws of aerodynamics will help them to build a plane and to fly it. Of course, they may ignore these Laws, thus exercising their freedom of choice. But if they do so, the plane will not fly, and the option of flying will be denied them. It seems, then, that freedom lies in deciding which of these two free choices to forgo. In general, certain combinations of choice are incompatible, and this is apparently a hard, irreducible fact. Now, one may build as if the Laws of aerodynamics did not exist, and forgo the second choice. But rightly or wrongly it is the common view that to do so is unreasonable, and that there is more benefit to be derived from flying than from constructing fantasies about space machines that require no fuel and never exhibit metal fatigue.

The foregoing illustration may be a false dichotomy. Further knowledge may show that it is indeed possible to exercise both choices; but arguably if this reconciliation were easy and obvious, it would have already been achieved, and new scientific Laws would be required to fulfill both. These new Laws, however, would themselves then be recognized as constraining forces.

Thus, two conclusions seem obvious. First, vis-à-vis any physical matter, the exercise of freedom consists not in defying scientific Laws but in either paying attention to them or not. A legislature might pass a law that π equals three, but that would frustrate attempts to calculate accurately the amount of paint needed to paint cylinders.

Second—and this point is more subtle—what we ordinarily mean by the exercise of freedom is the transfer of arbitrary choices from what may be perceived as a means to an end. There is a choice between choices. A person may either choose to empty the car's tank of gasoline, or allow it to be kept full and choose whether to use the car or not to go shopping. There is no totally free choice at both steps. The common attitude would be to feel freer if the gasoline tank were full and to be free to decide whether or not to drive. It is clear, however, that the second choice can in turn be treated as a means. To acquire certain commercial foods, there is no choice but to shop. We can say with some generality, however, that displacing the arbitrary choice from the means increases the range of arbitrary choices. This statement is true if the owner of the car goes shopping, which allows a wider range of choices than the limited choice of driving the car or not. It is also true in the world of knowledge. A person may choose not to learn to read but is thereby denied a wider range of arbitrary choices.

We may sketch out very briefly, and as an illustration rather than a coherent theory, what we may call the economy of freedom (Table 7.2). As we go from any particular level of achievement to a higher one, there is a price paid in effort and sacrifice of immediate liberty that is, or at least may be, rewarded by an enhanced scope for the operation of liberty and an expanding reward that may, so to speak, be reinvested in the short term in a yet more exacting payment for a still deeper liberty and thus greater scope for freedom. The dauntless who pursue the process steadily further may forget or despise the rewards of liberty yet acquire a taste for excellence of which those who cash their freedom early in exchange for liberty may never get to know or understand. But we must suppose that there are many who can see the more remote rewards but do not think them worth the effort. Such

Table 7.2. The Economy of Freedom

State	Liberty of Action	Price Paid	Freedom in Achievement	Example
Unstructured	High	Little	Low	Primitive life
Enjoyment				
Knowledge	Moderate (study; reasoning)	Increased	Increased	Scientific life
Art	Moderate (technique; esthetics)	Increased	Increased	Cultural life
Law	Moderate (obedience information)	Increased	Increased	Peace; security
Betterment				
Virtue	Much reduced	Cooperative effort	Much increased	Friendliness; community sense
Heroic virtue	Severely reduced	Austerity	Incalculable	Excellence; genius; holiness

judgments are different in kind from the judgments in those actually taking part in the struggle. We see the whole system as a Chinese box, with (at each stage) two levels: the existential struggle, and the judgment as to whether it is worthwhile to conserve freedom uncashed for the present. It is not difficult to think of higher levels. Most people are more or less content with what they have and are prepared to take no effort to get beyond it. Some, the talented, set their ambitions on higher levels of success, and having discovered a formula may rest content with that. The Mozarts and the Miltons may regard success as a snare and seek achievement, the success formula that transcends success formulas. The Beethovens and the Rembrandts are seeking something that is so far beyond achievement as to be uncanny. Yet we advocate nothing. The beat of Thoreau's other drummer (1854) is perhaps to be seen as a yet higher step in the Chinese box of freedom.

It is difficult to believe other than that enlightenment—using the word in a very general sense—liberates and darkness enslaves. But this liberating quality is not true of the physical world only. The notion of a physical property is an abstraction from a class; therefore, a "property unique to the individual" would be a contradiction in terms. If the human being can be said to have properties, then this implies at least some regularity among human beings too, which in turn implies a Law for the behavior of each (in the descriptive empirical sense).

It is in a sense true that the Law is different for each person, not because each has unique properties, but because each has a unique set of properties: the distinction is one between cardinality and dimensionality (q.v.). But how are individuals to decide what the Law is for them personally? The answer must either come from an adequately developed theory or from empirical studies. By *theory* is meant a formulation of the nature of human beings without appeal to experience; by *empirical studies* is meant reflective analysis of experience. Both present difficulties.

Where is a theory, divorced from experience, to come from? Is it even likely to be intelligible? Those who reject all prospect of supernatural revelation will have recourse to empiricism, which is beset with its own, and perhaps ultimately not very different, problems. There is uncertainty as to what the measure of achievement may be; there are the difficulties of conducting diachronic ("longitudinal") studies with no clear indication as to how long the observation of consequences should last; in the application of inferences to future conduct of the individual there are the well-known problems of finding a formula embodying the necessary and sufficient data to predict the best individual course.

But there are problems deeper than criteriology. Popper (1959) crystallized what is indeed the received tenet of scientific inquiry. One does not proceed by what he terms the Baconian principle that a sufficiency of unconnected facts will eventually lead to the truth. The exploration of the empirical is necessarily selective; and, from symmetry, the principles of the selection cannot be taken from the data themselves. The fact that in any systematic observation only a small fraction of sensory stimuli are admitted as relevant to any particular problem requires that behind it there lies at least the ghost of a theory, a gauge of relevancy; and any such theory is better to be explicitly stated than not. The whole failure of the Baconian endeavor shows the dangers of acting by other counsels.

The Law as a Mystery

It is granted that these are difficult matters; but we have little patience with the mystique of nihilism. To have failed so far to find one adequate formula is no good reason for supposing it does not exist, or that any Law is of its nature merely an irksome restriction on human freedom. A thousand failures may damp one's enthusiasm but furnish no proof of impossibility.

Revealed religion is quite foreign to our topic in this book. Nevertheless, it is in no way at odds with it. In the terms that we have spelled out earlier, the two are best seen (in the spirit of Example 7.11) as not disjoint, but simply independent. Nothing Ethical we have said about the Law (as an enlightenment and not as an enactment) clashes, or need clash, with its teachings.

A rational explanation of reasons for behaving in such and such a way in unintelligible terms would be of little help. The dangers of eating pork or shellfish would be difficult to explain in terms of microorganisms to a primitive society that knew nothing about microbiology and could not be persuaded that it is worth studying. But a proscription with external sanctions (much as one might reprimand a small child for playing with the fuse box, although to an older child a rational explanation would be better) is perhaps the best that experts in public health may aim for in the first encounter with a backward people.

CONCLUSION

Our thesis is that the Law is to be discovered, not invented; that it describes relationships between Things; and that it calls for Acts where there is a rational correspondence between behavior and insight into consequences, and not something totally other that the grammarians call the imperative.

We do not mean that the rational approach to behavior is self-sufficient; the full consequences of our Acts are not easily discerned. But if Ethics is the study of the relationships between human Acts and their consequences in the light of unaided reason, then it should be conceived as a descriptive process. As a result, the Ethical nature of an Act or a policy must include a knowledge of all the consequences, proximate and remote, so far as we can ever observe and know them. Nor do we imply that either knowledge or understanding (in the natural sense) guarantees freedom. Ultimately behavior is a mystery of physical indeterminacy, of the exercise of freedom and of other and deeper matters. But a free decision presupposes understanding and deliberative action.

8 Normality and Disease

Much, arguably too much, of current Medical Ethics revolves about notions of normality and disease. Such-and-such a treatment or protective step will be thought Ethical because it promotes normality and combats disease. But that merely prompts the question, What is normal and what is diseased? Insofar as that viewpoint is a casual description of what (by common, if poorly articulated, consent) is good practice, it can do little harm. But it is a fragile basis for exploring and resolving disputed opinions. Perhaps, like the chairman's gavel, that step is useful as a call to abandon idle chatter and get down to cases. But as a Logical step it is a parody of a bad style in deductive Logic used to solve practical problems. The Logical component is merely a ceremonial exchange, and the real substance (if any) is crammed into one premise, like a text that merely concatenates a long set of elaborate footnotes. The format may clarify the terms of the argument and suggest a proper procedure defining the field of discourse; but by itself it establishes nothing. Of course, if the proposition in the premise (e.g., the claim that such-and-such a condition is diseased) proves to be easy to establish, then formal syllogisms may be of use in bridging the gap between sound speculation and practical decision making.

There is a large Philosophical literature on biological normality that is safe from us, since most of it shows no serious engagement with Medicine or science at all. Even Reznek (1987), a psychiatrist with a professional commitment to Philosophy, seems to deal with the clinical material in a way totally foreign to us. What is equally disturbing, Vácha's brief but well-documented accounts (1985a, 1985b) of early thought (much of it German) on normality in Medicine are ignored, and so is the considerable but scattered literature in English. Fleck's text (1935), which Kuhn (1970) found so seminal, is also ignored. These comments must not be taken as a criticism of the Philosophical literature, which naturally has its own concerns and responsibilities; but it discourages us about the prospects of finding much of relevance to our analysis, the orientation of which is, as we have repeatedly stressed, Medical. Nowhere in this book is our resolve to avoid invading substantive Philosophy and Ethics so severely tested.

The topic of normality, in the terms in which we receive it, is both far-reaching and convoluted. In view of the difficulty of the analysis, we shall break with our usual expository pattern by furnishing a brief initial plan of the argument.

We must go about our task gently and painstakingly. Perhaps a careful unfolding of the evolution of the problem will gradually bring to light something of the nature of the undertaking. We use the term *evolution* rather than the more natural and appealing term *history* because, as so often in tracing out details of an idea, the history, the actual sequence of events of its definition, is almost totally at variance with how it is to be coherently presented. The starting point of the inquiry was not the basic elements. Rather, it was some sophisticated but unsupported and barely intelligible proposition that must be dismantled, edited, and (let us hope) put together again in explicit and useful terms.

We propose three ways of perceiving normality. First, we present it as a state of excellence in itself, totally ignoring any context or relationship to anything other than its various forms. This view will prove insufficient, but it does make for a less cluttered understanding of much of the ontology that must be accommodated in any final model. Second, we present normality as confrontational, as a contest with the exactions and assaults of the environment. Third, we portray it as a phenomenon that relates harmoniously with its environment. The point of view of the first is like Plato from the top of Mount Olympus; the second, like Charlemagne in all his glory; the third, like the mighty ones in the *Paradiso*. The reader will no doubt perceive that as the models succeed each other, the organism enjoying the normality becomes more and more engaged in the outside world. In the event, the boundaries separating the organism and the environment become thicker, fuzzier, and more protective. And that is the way we come to see it. In that fashion all manner of paradoxes and other intractable problems emerge as factitious. But it will make billiard-ball Ethics harder than ever to sustain.

The account ends with a brief note on how clinical intervention (where most of the Ethical problems are vested) may bear on the understanding and use of the notion of normality.

NORMALITY IN ISOLATION

It is probably believed by most that to recognize the normal is simple. And who are better qualified to do so than the physicians, who are supposed to be continually confronted by normality and disease? Their daily task is to see an unending string of patients who are to be sorted out into two groups: those who are diseased and need treatment, manipulation, palliation, and general care; and those who are healthy and may be reassured. At first blush this task, however complicated in detail and demanding as it is of skill, knowledge, and time, seems to be not only reasonable and natural but even obvious. Disease, we are to suppose, has high ontological density. More and more, as scientific knowledge expands, it becomes a white-box inquiry; and the scientific facts are much more elemental than the level at which the whole personality is integrated. There are, and will be, no Chinese boxes or kindred problems to grapple with.

It is a captivating myth, so captivating as to generate resentment toward any calling it into question. There are always those stalwarts who mistrust whatever purports to be enlightenment, who have learned their craft in a bitter school and resist any simplification. If this cry is fervent enough, it may obscure the fact that indeed simplification is progress and, given a chance, may lead to enlightenment and improved care; but oversimplification is heresy and in the end may lead to small advance at the price of much trouble and even suffering. To Einstein, apparently, belongs the dictum "Everything should be made as simple as possible and no simpler." For those with any serious commitment to the Ethical outlook, the proportions involved must demand cautious attention. As we shall see, there are complexities.

Normality and Disease Are Dynamic States

Normality is not a static equilibrium that, like the Parthenon, is at its best as the architect left it and retains its beauty only so long as it undergoes no change. Any state of a vital body that we can imagine, good or bad or indifferent, must represent the totality, the algebraic sum, as it were, of a congeries of conflicting and competing mechanisms; it is the resultant of a great diversity of active forces. In conditions that we call healthy, we invoke the idea of a dynamic equilibrium, which implies that the various components are balanced in such a way as to maintain something close to a steady state of well-being. For instance, the intake of energy is effectively balanced by expenditure of energy, intake of water by loss of water, generation of heat by dissipation of heat. But, of course, over time there may ensue continual change in the components of the system with no new equilibrium being reached, so that the condition of the system is shifting from a state of balance to one of defective balance (as in a person dying of starvation or one developing heat stroke).

The onset of disease may be instantaneous in an earthquake, a gunshot, a decapitation; or by disruption of a vital system as in ventricular fibrillation. But most commonly the onset is not abrupt but gradual. People do not starve, become uremic, or go into liver failure instantaneously. Such changes rarely come about by severe imbalance in load among factors that should be in balance; rather, they come from minor imbalances that accumulate over time until they eventually exceed the tolerances of the system. No conspicuous onset of disease may occur at all. Gradual disruption in the day-to-day life, increased preoccupations with distorted relationships among persons, and disturbances of sleep all take their toll. Now, there is a general belief that early Diagnosis provides the best way of aborting the disease at a stage at which permanent cure has the best chance. But early Diagnosis usually depends on scarce and unobtrusive evidence, and hence compromises that certainty in Diagnosis that is desirable whenever serious decisions on treatment are to be made. Whether the particular diagnosis is favorable or not, the inevitable price paid lies in erroneous decisions, a price that would not arise if we were to forfeit speedy Diagnosis and (in the extreme case) let the disease run its course, or the health continue, as the case may be. Again, Medical Ethics must be concerned with how to strike the balance between the two kinds of error, a matter we address in Chapter 10.

Ontological Density

Unsettling as these problems may be, however, there is a much more fundamental difficulty, that of the categorization itself into competing classes. This is the phenomenon of ontological density (see Chapter 5). Let us start with two simple and completely neutral illustrations from ordinary experience.

EXAMPLE 8.1. Ponies fall into two fairly clear types, male and female. However, the term *pony* itself may be applied to any small horse. Putting ponies into a category of their own, separate from horses, may be commercially useful, but the fact that they can be conveniently so categorized does not necessarily correspond to any particular biological factor. They are not, for instance, a separate species of animal. The fact that animals may form a group in the wild, so that there are recognizable groups like Shetland ponies, does not disprove that they are nonetheless horses.

EXAMPLE 8.2. An even more striking example would be the large number of varieties of dogs that have been artificially bred. When dogs win prizes at shows for the excellence with which they exhibit the characteristics of their variety, it is well to remember that these characteristics are artificially defined because of supposed advantages in certain activities (hunting various types of prey, sheepherding, manipulating bulls, recovering waterfowl) and not in any sense spontaneously set as the result of the operation of natural genetic selection.

Let us move on to some clinical illustrations.

EXAMPLE 8.3. Suppose that on routine annual chest X-ray of a nurse a shadow in the lung field is found that may be an early tuberculous lesion. A decision about diagnosis and management at this early stage may anticipate serious disease. This decision may be medical therapy or perhaps a localized resection, neither of them a small matter should the shadow in fact represent some trivial nontuberculous anomaly. If treatment is withheld, the doubt will be resolved in time, but the price may be the risk of more extensive and dangerous damage. In a word, error of diagnosis either way, false positive or false negative, will exact a penalty.

EXAMPLE 8.4. When we consider patients with tuberculosis, for instance, we behave as if they were without dispute members of a perfectly distinct category that is diseased. There are, of course, patients in whom the diagnosis is doubtful; but that doubt arises merely because of the indirect (and therefore the noisy and fallible) nature of the means of Diagnosis available. In brief, the problems of uncertainty are purely epistemic. Let us for the time being take that to be a reasonable supposition.

Plenty of instances might make us wonder about the nature of Diagnosis. Is it really like deciding chemically whether a piece of metal is pure iron or pure tin? Or is it like a horse breeder telling the difference between a pony and a horse?

EXAMPLE 8.5. Intrepid attempts have been made to demonstrate that *hypertension,* a term of perhaps some practical utility, is to be put in a clean clinical category. Despite occasional minor successes from the empirical side—in porphyria, polycystic kidney, hereditary forms of pheochromocytoma—the promise is so far unfulfilled. Most of the patients thought to have hypertension have no such distinctive anomaly. Nor have we reason to be surprised, for blood pressure is considered to be regulated, or at least seriously influenced, by many factors, by no means all of them genetic.[1]

How well we may eventually fare in our search for an ontologically dense disease hypertension remains to be seen. But at the present time it does not appear to be a useful category from the standpoint of elucidating the pathogenesis of any disease, or curing it.

Ontological cohesion is not simple to attain even in the case of a fairly well defined genetic disorder.

EXAMPLE 8.6. The Ellis–van Crevald syndrome, or EVCS (McKusick et al. 1964), is one of the few disorders in which (short of chemical identification of a specific gene) an intrinsic reason exists for dividing people into two distinct groups. One of the most striking features is short stature evident when the patient is standing, but much less so when sitting. (Much of

1. To the Medical scientist, the best hopes of demonstrating a convincing category of high ontological density lie in seeking a single causative gene, which is inherited as a binary trait, such as porphyria; or a specific infection, as in pyelonephritis; or a specific dietary factor, such as deficiency of vitamin B. All these conditions are listed as causes of hypertension.

the shortening lies in the length of the tibias). But there are other notable features: a defect, often gross, in the interatrial septum; six fingers on the hands and sometimes six toes on the feet. The substance of the disorder has been traced in particular pedigrees for more than thirteen generations, and the genetic analysis strongly suggests that the inheritance is autosomal recessive. However, no causal gene anomaly has yet been chemically identified that would cut the ontological Gordian knot.

Now, in general, there may be no more meaning in dividing people into short and tall than in dividing horses from ponies. Arguments from breeding are widely used, but often with lamentable misunderstanding of how to interpret the results. Much is made of the fact that children resemble their parents, which after all is not to be wondered at for many reasons other than genetics. Indeed (what to many may seem paradoxical), insofar as EVCS and such conditions are regarded as genetic disorders, *the greater the contrast between the heights of the parents and of the child, the more likely it is that a Mendelian disorder is involved, and hence that a true, distinct category exists.*

EXAMPLE 8.7. However, every clinical geneticist is familiar with the (perhaps wholly figmented) problem of "constitutional short stature": a person's height of five feet might reflect some sort of malnutrition, or endocrinopathy, or Mendelian disorder of growth, but the case leaves misgivings in the diagnostician's mind when the person's parents also are short.

Even in the supposedly cleaner, clearer framework of biochemistry, the normal healthy state is not easy to define.

EXAMPLE 8.8. Particular metal ions are obligatory in catalytic or structural roles in a wide range of the cell's chemistry. Nearly all known structures and reactions involving nucleic acids are supported by diverse metals —calcium, magnesium, manganese, copper, zinc, and others (Butzow, Eichhorn, and Shin 1990). Even with the same species of DNA, RNA, or nucleotide, one range of concentration in a metal ion may stabilize a structure or promote a particular reaction, while another may inhibit the reaction or lead to degradation of structure.

Connotations of the Word *Abnormal*

A major problem is one common to all measurable characteristics that display a distribution, that is, variation among members of the putative class. *Somebody* must lie at the extreme known values. There must be one person in a million who is the one-in-a-million person. There seems little reason for deciding that persons are "abnormal" simply because they are individually unusual.

Of course, it can be argued that this deprecating attitude is overreacting to an arbitrary usage of the word *abnormal*. What is wrong with arbitrarily labeling the unusual person abnormal? On the face of it, nothing. But that is not the way that a language may safely be used in practice. It is perhaps an irritating affectation to say that Isaac Newton was an "abnormally clever man," but at one level it is harmless. *Normal* and *abnormal* are, however, words of which the meaning (as understood and, more dangerously, felt) is difficult to control. And against this use, the plea that "it was not intended in that sense" is scarcely a defense. It has been pointed out (Murphy 1997) that in the common medical context alone there are at least seven major meanings attached to the word *normal*, some of them devoid of value judgment ("The distribution of blood cholesterol levels in middle-aged white males is not normal," i.e., not Gaussian), and some heavily loaded with obligation to react ("When the cholecystogram is not normal, many surgeons recommend elective removal of the gall bladder"). In the use of such a word, even in a specially and clearly defined sense, confusion of meaning can easily arise, even in the course of a single argument.

Besides, it is evident that merely extreme performance does not impel us to any activity whatsoever.

EXAMPLE 8.9. A child may be given remedial training to improve a memory that is unusually poor; but a child with a memory that is unusually good (a quality just as common) would not be given remedial training to forget.

It seems to be impossible to attach any purely scientific meaning to "the normal" that is of any help in making decisions (Murphy 1966), at least Medical and Ethical decisions. Those who may wish to preserve the notion of the normal must have recourse to some kind of desirable characteristics (the optatives) that lie outside the domain of the purely empirical. The difficulty is well known to any eugenicists who have attempted to deal with the broad, as distinct from the technical, aspects of their subject. Although a great body of expertise about the methods of animal breeding has been built up, so that one can breed sheep with a heavy yield of wool or cattle with meat having some desired content of fat, all this would be of little interest other than commercial value. The analogy is to the point when the broader implications of genetic counseling are considered: the interests of the individual may be in conflict with those of the rest of the family, and both may damage the interests of the human race. There are matters over which (in the present state of our knowledge and ignorance) there would be no dispute. But such cases are rare and contribute little to the general elucidation of the problem.

EXAMPLE 8.10. It is difficult to see that there could be any reason for promoting the number of fetuses with anencephaly. Even there, however, formulating any policy whatsoever is open to the (admittedly formal) objection of due process that there is no lobby, or even pretended lobby, to campaign for the affected fetuses and to uphold whatever rights they may have or considerations of which they are worthy.

Eugenic Issues

In our first representation of normality, there is no opportunity for any eugenic issue other than the number and qualities of the offspring. Even ignoring the impact of competing species, the survival of the population is necessarily in some doubt. High fertility in the short term will make extinction less likely, but the demands of food and the care of the defective (if the stock is sickly) may offset some of these genetic advantages. In the long run, the increasing size of the population may lead to want and starvation even if the farming and production are of the best quality.

A particular conflict bearing on the desiderata and the notion of the normal is seen in comparing the abilities of a population to meet present and future genetic demands. There is a growing awareness that at least some disorders are, from the eugenic standpoint, the result of a kind of premium paid to insure the corporate population against future risks. There exist genes that when inherited from one parent only (i.e., where they are in *heterozygous state*) appear to confer not merely equal but even superior resistance against specific infections. Even after many years of searching, the claims for the existence in human beings of these so-called balanced polymorphisms remain meager; but the reality of *hybrid vigor* is well known to both animal and plant breeders. Many of the threats from dangerously shallow analysis of these difficult interlocking problems may be more or less remote at the present time, but it is certain that they have repeatedly occurred in the past (although recognized, if at all, mostly in hindsight). No doubt these dangers will recur in the future; and we have every reason to suspect that they may be occurring at the present time, although they may be too intimately part of our lives for us to recognize them. It seems tautologously, even trivially, true that if the genetic structure of the population is perfectly and narrowly adapted to the exigencies of the present time, it must be less well adapted to the inevitable changes of the future. The wisdom of market investment counsels judicious diversification. The wisest population policy is one in which there is a balance between the demands of the immediate present and those of the more or less remote future. However, the key word is *judicious*. There is no reasonable proposal that a genetic condition with gross disablement and early death, such as Tay-Sachs disease, will ever be accepted as normal.

Too many instances are encountered in which superficial judgments are made about the normal for no better reason than an urge to sort subjects into categories. Categorization may be desirable where there is no hint that the classes are of differing merits: by sex, for one, or by blood group, for another. It must be admitted, however, that even at this subdued level, traditional standards may often be wrong. New standards devised to replace them may be an improvement; but being less thoroughly tried, they may eventually prove little better or even quite wrong.

Often there is no acceptable way to decide who may be the best judge. Psychiatrists and psychologists commonly see the results of deplorable patterns of behavior imposed by adults upon their children; the children, in turn, impose them on their own children. A similar cycle may occur between teachers and students. Those who impose these patterns thus perpetuate what may be a disorder, all the while convinced, no doubt, that they themselves are behaving normally. We mentioned earlier the harm done by insisting that the student must not write with the left hand. The penalty is not merely the distress to the student but also the withering of compassion in the teachers who impose the prohibition.

Such cases, one might suppose, are to be defended on the grounds that, however mistaken and however harsh, they are at least sincerely directed to promoting the best. But (a recurrent theme) the desideratum is not only the pursuit of one optimal state but the pursuit of the optimal diversity. Children vary, and variation is often desirable. But discipline is also necessary. Neglect of either quality may impoverish. What may be desirable in one situation is often undesirable in another, and it requires considerable wisdom not to err over impositions. In brief, the error is precisely the cultural homologue of the animal breeder whose strategy is to deal with inbred lines homozygous at all loci, as if the variability of the environment did not impose its own often highly diverse and unforeseen needs.

EXAMPLE 8.11. In the minds of the laity and of many clinicians, the word *malnourished* almost always connotes insufficient food intake. In the most prosperous societies, most malnutrition (i.e., literally "bad nourishment") is of quite the opposite kind. Especially in adults, the widespread and major clinical problems are overeating or eating too much of certain foods. The claim that much of atherosclerosis is due to unbalanced diet has a respectable body of black-box empirical support. Actuarial figures show that those with weights somewhat less than average for their heights and ages have a longer expectation of life than those over. Little attention is given to this evidence in popular images of health. The baby shows in vogue between the world wars favored the plump and the smiling. Modern beauty contests and athletics (notably gymnastics), at the other extreme, idolize the thin. These standards too have risks. They may cause anorexia nervosa, which is harmful and sometimes even fatal. What is more, no permanent pattern of good nutrition is cultivated, and later in life there may be bulimia and obesity. Both sexes are liable to these ill effects.

G. K. Chesterton, of his wisdom, recommended that before we abolish a custom we should try first to discover what its origin may be. If it is known to have been based on what is now shown to be untrue, then clearly it is untenable. If it is *known* to be harmful, it must stop. But it is arrogant to tamper with custom simply because it is ancient and to replace it by a hastily thought-out scheme unsupported by either deep argument or sound empirical verification, the principal quality being novelty. Likewise, although an uncritical appeal to the "wisdom of Mother Nature" may be foolish, those who would fiddle with the manifest successes in surviving of a process operating successfully for three billion years or so had better know what they are about.

The definition of such categories as *normal* and *diseased* may easily entail gross personal or group bias. It is, for instance, too easily supposed that the mentally dull, the backward, have nothing to contribute to society. Scholars, accustomed to mistrusting the impartiality of personal judgments and explicitly recognizing that they themselves make biased judgments, might well have misgivings wherever the matter to be judged is the human species of which they themselves are members. The very wish to reproduce resides in a more or less conscious urge to replicate one's own image, a trait that Leonardo recognized in the operations of the painter (Schwartz 1995). But then naturally it will be the thoughtful who do the thinking and vote for their own kind. The wisdom is that democracy acts as a counterpoise to the unbridled power of an elite who may themselves, in other ways, fail.

Open-and-shut illustrations notwithstanding, the answer as to what is normal is rarely obvious, especially when the judgment is strictly out of context. Indeed, we are almost provoked into a discussion of what *obvious* means. However, it is at least clear that even the most blatant obviousness can never amount to a formal proof of anything, even where there is consensus among reasonable minds.

NORMALITY AS CONFRONTATIONAL

So far the discussion has dealt with the question of normality as if it were an intrinsic attribute of the organism. There are formidable difficulties about the meaning of *normality* in this context. It seems unreasonable to suppose that some equatorial animal, say an African elephant, by the fact of migrating steadily north and nothing else, becomes progressively abnormal as it goes. A more promising and illuminating approach may be to examine the relationship between the organism and its environment. However, this task is more complex.

The survival of a species depends on two basic matters: the conditions in which it can operate, and the circumstances in which it exists. Both vary considerably. Some organisms thrive only when oxygen is abundant, others when there is no oxygen at all. Jellyfish flourish in warm water, the Atlantic (big-clawed) lobster in cold water. The very fact that various species exist is proof that these diverse environments are available.

Genetic selection and, in the long run, Darwinian evolution depend on how much the most favorable operating conditions for the inner workings *(milieu intérieur)* of the organism differ or may differ from the actual conditions that the environment offers. With very elementary organisms, this tension is simple: in a suitable environment the organism thrives. Otherwise it dies. Clearly it is an advantage for organisms to have means that will buffer somewhat the effects of the environment. Systems for doing so seem to be of six principal kinds: transformation, selective adaptation, homeostasis, instinctive action, calculated protection, and migration.

Transformation

Where threatened, the organism may suspend all effort to maintain ordinary functioning, and until the conditions are more favorable settle for a secondary state in which at least survival may be assured. This metamorphosis occurs in viruses that may survive indefinitely in crystalline form; in unicellular organisms that may change into spores when challenged by extremes of heat and cold; in sequestration of desert spiders against extreme drought; in an elaborate form, in the hibernation of certain mammals. The phenomenon of "heat shock," more generally a sudden change in any of a variety of environmental conditions in cell culture, has been shown to involve a class of gene responses that change cellular metabolism including increased synthesis of protective chaperon proteins (Pardue, Feramisco, and Lindquist 1988). This process most typically affects the individual rather than the species.

Selective Adaptation

Strains of the organisms that have a particular advantage against the habitual environment will be selected for. Cases in point are commonplace —for instance, the blubber in the whale is an excellent insulator against cold. In the gross, of course, such changes are evolutionary (adapting the species) rather than physiological (adapting the individual). However, there are, for instance, seasonal bodily changes of an anticipatory character. In animals bearing fur or wool, the effect of cold over a prolonged period of time is to increase the thickness of the coat. Many organisms, including human beings, increase body fat at the onset of winter or before, which acts as both an insulation against cold and (in so-called warm-blooded animals) a source of enhanced metabolism as needed.

Homeostasis

With more elaborate organisms, at least, there are various mechanisms, mostly reflex and in that sense automatic, that tend to anticipate and to offset perturbations in the interior milieu caused by outside forces. Unlike organisms undergoing transformation, they attempt to maintain full operation, and when this goal imposes an excessive strain, the whole organism suffers.

Homeostasis differs from selective adaptation in two major ways. First, it does not *anticipate* needs but responds to needs already felt.

EXAMPLE 8.12. Cold, for instance, leads to shivering, which by driving the blood from the skin reduces a major portal of heat loss; to the inhibition of sweating, another device for heat loss; and to increasing metabolism. Details of these changes, of course, occur in the broad genetic context. Fur-bearing animals, for instance, do not sweat, so that is one thermostatic mechanism denied them; but they may make their bodily hairs more erect, increasing the depth of the insulating coat. Birds fluff their feathers to the same effect.

Second, homeostasis is *cybernetic.* There is a preferred value for the trait to take (the *homing value*). The vigor with which the response tries to restore the displacement is regulated by a *response function,* which is some kind of mathematical relationship of the degree of *discrepancy*—that is, the (signed) difference between the actual current value and the homing value—and by a constant of proportionality, termed the *restoration constant.* The rate of response might, for instance, be three times the cube of the discrepancy.

The repertoire of the qualities of homeostatic mechanisms is remarkable in its economy and scope. As a primordial mechanism on which it draws, the reflex arc calls for our first attention.

The reflex arc. The reflex arc comprises a set of five components (Figure 8.1). First, a specific *sensor* gauges the state of the system being regulated. Second, an *afferent path* carries information from the sensor to the third component, a *control mechanism* that assesses the discrepancy and responds with a suitable size and sign of correction to be applied. Fourth, there is an *efferent path* that carries the information about responding from the control mechanism to the fifth component, the *executive mechanism.*

As may be imagined, response takes time. The interval between the perturbation and the response to it is termed the *lag time.* Much of the detail of the simple system depends critically on three factors: the length of the lag time *(L),* the size of the restoration constant *(b),* and the form of the restoration function *(F).* But some of the pertinent features are that in lagged systems the process may break down either because it is insufficiently vigorous (so that effects of recurrent perturbations may accumulate faster than they are corrected) or because it is too vigorous (and uncontrol-

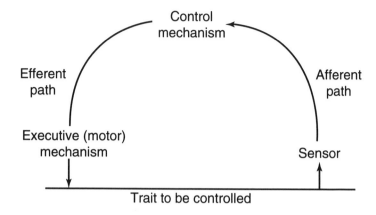

Figure 8.1   The basic components of a simple reflex

lable and lethal oscillation may result). Restoration functions of fractional order (i.e., having response proportional to the discrepancy raised to a positive power less than unity) permanently oscillate rhythmically, which itself may be a valuable property, although a perpetually oscillating process largely vitiates the primordial, purely restorative, goal of homeostasis. The smallest cost for correcting a perturbation is attained by intermediate degrees of control. The topic of physiological homeostasis is a complicated one with a small literature in biology (Wiener 1948; Ogata 1970; N. Macdonald 1978; Murphy and Pyeritz 1986; Murphy and Berger 1987).

EXAMPLE 8.13. In the knee jerk (itself a reflex but not homeostatic), the lag time depends on little more than how fast the message may take traveling the circuit and how fast it takes the muscles to contract. The length of time is greater in the long distal arcs (e.g., the ankle jerks) than in the shorter pathways in the arm reflexes (Iansik 1986). The peculiarity of the effect of the lag may explain the rare property among oscillating responses that clonus may be sustained for a few beats only (Murphy 1990).

EXAMPLE 8.14. In the response to the load of carbohydrate taken during a meal, the lag time may involve not only the time to start the release of stored insulin from the pancreas but the synthesis of new insulin, which may take thirty minutes or more (Yallow and Bersen 1960).

Simple homeostatic processes of this kind are not only important in the immediate light they may throw on the problem of cybernetic control and its relationship to disease. There is deeper insight to be gained from realizing that homeostatic circuits may be nested one inside another. This phenomenon opens up a hierarchy of processes with no natural limit. It may lead to a system of enormous subtlety and complexity, and even to an autonomous artificial intelligence.

We shall have to be content with one elaboration. The demands of the physiology may make it necessary to be able to adjust the three quantities L, b, and F.

EXAMPLE 8.15. In the disorder non-insulin-dependent diabetes mellitus (NIDDM) there is a high blood glucose level that has untoward effects due apparently to failure in handling a carbohydrate load. Indeed, there is old evidence in NIDDM (Yellow and Bersen 1960; Selzer et al. 1967; Cerasi, Efendic, and Luft 1973) that L is large, and so is the product Lb, even before there is ordinary clinical evidence of the overt disease. A danger, then, is that Lb is large enough to cause uncontrollable oscillation in the blood glucose level. If L cannot be lowered, then b must be. How can that happen? Well, one method is for the number of insulin receptors to be reduced, a change that is indeed a well-known phenomenon in diabetes mellitus (Olefsky 1976, 1984).

We need not go into details, but it is clear that here, because of the mechanism for cybernetically adjusting the correction parameter, we have a second homeostatic loop (a *retreat mechanism*) that changes the initial one. Nor is that the end, for the retreat loop is likely to be a response to some other sensor mechanism distinct from the first; and there may in turn be other sensors that operate on the first retreat loop; and so on indefinitely.

EXAMPLE 8.16. Many processes of hormone control and their aberrant forms operate homeostatically through the pituitary gland, which generates a class of trophic hormones. The menstrual cycle—which is a major device in regulating fertility, both spontaneously and artificially—is one such system, with two major regulators. However, the pituitary gland is in turn under the influence of a second retreat loop involving the hypothalamus. Moreover, there is evidence of at least a third retreat loop; and general metabolic factors (e.g., starvation and fanatical weight reduction), psychic factors (anorexia nervosa), and even social factors (women living in a community) may impinge on, for instance, the timing of menstruation. So far as we know, at the time of writing, there has been little theoretical exploration of the properties of such systems.

The simulation of homeostasis. We have said that the homeostatic process is cybernetic; that is, it aims to restore to initial functioning a system that has been perturbed. It is essentially dynamic and may be called upon any number of times. Sometimes in the course of a disease the sequelae may involve a disablement that is nevertheless beneficial and may create the illusion of purposive compensation. We illustrate such an event in the next two examples.

EXAMPLE 8.17. The connective tissue of higher animals and humans is formed from fibers of the multistranded protein collagen, which is laid down extracellularly. Initially it is weak and pliable, but in time and with age it becomes tougher and more rigid. The advantage of toughness gives way to the disadvantage of stiffness in cartilage, the joints, and elsewhere. It has been known for some time that these physical changes stem from chemical crosslinks built between adjacent strands of collagen, and that the number of such crosslinks increases with age (Butzow and Eichhorn 1968). It was surmised that the measured age-dependent increase was due to a continuous buildup in crosslinking. The enzyme lysyl oxidase, which is released extracellularly, is a main component in physiological crosslinking of collagen, and is perhaps implicated in the crosslinking that occurs in atherosclerosis and the fibrosis of liver and lung (Nagan and Kagan 1994). However, older tissue contains lower levels of lysyl oxidase than younger. The increased crosslinking with age thus appears to be a net effect of at least two active processes: continued crosslinking, and continued preferential proteolysis of the less crosslinked material (Kagan and Trackman 1991).

We may note in this connection that there are heritable disorders of connective tissue traceable to deficiency in lysyl oxidase (McKusick 1994: entry *153455). They include the disorders cutis laxa and Ehlers-Danlos syndrome type X1.

EXAMPLE 8.18. There is a hereditary disorder, familial prolapse of the mitral valve of the heart, known by the acronym the MASS syndrome (Glesby and Pyeritz 1989). It has some of the features of the Marfan syndrome. Extensive experience has shown that the overt cardiac features are rare in the young and the old (Devereux and Horan 1992; Strahan et al. 1983), and Devereux has suggested that the age-dependence in appearance is due to stretching of the valve. The signs subsequently disappear because the valve is no longer lax but hardened by deposition of calcium, or perhaps by induration of the collagen such as was discussed in Example 8.17. A stochastic model that takes that sequence of events into account gives a more satisfactory fit to the Mendelian hypothesis (Strahan et al. 1983). We reasonably conclude that the trait of valve prolapse, hidden at birth, is brought to light by some process of wear and tear, but later it is hidden, perhaps by toughening of the fibrous tissue. However, although this latter change is beneficial, it is so by the chance cancellation of two effects. It is not suggested that if prolapse were in some way to recur, the further sclerosing of the tissue would again rescue the patient. In that sense it is not a true homeostasis. Note also that under other circumstances (e.g., the sclerosis of the aortic valve) the "correcting" process is in fact harmful.

Instinctive Action

By *instinctive action* we mean the responses to a disturbance made unreflectingly and naturally by members of a species. Thus, mammals that are cold tend to curl up and to huddle together, actions that diminish the surface area and hence reduce the heat loss of the whole group. Hungry babies instinctively suck if offered a nipple. The young, when frightened, try to escape, cry, and otherwise seek parental protection.

Such responses are roughly analogous to homeostasis, but they differ in several important ways. For one thing, they are executed by quite different anatomical mechanisms, by striped muscle rather than splanchnic muscle; and by different parts of the nervous system, notably the so-called voluntary rather than the autonomic nervous system. It is important to address two natural criticisms of this formulation of instinct.

The first criticism is that the words used (*voluntary, autonomic,* etc.) may suggest that, into what purports to be fact, scientists are intruding gratuitous interpretations that hint at qualitatively different processes. Eliminative materialists such as Churchland (1984) will quarrel not only with the opinion but also with the insinuation of these nuanced words. The discussion of Searle (1992), though he holds strong and frank opinions of his own, lays out the views. There is point to that complaint. However, there is no dispute that, call them what you will, the mechanisms involved in homeostasis and in these instinctive reactions are different. Instinctive behavior is generally more elaborately organized, and therefore neither so stereotyped nor so predictable as the homeostatic. Moreover, in higher organisms, at least, instinctive behavior invades consciousness and appears as purposive. It constitutes what is widely recognized as *behavior.* Thus, the means of reducing bodily heat loss may be highly diversified and opportunistic, that is, exploiting peculiar, even unique, mechanisms for which the organism cannot have been prepared by evolutionary mechanisms or even previous experience.

The second criticism is that calling any form of behavior *instinctive* does not explain anything at all. Doing so merely tries to make a putative mechanism out of a mere gap in our understanding (Bateson 1972). It is an intensely black box. We do not dispute that criticism. It is difficult even to imagine how instinctive behavior can operate or (to cast the challenge in the very strongest confrontational terms) how it can be coded for genetically; and how in turn the code might be translated reliably, and efficiently converted into credible existential terms. Here there is every reason to be suspicious about facile reductionism, rich in assurance and poor in specific models. But we can merely repeat that whatever the mechanisms (and they may be of many quite different kinds), at the present time the evidence shows the most convincing signs of their being quite different from homeostasis. If nothing else, this category defines a major area awaiting inquiry.

Calculated Protection

The advent of the intelligent organism allows highly organized behavior to be used for engineering (by the beaver, for instance); for collective strategic hunting (as among jackals); for protection against the cold by various elaborate devices. Use of fire and the wearing of clothes seem to be distinctively human devices. But the ability to abstract allows planning and execution of long-range undertakings. The discovery of the theories for projecting the outcome without appeal to pragmatic experience allows unlimited extensions (such as central heating, air-conditioning, and refrigeration).

Migration

Organisms may migrate in search of new food, or as a protection against the weather, or to escape predators, or for various other motives or reasons. Migration is widespread in higher organisms with diverse elaborateness and subtlety, from the seasonal migration of birds to the wonders of the travel agency.

A Psychic Analogue

The foregoing illustrations are mostly devices of the physical body. In higher organisms the mind too has its needs and gratifications. They arise in the course of ordinary stimulation and as concomitants of the experience of annoyance, alert, or alarm in psychic activity, whether conscious or unconscious (see Appendix 1). Some of the responses are dramatic (hysteria, mania, depression, dissociation, compulsion, and obsession). The extent of the disturbance may be gauged by the Medical needs, which may range from outpatient visits to commitment to hospital. We are intrigued by a buffering system, analogous to physiological homeostasis, that enables the mind to function in the face of diverse endowments, conventionally called "genetic," and in a physical environment that is sometimes hostile. The responses are by no means unalloyed, but they may tide the troubled mind over what might otherwise be an overwhelming experience, until a more pleasant and harmonious accommodation is reached. We may briefly sketch some of the devices involved.

1. *Transformation into processes of defense:* Simply stated, there are four principal lines of defense: acting-out behavior; psychophysiologic and psychosomatic reactions; psychoneurosis; and psychosis. There is active research aimed to delineate on the one hand etiology, both genetic and environmental, and from the pathological standpoint, pathogenetic mechanisms, such as those in depression.

2. *Sublimation:* The capacity of the human being to deal with the stress of life includes the solace of a wide repertoire of devices: cultural (including ceremonial, festivities, enjoyment of the arts and humanities), recreational (sports, travel, health cults), and many spiritual and transcendental activities.

3. *Homeostasis:* Particularly in matters of mood, the mind shows ability to adjust itself to what at first may be damaging encounters: grief and the trauma of disappointments, for instance. We may also mention here the oscillating character of lagged homeostatic systems of fractional power and their possible relationship to the clinical diversity of bipolar mood disorders (Murphy 1987).

4. *Instinct:* The capacity of the mind to manage successfully, or to tolerate or even repress, painful or destructive conflict is inborn and akin to instinct.

Eugenic Issues

The emphasis under this confrontational picture of normality is rather different from that of normality in isolation described in the first section. There is a sense here that the organism is no longer a helpless victim of the environment but can, with ingenuity, by putting up a struggle of some kind, improve the chances of survival. Moreover, in part the environment comprises other organisms of the same or kindred species (although differing in allelic content so that they are competing in the same domain), and of more different types that may be prey, predators, and symbionts such as saprophytes and parasites. In more developed interactions there may be whole ecologies with a richly complex dynamics, the representation and understanding of which may extend far beyond available methods of mathematics and may beggar the resources of even the most elaborate computers. The trend of evolution is much more elaborate than earlier. There are conflicting qualities in the aspects of survival, special premiums attached to variation as well as excellence of the standard type; to efficiency of the entire reproductive process as well as high fertility (Murphy 1978b; Murphy, Krush, et al. 1980); to moderation of conquest that does not threaten the ecology; to unrestricted cropping and hunting; to camouflage and cunning as well as to aggressive strength and speed of pursuit.

Commentary

These complex mechanisms, and perhaps others, vastly complicate the Ethical underpinning of normality and disease. No longer is there a simple tension between the native endowment of the organism and the environment in which it finds itself by chance; rather, there is a complicated series of interactions among the various buffering mechanisms one with another and with the interior and exterior milieux. It seems evident that the greater the discrepancy between the two milieux, the more strenuously the protecting mechanisms are taxed. We may summarize these considerations using cold as a substantive illustration. There are four broad basic components: the *interior milieu,* which is the zone of operation of the vital process; *insulation,* which is the set of involuntary mechanisms in response to challenge from the environment; *protection,* which comprises the voluntary mechanisms of responding to environmental changes; and the *exterior milieu.* The responses to harmful changes in the environment may be classified accordingly. They may also be grouped as tactical (or immediate) responses and strategic (or long-term) responses.

First, there are the changes in the interior milieu. Simple arrest of function is the immediate response. Presumably it is mainly a physicochemical phenomenon. Indeed, it is somewhat contrived to regard it as a response at all and not, perhaps, a passive consequence. This process will depend on the native endowment of the organism. Hence, its perpetuation is mainly a matter of genetic selection. The interior milieu may also respond strategically by undergoing metamorphosis, a matter of physiology. Again the capacity to undergo this change is no doubt largely maintained by genetic selection.

Second, insulation is of two types. There are diverse tactical devices of homeostasis, which are restorative mechanisms in response to discrepancy between the interior and the exterior milieus and hence physiological processes of a cybernetic character. The strategic aspects of insulation are analogous. Both mechanisms are controlled by the vegetative nervous system and, since they cannot be voluntarily manipulated, are presumably subjected to genetic selection.

Third, there is protection, those responses that are mediated through the voluntary nervous system. Instinctive responses are tactical in character: in insects they seem to be wholly inborn and genetic, whereas in higher organisms much is experiential and learned under the guidance of the parents. While instinctive behavior is elastic, nevertheless it shows little true inventiveness. The engineering, the strategic component of protection, is deliberative manipulation of the environment. By its very nature this third group comprises almost exclusively cultural forms (often rudimentary). It occurs in some animals (e.g., dam-building by beavers).

In all of the foregoing, the organism remains in its environment and protects itself as it may.

A fourth device addresses the exterior milieu more immediately. Inadequacies may be lessened by evading harmful outside challenges. The means are physiological and intellectual, preserved mainly by genetics and culture, respectively. The tactical response is flight, as in climbing a tree for safety from flood, or seeking shelter from the cold. The strategic response is either permanent or seasonal migration. The historical development of systematic reasoning and the habit of making judgments and exercising prudent choice greatly extended the scope of engineering and migration.

Clearly, survival is a complex interaction between these four components and diverse mechanisms, which makes the Ethics more intricate. What is the advantage of having all these complicated means of mitigating selection? We know of two, both showing the uses of elasticity.

One advantage is specialized control over the environment. The environment acceptable to the naive organism may be a restricted one. Humans are the species with the widest geographical distribution because, unlike the jellyfish, they may carry their own environment around with them. Most complicated processes such as thought seem to operate best over a narrow temperature range. To maintain the brain temperature within narrow optimal tolerances calls for elaborate devices.

The other advantage is the provision of genetic resources. The life of the single organism is usually short compared with that of the species; and over the lifetime of a species, big environmental changes occur. What is the best genotype may vary widely over that interval. Now, since most mutations are harmful, the genetic process is perforce intensely conservative. But in times of rapid environmental change, conservatism may be the undoing of the species. The species may need a means of changing genetic composition far faster perhaps than the speed of useful mutation allows. The needed genetic material must come from a ready store of mutations, often ugly, now beneficial though formerly detrimental. There are several genetic devices for hiding them until useful: recessivity, hypostasis, incomplete penetrance, and, in a more complicated fashion, multilocal systems. In the transition, a recessive trait hitherto regarded as harmful, although safe when hidden by a dominant allele, now becomes a normal trait, still recessive, while the abnormal trait is a dominant diseased state and rapidly eliminated.

NORMALITY AS HARMONY

With very simple organisms, the notion of normality might reduce itself quite simply to conformity of the organism to its environment. Such a state must be acceptable, since little can be demanded of a simple organism except to survive long enough to reproduce. In particular, there would be no question of deontology. In a particular environment, the organism would either be normal and survive or be abnormal and die. But this meaning of *normal* is a hypallage, a transferred meaning, properly predicated not of the organism but of its relationship to the environment. Icy cold water is not abnormal; neither are all jellyfish. The abnormality lies in the incongruity of a jellyfish and icy water. Normality is a matter of the harmonious interrelation between the two. Icy cold water might be a natural habitat for polar bears, while jellyfish might survive perfectly in the waters of the South Seas.

This notion of normality as harmony between the organism and its environment can be extended to somewhat more complicated organisms, though with mounting ambiguities. Now, because of insulation, there is ambiguity as to what is meant by "the environment." Claude Bernard (1872) made the classic distinction between the internal environment of the organism and its external environment; and Cannon (1932) formulated this relationship in terms of homeostasis. Insulation in the first place is a mechanism for creating a buffer between the two; but at a certain stage of evolution it starts to acquire some independence of function, which makes it an object of selection in its own right so that it is ordinarily present in diverse form.

EXAMPLE 8.19. The human higher centers of organization function best when the temperature of the interior milieu is about 37 degrees centigrade. Now, this temperature could be maintained artificially by living in an environment that has that temperature without benefit of homeostatic mechanisms that preserve the temperature of the interior milieu. But, of course, in practice the matter is more complicated; homeostatic mechanisms have a certain persistence. Living requires expenditure of energy that must be dissipated. Human beings at an external temperature of 37 degrees centigrade are uncomfortable, and body physiology uses certain devices such as sweating to reduce the body temperature somewhat.

In attempts to apply the criterion of normality as harmony to the most elaborate organisms, the notion that the normal is the state ideally suited to the environment breaks down at three major points.

First, the environment is not absolutely constant. Yet the intuitive notion of the normal is that it has a certain stability not to be conceived of as fluctuating rapidly as a result of external causes. The idea of a person living in a desert who was normal in the daytime and inexorably abnormal at night seems absurd. We find it necessary to suppose that the notion of the normal is not simply a fixed state but a certain range of congruities between the organism and the environment. In the same way, certain psychic changes in the individual may be perfectly appropriate responses to disturbing experiences. We may argue that it is normal to be afraid when chased by a tiger; or to be indolent when hungry or tired; or to feel angry when attacked. Behavior that is acceptable in an infant may be unacceptable in a child, and so on through ordinary development and maturation.

Second, cybernetic mechanisms (mechanisms that automatically tend to repair departures from the habitual or homing value) can only be triggered by some departure from the optimal value (although the minimum perceptible departure may be small). Some range of values must needs be accepted as normal.

Third, as we have seen above, there is conflict between the interests of the individual and the interests of the species. Not, to be sure, a major conflict; but the short-term demands of the individual can perhaps be met only at the expense of long-term jeopardy to the species. Natural selection impinges more on the species than on the individual, and hence every organism inherits much genetic material that to the individual is useless, or even possibly harmful; and that material is offset by various mechanisms for assuaging its effect, the main value of which is to conserve a variety of genetic blueprints any one of which may prove useful at a much later date. So yet again there is reason to believe that the very complicatedness of the organism requires the outlines for the notion of the normal to be somewhat softened to accommodate a range of normal values.

When we attempt to apply these principles to the most highly evolved organisms, especially human beings, the situation is yet further complicated. Discrepancies between the organism and its environment that lie quite beyond the cybernetic powers of homeostasis may still be dealt with by the methods of protection. Among the mammals, humans (being virtually devoid of body hair and of blubber) are perhaps the least well adapted to live in a cold climate. Current views suggest that the human species arose in central Africa perhaps three or four million years ago; no doubt the climate was warm, and complex methods to conserve body temperature within tolerable levels were unnecessary. But by elaborating the processes of protection (fire, clothing, housing, and finally central heating), human beings have been able to migrate further and further from the ancestral place of origin. Persons living at the North Pole without any of these means of protection would be in a very abnormal relationship indeed. Yet in common usage of the term, at least, the Inuit are not regarded as abnormal. Of course, this capacity to withstand cold is not exclusively a matter of protection, and some persons, as a result of education, training, and habituation, are better able to withstand cold climates than others. The outcome of using all these different mechanisms is to widen the range of circumstances in which the body will work fairly well. The naked preserve themselves against the cold by shivering and by vasoconstriction of skin; but when protection is added, it reduces the demands on homeostatic mechanisms. Thus, there is a kind of reciprocal relationship among the three determinants of efficient functioning (i.e., the interior milieu, insulation, and protection). The more the burden is taken by the one system, the less it is imposed on the others. If we envision the normal as an arbitrary range of incongruity between the organism and its environment, it seems clear that the acceptable range would be wider in the presence of protection than in its absence and where there is efficient homeostasis than where there is not.

The Properties of the Multilocal System

The other conflict that imposes the need for a range of normal values is that between the immediate needs of the organism and the long-term needs of the species. Several of the genetic mechanisms that attempt to reconcile this conflict (recessiveness, hypostasis, and incomplete penetrance) have already been mentioned and are widely recognized. But there is a further mechanism that has not really received the attention it deserves from the population geneticists, namely, the virtues of the multilocal system (Murphy 1966). There is reason to believe that characters such as height, intelligence, blood pressure, and blood cholesterol level are not under the control of single genetic loci but reflect the composite effect of contributions from many loci. Suppose that the effect depends upon the Random and more or less independent assortment of a large number of factors. Given a fixed overall mean, as the number of independent, equally important, contributing loci with additive effects increases, the variance of the trait (roughly, the dispersion of the results) falls. As a result, a larger proportion of the organisms will by chance fall close to the optimal state; and this has indeed been shown to be true, for certain systems of selection, at least. It was noted that in some conditions in human beings there is evidence that the carrier state is more fit than either of the homozygous states. Such a system (the so-called *balanced polymorphism*) has certain advantages, but it may involve a heavy toll of deaths from genetic disease. Furthermore, such a system is somewhat unstable: a temporary but severe change in the environment may lead to permanent extinction of one or another of the alleles.

In contrast, multifactorial traits enjoy three advantages. First, they tend to cluster around the optimal value, and few individuals will drift far from it. Second, should the environment change, a new optimal value will emerge around which the organisms would again cluster, but as a result of change in gene frequencies *with little threat to any contributing genes at the pertinent loci that might later prove beneficial*. Third, with a larger number of genes making proportionately smaller contributions, a finer gradation of phenotypes is possible. These three advantages may explain why so many important traits in higher organisms are under the corporate control of many loci. But illustrations explicit in every detail are difficult to discover in human beings. They are, of course, well documented in commercial stock, animal and vegetable.

A Note on Selection of Homeostasis

The genetic aspects of this vital topic have so far received embarrassingly little attention, perhaps because quantitative geneticists have little interest in physiology and physiologists little in genetics. Yet there are important implications and reasonable warrant for expecting new insights into what in classical quantitative genetics have been intractable puzzles.

EXAMPLE 8.20. It is easy to grasp why and how selection should drive the mean close to the optimal; but since it is the outliers that are selected against, it is hard to see why the scatter is not more ruthlessly selected against. Theory shows that in a multilocal system the minimum scatter due to genetic segregation is zero.[2] Yet the variation remains large, and one might wonder whether it is being actively supported. But while the usual theory has weak speculation and little evidence, theory of homeostasis shows that the values of the specifications that produce either too tight a control or too lax a control are each in their own way harmful (Renie and Murphy 1983). The intermediate combinations will be stably selected for, and, as a consequence, that component of the variation determined by the effect of Random environmental perturbations will be maintained at a level that overrides the effect of genetic selection on the means.

To questions about the behavior of selection on more complex homeostatic systems, there are scarcely any answers. Preliminary studies show that there is an analogous conservation of variance in systems with one retreat loop that will drive the behavior away from both extremes: laxity and wild oscillation (Murphy n.d.-c).

Eugenic Issues

The more complex view of normality as harmony makes the optimal phenotype harder and harder to define, partly because of the increasing difficulty in distinguishing the organism from the environment; and partly because the interactions are so intricate that any attempt to improve the population is likely to have all manner of side effects that cannot be foreseen and that may be seriously harmful. As might be imagined, the more intricate the protective devices, the less the impact of external selection. But one of the powerful sources of external selection is artificial breeding. It is not, then, surprising that these protective devices make it progressively more difficult to nudge phenotypes toward a goal, even if the goal could be defined. That task has a much better prospect with genetic engineering: introducing ge-

2. This minimum is reached when in a closed mating population there is fixation (homozygosity) at all the participating loci and mutation is negligible.

netic material deliberately rather than waiting for appropriate new mutants to occur by chance. However, that course still does not relieve the geneticist of the need to understand the ontogenetic and pathogenetic aspects of the relationship between genotype and phenotype. Indeed, overcoming natural protective barriers as genetic engineering would do makes the need to understand the causal relationships more important than ever. It is one matter to detect the seriously harmful traits and, if the causes are known, to take reasonable preventive measures. That is a common concern in genetic counseling. However, despite some minor attitudinizing, that is not what is usually meant by *eugenics,* the search for the super-race.

A Qualifying Note

One feature that is persistently overlooked is the real (though rather unobtrusive) conflict between Darwinian evolution and dynamic population genetics as addressed by their respective students.

Evolution is studied on a very long time scale; although much of its material includes the fossil record, the unifying idea underlying it is what survives in the sense of perpetuating its line of descent, and therefore by definition has an evolutionary and hence relative genetic fitness greater than unity. The cardinal tenet of Darwinism is precisely that in the main sweep there is no equilibrium. Insofar as a species neither evolves nor dies out—as seems to have been true for many millions of years in many of the mollusks—it is (tautologously) not undergoing evolution. Again, evolution does not address lines of descent of individuals, although (in a kind of rough analogy) it studies lines of descent of species; as a consequence (looked at Statistically), the sample space is not defined, and no formal tests of (Statistical) hypotheses are possible.

In contrast, dynamic population genetics (i.e., the diachronic study of those phenomena such as mutation, migration, selection, Random drift, and biased drift that bear on the genetic composition of a population) is a relatively short-scale study that in human beings seldom extends for more than five or six generations even for hearsay evidence; the sample space is usually better defined (although to the fastidious standards of the Statistician often inadequately); and, in the domain of Medical genetics, there is concern with both evolutionary and relative genetic fitness less than unity. Much of this field (notably the usual, indirect methods of estimating the mutation rate for recessive traits) is inferential rather than observed, so that a key assumption is that an equilibrium exists between the rate of new mutation and the payment of mutational debt.

It is clear that there is a clash between the scope of the two fields over the issue of equilibrium. The clash may be resolved by supposing either that the subject matters of the two fields differ or that the departure from equilibrium necessary to give substance to Darwinism has only a trifling impact on the population geneticist's analysis. The other alternative—to divorce the two fields as incommensurable, much as mechanical engineering is divorced from particle physics or semantic analysis is divorced from journalism—seems too distasteful and too discouraging at the present time to be seriously considered.

However, these comfortable assumptions are in some difficulty in view of the growing interest in the phenomena of punctuated evolution (Stanley 1996): the idea that mutation is nothing like a homogeneous Poisson process, a phenomenon operating at constant risk, but instead exhibits conspicuously higher rates in some eras and lower rates in others. The mechanism is still disputed, but there is convincing evidence in the fossil record, which has been a thorn in the side of the Darwinians throughout the last century.

The evolution of the human species is at present under radical dispute. In recent years the length of time has been increased by nearly an order of magnitude. The evidence is almost wholly physical, and the available evidence about cultural patterns (social life, speech, manufacture of artifacts, cults, etc.) is inevitably indirect, fragmentary, conjectural, and confined to a small fraction of that long history. For instance, the precise relationship between Neanderthal and Cro-Magnon is unclear and indeed something of a mystery. It is supposed that Cro-Magnon won in the long run because of greater intelligence. There is clear current assurance that the human species has an elaborate capacity to reason; to grapple with values and make moral judgments (indeed, the ultimate driving force behind this book); to record history by storytelling, by myth, and eventually by permanent written records and the like. These latter changes have been so fundamental in the evolutionary path that (like the pathologist, the educator, and the Philosopher) we are obliged for the present, at least, and probably long into the future, to acknowledge that there is a hiatus that must be respected. Being part of the system ourselves, we may ultimately lack the analytical wherewithal to bridge that hiatus. To say the least, it seems pretentious to suppose that constructing an unbroken chain of mechanisms that will vindicate the deconstructive materialists is nothing more than an extended technical exercise.

THE DEFINITION OF THE NORMAL

It has been pointed out elsewhere (Murphy 1997) that the word *normal* has a great many different meanings, some quite neutral in tone and some involving more or less personal preference. In the present analysis of the normal we avoid entirely all questions of merit. As in the other chapters of this book, we are attempting simply to analyze the meaning of certain fundamental ideas; to try to determine how far they correspond to natural phenomena; and to assess the extent to which they are simply arbitrary judgments, the use of which in cogent Ethical arguments may be somewhat brittle.

The analysis presented above seems to suggest that the notion of the normal is at best a vague one and not to be unambiguously inferred from any natural juxtaposition of phenomena. How, then, is it possible to attempt to distinguish between the normal and the diseased states? Apparently this can be done by appeal to two broad mechanisms:

1. What is to be considered normal in an Ethical sense may be determined by appeal to some field other than empirical science. The notion of the normal might be sought from metaphysics, Morals, esthetics, politics, theology, or elsewhere. Given that the desired states can be furnished by such areas, there are formal scientific criteria (so far, overwhelmingly Statistical in character) that furnish a means of relating measurements to the prescribed normal.
2. More directly, the state of the normal may be determined by defining some desirable outcome and deciding how this is to be attained. Again, however, there is at least an implicit appeal to something that is other than a neutral description of objectively demonstrable fact; and this is a matter that is taken up in greater detail in Chapters 10 and 11, on the making of decisions and on biological viability.

THE DEFINITION OF DISEASE

The definition of disease is a large and intricate topic. Disease by convention among pathologists is (like health) a dynamic processes, and therefore (like it) a phenomenon of living systems only. A disease cannot occur in a cadaver, although the evidence of it may remain. The word itself, *dis-ease,* originally implied discomfort or distress of some kind, but this requirement has long since been waived. Clinicians happily talk about the "preclinical disease," denoting a stage at which perhaps the fate of the patient is already sealed but the patient has no symptoms. Such a denotation makes good sense in a few instances: in Tay-Sachs disease or other lethal but age-dependent genetic disorders; or cancer with widespread metastases; or, latterly, AIDS. But when Diagnosis is to be pushed back earlier and earlier, there comes a stage when no decisive statement can be made, even if there were in principle no limitations to the inquiry that can be undertaken. At that stage the doubt about the disease is not by any stretch to be seen as epistemic but ontological.

EXAMPLE 8.21. Tuberculosis must start with the *Mycobacterium tuberculosis* entering the body. But that entry in itself cannot be usefully taken as sufficient to constitute a disease; otherwise, many people living lives of robust well-being would be diseased much of the time. That objection is even more searching when the organism is a common body saprophyte. There are organisms in virtually every bowel that in adverse circumstances may attack the body (notably *E. coli*). For an infectious disease there has to be some preliminary skirmish in which the body sustains some kind and degree of injury.

It will be easily seen that many minute and commonplace factors in the environment, each in isolation having negligible impact, may in aggregate threaten or overwhelm life—anthracite, asbestos, allergens, copper, lead, and thousands of others. At what stage is it useful to treat the accumulation of, say, mercury from tuna fish as mercury poisoning? Is it reasonable to regard the notion of disease as inexorably quantitative—to suppose that there is no natural threshold at which a *normal* accumulation of poison becomes a *diseased* accumulation? The same question arose in Chapter 3. We have no facile answer.

Another matter must be raised. Do the states *healthy* and *diseased* exhaust the possibilities? Is there some neutral territory that perhaps merits attention? Should clinicians—at least acting as agents of society on whom the responsibility rests—be diagnosing the disablement of disease (what is currently seen as the clinician's function); diagnosing health and reassuring those who enjoy it; and identifying in what way the intermediate persons could be led to enjoy better health and have the benefits of strenuous application of what is called preventive Medicine? What Ethical problems would be introduced by the solemnization of that third group? Is there an Ethical imperative to acquire an adequate body of information on which this preventive Medicine might draw? Where in all this array of problems are such disabling conditions as grief, disappointment, discouragement, vice, and crime to be accommodated?

Having taken note of these caveats, let us attempt to lay out some ontological types of disease. The word *disease* as it is ordinarily employed has at least two major meanings. First, it covers both the effects of a hostile environment and the attempts of the organism to cope with it. For instance, frostbite is the consequence of extreme cold, whereas most of the manifestations of pneumonia are an attempt to counteract the consequences of invasion of the lung by a hostile organism.

However, there is another important sense of the term, and a much more sinister one, denoting some defect in the operation of a homeostatic system. These disturbances fall into four broad categories:

1.   The homeostatic system may simply be incapable of coping with the ordinary challenges with which it is confronted. The disease that we know as surgical shock perhaps falls into this class.

2. Homeostasis may be highly efficient but be misdirected to the maintenance of a deleterious state.

EXAMPLE 8.22. In patients whose blood pressure is dangerously high, therapeutic attempts to lower the blood pressure are not, so to speak, welcomed by an embattled physiology as a support but are actively combated by the very homeostatic mechanisms they are intended to help. Such organisms will in general be less genetically fit and will tend to be eliminated by genetic selection. Adequate Medical treatment then allows them to be healthy and able to reproduce. Hence, treatment will assuage somewhat the force of genetic selection and tend to keep such stock alive.

EXAMPLE 8.23. Lactation is commonly but not invariably associated with infertility. Now, one could make a reasonable case that since both pregnancy and lactation draw heavily on the maternal nutritional reserves, it is abnormal that they should be competing with each other. If that is so, should fertility during lactation be more securely depressed by medication to ensure that pregnancy does not occur?

3. The characteristic of interest (e.g., body temperature) may be carried outside the *zone of convergence* of the homeostatic system (i.e., the range of values within which homeostasis can even attempt to return the value to desirable levels). This appears to be the case in heat stroke, and perhaps in severe irreversible shock. Extreme psychologic stress is another example.
4. The disease process may represent an anarchy on which the homeostatic system can have no impact at all. Cancer is a classic example.

It might be argued that where any of the above four mechanisms is known to be operating, we may take this state prima facie as a diseased one and to be treated as unconditionally abnormal.

PROSPECTS FOR PREVENTION AND INTERVENTION

It will be convenient here to list the ways in which the relationship between the organism and its environment may be deliberately manipulated. By doing so, we are not endorsing any of them. To the contrary, we *prescind* entirely from any Ethical matters that arise with deliberate interventions. We group them according to the interior milieu, insulation, protection, and the exterior milieu.

With the *interior milieu,* the essentials are the genotypes and their state of operation; social, educational, and cumulative experience; immunity;

and so on. Intervention in this area can also be considered from the standpoint of the individual organism, or from the society of which it is a member. The possible interventions[3] include three major steps:

1. Only those organisms deemed "fit" would be encouraged, or even allowed, to survive and reproduce. In practice, a variety of methods have been used, such as abortion of fetuses or killing newborn having certain phenotypes, the deliberate withholding of lifesaving treatment, and sterilization of the unfit.
2. The genetic endowment of the organism may be specially modified by the methods that are usually referred to as genetic engineering, that is, the introduction of foreign genetic material into some or all of the body cells. This phenomenon *(transduction)* is well known in microorganisms, and within a matter of years it will no doubt be effectively practiced in the higher organisms.
3. Deficits in the interior milieu may be replaced by substitution therapy (e.g., for deficient hormones). The latter step is directed at the individual only and confers no direct transmissible benefit on society in general.

As to *insulation,* defective homeostasis and its consequences may be adjusted by the use of (e.g.) antimalarial drugs, corrective surgery, and the like, which it would be pointless to discuss in general.

Protection may be directed either mainly to the external structural environment (e.g., providing warm houses for all); or primarily to support of fragile organisms (e.g., by enriched nutritional culture or, for higher organisms, special diets in hereditary disorders of metabolism).

The *exterior milieu,* finally, may be deliberately manipulated by methods which properly belong to the domain of ecological engineering.

It is evident that the more manipulation is applied to one of these areas, the less there is need for manipulation in another. Special diets for phenylketonuria (protection) would not be necessary if progeny homozygous for this condition did not survive.

CONCLUSION

In the course of history, investigation of the normal has so far gone through three stages.

The first surmise was that the ambiguity in phenotypes is epistemic: the data are noisy perhaps because what is of Ethical interest is far re-

---

3. These are possible interventions. Their merits fall within the domain of Ethics and are not analyzed here.

moved from the fundamental defect, and progress will come from more refined phenotyping or causal analysis. That view has led to a very few spectacular results. However, it seems they are far from typical. The usual pattern of inquiry meant a progressive estrangement from the root inquiry. So conspicuous a disorder as the heart attack became progressively recast as myocardial infarction; then as coronary atherosclerosis; then as hypercholesterolemia; then as a variety of inborn errors of metabolism; then as disordered HMG coenzyme A reductase. The refinement was impressive, but it had less and less to do with heart attacks. No doubt the latter are indeed a diverse group of disorders, and perhaps that is the correct perspective; and if there is an Ethical interface, it should deal with the basic chemical defects. But since these chemical anomalies do not invariably lead to clinical disaster, the conclusion is open to the charge of trivializing the Ethics. It may be pointed out that disorders of cholesterol are by no means the only line of refinement. Heart attacks occur, for instance, from a chemically refined (if rare) inborn error of metabolism, homocystinuria; from a disorder of coagulation, Antithrombin III deficiency; from disorders of the arterial wall as in pseudoxanthoma elasticum; and various other causes.

The second surmise about the difficulties in investigating normality (to which the outcomes of the first gave way) is ontological. The original question had not been stated correctly: it was based on the implicit assumption that the heart attack has a high enough ontological density to be a coherent topic of discourse. There are indeed many more striking "diseases" where this claim has been so undermined that the term has virtually ceased to exist: dropsy, apoplexy, the falling sickness, brain fever, the vapors, the decline, ague, the founder.

The third surmise has had its origin from several lines of thought that at first may have seemed almost wholly unrelated but that have been gradually amalgamated by clinicians constructively exposed to Statistics and the quantitative revolution in Medicine; to the consequences of the controversy between Galtonian and Mendelian genetics, Fisher's masterly reconciliation (1918), and the rise of quantitative genetics; and to the neo-Darwinian revolution of Fisher (1918), Sewall Wright (1969), and others (Dobzhansky et al. 1977). From this syncrisis is slowly emerging the perception that the fuzziness of the phenotype is not an epistemic or even an ontological defect but a quality that has been bred by its selective advantage. Attempts to elucidate the components of this complexity in the internal and external ecology are to be applauded and indeed must be pursued if there is to be any hope of understanding the whole. But to try to grasp the nature of the whole emergent structure by imposing an artificial and highly misleading emphasis on some one element is as mistaken as to suppose that the ensemble of an orchestra is faithfully represented by the skill of the flute player or the agility of the concertmaster. Evolution, it seems, is not a reductionist; and surely Ethics should not be either. But this leads us more than ever to deplore and mistrust billiard-ball Ethics. Everything should indeed be made as simple as possible and no simpler.

Where this inquiry will eventually lead remains to be seen. Ethicists, however academic, are obliged somehow to deal with real-time problems that can no more be suspended until the perfect solution is obtained than emergency operations or treatment of diabetic coma can. But prudence seems to demand, however, that in their endeavors they be excruciatingly careful not to mortgage their future by supposing the current perception of Medicine to be a fair and accurate account of its true nature.

9 Probability, Certainty, and Certitude

To suppose that any course of behavior, and in particular Ethical behavior, is based on complete knowledge about the issues involved is a gross, and indeed a dangerous, oversimplification. Even when the gaps are large and obvious, courses of action are often decided as if none of the key issues has been overlooked. No further assurance is gained by mere possession of data alone, for the data themselves may be neither firm nor clearly defined. Scholarly people who conscientiously collect their information before taking action, and have good reason to suppose their judgment sound, do not in general treat their information as above criticism. They implicitly accept the limitation and indefiniteness, whether subjective or objective. A surgeon, for example, in planning an operation on a patient may believe that cure is impossible, improbable, possible, probable, certain. These crude groupings represent a continuum from impossibility to certainty.

THE FORMAL APPARATUS OF PROBABILITY

At the outset we must distinguish clearly among three separate approaches. They correspond to the three facets of scientific discovery, namely, the *experiential,* the *analytic,* and the *conjectural.* In the end all are equally important in the sense that without any of them, no science is possible. To speculate without reference to empirical data may lead to great matters and important conclusions, but they are not science. The medieval approach to science (at least up to the revolutions of Albertus and Roger Bacon) was, not to *exclude* experience from the speculation, but to suppose that it required no formal attention and could afford to be treated casually. This attitude we previously encountered in Example 6.2 and the commentary in dealing with the *McNaughton* rules for the defense at criminal law on grounds of insanity. On the other hand, to collect data without any commitment to some known, or surmised, order leads to what Popper (1959) identifies as a misdirection in the science of Francis Bacon. Popper's perception is not surprising, and is indeed commonplace. It would be false to see the division as one among speculation, epistemology, and ontology, since all are ultimately indispensable for all three approaches. But the current drive of science is to regard the main discipline of collecting and analyzing empirical data as provenient; the interpreting of data as mathematics of secondary importance; and the imaginative expression of their meaning and implications as an occasional expression of curiosity.

Now, these broad matters lie at the very heart of the confusion surrounding Probability, which it is our business to explore in this chapter. The whole topic has to be examined under all three rubrics: provenient, analytic, and conjectural. There is nothing very revolutionary about the basic idea in, say, physics. There, it is universally accepted that experimental physicists do experiments or (e.g., in astrophysics) make precise observations without the manipulation that we attach to the word *experiment*. They do so under the guidance of the theoretical physicists who analyze the data and continually develop their models. These models are sometimes far-reaching but arcane speculation that is formal but may be beyond the bounds of imagination. The theorists then sound them out on the data, modify them as need be, and propose new experiments or observations that will help the next round of inference. The main difficulty in biology and Medicine is that there is a superabundance of data about a vast multiplicity of entities. Biologists cultivate too little of the imagination that produced Mendel's original insight, the Watson-Crick model, and the theory of antibody formation; and (partly from the difficulties of the subject and partly from disinclination) formal theoretical biology and Medicine remain underdeveloped.[1]

The theory of Probability is a branch of mathematics (or, if you like, applied mathematics) based on certain minimum axioms defined in advance. It is not the business of mathematicians to justify the axioms, except to make sure that they are consistent and sufficiently complete for a particular inquiry. Nor is it their responsibility to devise methods of verifying either the axioms or the conclusions in the empirical world. Verification lies in the domain of their scientific counterparts, the Statisticians; and the circle is closed by the ontological concerns of the scientist. That, of course, does not exclude the Probabilists from being interested in applications; nor does it mean that the Statisticians may not become involved in their own mathematically demanding details; nor that the scientists can safely afford to ignore either.[2] The distinction in their offices is rather one of *ultimate*

---

1. We mean, not that there is any shortage of speculation in our disciplines, but that it is at a very low level of resolution and coherence; for the most part it is not amenable to decisive testing. Many examples of these weaknesses will emerge in what follows.

2. It is chastening to recall that Archimedes, Newton, and Gauss, by common consent the three greatest mathematicians, all made contributions to physics that were of the first rank. Gauss (after whom the physical unit of magnetic flux density is named) completed the hat trick by inventing the first general Statistical estimator, the method of least squares. So much for purity of purpose.

allegiance and responsibility. Much of the perplexity over this topic of uncertainties stems from confusing these three quite distinct fields. Presented with the mathematician's idealized model of how such and such a Probabilistic system will behave, the Statistician builds up a distinct model that is centered on the problems of making inferences about Probabilities from some experience of the empirical world.

The scientist, the third party to the transaction, is neither a speculative nor an inferential theorist but a person whose allegiance is to the actual nature of the phenomena in a particular field. The scientist's task includes asking certain kinds of questions in the first place; searching for possible approaches to them; devising appropriate empirical methods; collecting data either by manipulative experiments or by observation; building up a surmise as to what the data indicate; seeking from the Probabilist what may be a Probabilistic model that describes the conjectured process; and consulting the Statistician for an approach to inference, hypothesis testing, and decision making.

Thus, we have three fields of expertise: the Probabilist with the mathematical model, the Statistician with the inferential model, and the scientist with the scientific model. The goal is to set up, as it were, diplomatic relations among these three fields. The task is not hopeless. Neither is it straightforward. Least of all is it a nonproblem, an unnecessary multiplication of entities. Once these principles are grasped, we may be assured, not that the task will be simple, but that it will at least be coherent. Ideally applied, this scheme will also act as an important source of diplomatic harmony. The scientist will not make belligerent accusations about the unrealistic character of the Probabilist's model. For the Probabilist is trying to be mathematically sound and illuminating, not experimental. The mathematician will not deplore the axiomatic messiness of Statistics, which is occasioned by the arduous role of matchmaker. And so for all possible combinations of experts. Shortcomings should be seen as residing not in the quality of the expertise but in the inappropriateness of the choice of a model. But if the sovereignty of the other expert is to be respected, so should one's own. A Statistician should not—and, if wise, in practice does not—tell the scientist how data should be analyzed, but rather will be content to offer or invent methods with known properties for use in cases where that method is appropriate (e.g., where certain assumptions are met). One needs little experience of any of the three fields to realize that useful and sound answers are rarely available ready-made for particular consultations; and indeed, one should be suspicious of those that are. What is gained from a good consultation is much more a matter of wisdom and a sense of the kinds of approach that might help than an outlet for providing do-it-yourself assembly kits.

These preliminary remarks are vitally important to what follows; but they may seem rather formidable. Let us take a simple example to illustrate something of the process.

EXAMPLE 9.1. A surgeon has performed a standard operation one hundred times, successfully in sixty-four, and wants to know what his success rate is. The question is Ethically important because part of the requirement for full consent is that the patient be given an honest statement about the risks involved—not the risk in the hands of the world's leading expert operating on the world's healthiest athlete, but *this* surgeon operating on *this* patient. Without more to do, the answer may be given, as a child of nine would compute it, as 64%, or 0.64. However, the real question may deal with something rather deeper. Every physician realizes that it is not always the healthiest patients who do best on treatment. The results show signs of factors that may be called "bad luck" or "randomness" or "rationalization." The results in the first fifty operations, especially for the male patients, were better than for the second fifty. The surgeon is, perhaps, interested in some less capricious assessment of all manner of factors. The Statistician, consulted, suggests grouping the data by sex, by age, perhaps by stage of the disease, and so on. Perhaps the failure rate will be affected by these factors. The Statistician may then suggest the use of the binomial model or the multinomial model. These two Probabilist's models predict that the number of successes in batches of one hundred data from a homogeneous process will vary in a particular fashion and enable the Statistician to make some kind of a statement about the accuracy of that figure 64%. The scientist (surgeon) will wonder whether the binomial model is a suitable one, in view of the stringent character of the assumptions involved for that model (e.g., that all outcomes are mutually independent, that the risk is the same for each subject); and it is the business of the Statistician to examine the robustness (i.e., how much the results would change if the assumptions were not quite true); and so on. The outcome may involve publishing the results; and perhaps all are agreed that a further study should be done with much more careful attention to the risk factors both major and minor. The whole process will be repeated, perhaps this time using a compound binomial model and multiple regression analysis; and so forth, with a new model and a more efficient study each time. By the end of the inquiry, no doubt the scientist's questions will have become much more penetrating. It will be clear that ideally, at each round there will be a playoff among the participating experts.

Let us take a more subtle problem.

EXAMPLE 9.2. In a modern military siege of a town many people may be killed by sniper fire. Where are the casualties concentrated? The question bears not only on risk but also on the Ethical issue of how surgical services should be deployed. Now, the chief surgeon may have formed the impression that the gunfire is so ill-directed that there is no undue concentration in casualties at all; the number injured in a region is simply determined by the concentration of population in it. Perhaps the best policy is to disperse population concentrations and surgical services. The Statistician will perhaps say that the problem corresponds at least roughly to the Probabilist's model known as the Poisson distribution (the homogeneous-risk model), the theory of which has been well worked out. There are well-defined methods of constructing what the distribution of cases should be from the data, and testing for goodness-of-fit of the model. But there are certain flaws in the demographic structure, and the Probabilist may be pressed into service to set up a more elaborate, heterogeneous-risk, model.

EXAMPLE 9.3. In fact, something closely analogous to this problem was the subject of a study by Lewitus and Neumann (1957). (See also Murphy 1979b, 1982, for calculations.) The issue was whether in a study (conducted over four and a half years) there was seasonal variation in the rate of attacks of coronary thrombosis in Israel. The question is rather like that posed in Example 9.2, except that here the scattering is occurring in time rather than in space. The Ethical issue now would be whether resources— which are granted to be limited—should be concentrated in some seasons at the expense of others. On about three out of four days there were no attacks at all; on about one out of two hundred days there were four attacks each. There was an excellent fit of the data to the predictions of the model and no persuasive evidence of seasonal clustering. But the Statistician has to be concerned that the field of observation does not accurately fit the assumptions underlying the Poisson model. Does that make any important difference in interpreting the results? If there is a seasonal clustering, how easily would the analysis have detected it? The Philosopher will wonder in this example, as in the two earlier ones, how (if at all) the Probabilities predicted under the Poisson model correspond to the Probabilities that the Statistician is estimating and using.

THE NATURE OF A PROBABILIST'S PROBABILITY

So far, we have just been using the words as tokens, as if they were heights or ages or atomic weights. We must now try to deal with them more coherently.

Following the usual tradition, we may represent the size of the chance of an event occurring as a point on a line extending from 0 to 1. The value 0 indicates that the event is impossible; 1, that it is certain. Intermediate points represent steadily mounting degrees of plausibility, from implausible to possible to likely to probable to almost certain. The scale 0–1 is arbitrary, that is, chosen after due thought because it has certain convenient properties. It is a Probabilist's scale, and its relationship to the real world is interesting.

Mathematicians treat Probability as a measure with no concern about what its counterparts (if any) may be in empirical reality. One feature they do preserve is the *notion of equal Probability*.

EXAMPLE 9.4. A common device of chance, the tossing of a coin, has proved so seminal that it has been recast as an abstract statement for mathematical use about a theoretically perfect coin that does not wear and change during use, tossed by a theoretically perfect hand that does not vary in its performance but is unfailingly Random. The coin is a *fair* one, meaning that when tossed it has the same chances of coming down heads and tails. We may not know what the chances are, but we may nevertheless choose to suppose—perhaps for reasons of symmetry—that they are equal. If we rule out other, frankly bizarre, outcomes (that the coin disintegrates in midair, or is lost, or lands and stays on its edge), then since the total Probability of all the outcomes must be 1—for it is certain that there must be some outcome—then the Probability of heads is ½. But it is not the concern of the Probabilist to attempt to verify that outcome. In the same way a fair die ("dice") has six faces all having equal Probabilities of being on top in any throw and, on the same argument, each with a Probability of ⅙. One may devise endless instances of such idealized representations of Probability such as blindfold shots at a target divided into arbitrary regions where area is the gauge of Probability (Murphy 1985).

There is nothing about the Probabilist's general meaning of *Probability* that demands that all events considered have equal Probabilities, or Probabilities that may be represented as multiples of some basic unit of Probability. What matters is that the relative Probabilities of two events can always be represented by the ratio of their two magnitudes.

EXAMPLE 9.5. For instance, on a circular target of radius two meters there is a square drawn of side one meter. Of shots uniformly scattered in all directions that hit the target, the Probability that the square is hit is $1/(4\pi)$, an irrational number.

For good reason some of the technically possible outcomes may be peremptorily discarded. When all the admissible events have been listed, the remaining Probabilities may be added and used to rescale the system in such a way that the total adds to unity (i.e., the Probability that one or the other of the allowed possibilities happened must amount to a certainty). This rescaling process is known as *normalization*. This step is used frequently in genetic counseling (Murphy and Chase 1975).

EXAMPLE 9.6. Suppose that a woman has a son with color-blindness, a virtually harmless X-linked trait. What is the Probability that her next son will inherit the trait as well? There are three possibilities about its origin. The mother may be homozygous (and so herself color-blind), in which case the recurrence risk is 1; or she may be a carrier, which would mean a recurrence risk of ½; or she may have no affected genes, in which case her affected son is a new mutant and the recurrence risk is the mutation rate and therefore minute. (For an X-linked trait, the father, who does not transmit an X chromosome to his son, has no impact on his son's phenotype.)

EXAMPLE 9.7. Suppose now the same pattern prevails, except that the trait is an X-linked lethal (e.g., Duchenne's muscular dystrophy). The first possibility must be excluded because the mother, if homozygous, would have the lethal phenotype and could not have had children. We are left with two choices: the son is a new mutant, or the mother is a carrier (also a rare event) and the son inherited the trait from her.

EXAMPLE 9.8. In Holmes's dictum to Watson (Doyle 1890), whenever all other explanations have been excluded, what remains, however unlikely, must be true. New mutation is a very rare event, perhaps 1 in 10^5 to 1 in 10^7. But if there is no other source of the gene—neither parent has it, and nonpaternity and nonmaternity have been excluded—then mutation must have happened. For instance, if in Example 9.6 there was a perfect test for the carrier state and the mother was found not to be a carrier, then by exclusion we conclude that the son is a new mutant.[3]

DEFINITION OF THE PROBABILIST'S PROBABILITY

Let us try to reformulate the idea in somewhat more refined terms. Historically there have been three main attempts to attach a formal meaning to the notion "the Probability of a (future) event."

DEFINITION 1.   The *Probability of an event* is the limit of the proportion of times that the event occurs when some well-defined operation is performed an indefinitely large number of times.

EXAMPLE 9.9. The Probability that a future child will be male would be the value that the proportion of all such outcomes among births assumes

---

3. Certain minute technical refinements have been ignored in this argument.

in a sample, as the size of the sample becomes infinite. (Extensive studies show that it is about 0.52.)

This definition, which works admirably in some cases, gives rise to more or less greater difficulties in practical cases. For example, from a practical standpoint we cannot study an infinite sample of births, and a strict constructionist would say that we cannot have a definition that depends on an operation that cannot be performed.

A more serious problem is that this formulation of Probability makes no provision for the unique case. That does not in principle create any scientific problem, because, in general, science deals with general properties that classes share in common (Murphy 1981c). But there are many Ethical problems that might not be so tidily dealt with. It seems doubtful that a clone of Mozarts, all busy producing the same kind of music, would have much interest to the musician, however many theories of intelligence it illuminated. Yet the uniquely excellent would certainly have considerable weight in Ethical arguments about (say) the allocation of scarce resources.

Again, there are difficulties of various kinds, Statistical, provenient, and ontological, about applying results in particular cases. One of the difficulties is the estimation of parameters (a Statistical problem) when it is possible that they are changing.

EXAMPLE 9.10. A problem arises (Murphy 1985) as to whether the spontaneous movements in rheumatic chorea are random or not, a question that may bear on pathogenesis. In the first place, it takes great skill and experience to distinguish these movements from true purposive movements; and there is no doubt that their frequency varies as the attack starts, reaches its peak, and gradually subsides over a period of weeks. If the process is truly Random (which demands, among other matters, that there be a distribution function to which the timing of the movements converges), its characteristic parameters must be changing. Moreover, the issue is behavior in a particular patient, and evidence from other patients is at best weakly corroborative.

There are many other difficulties that are of a highly technical nature.

COMMENT. This formulation of a Probabilist's probability is a good way of getting at its notional meaning, but it provides an unsatisfactory definition and a wholly impracticable criterion. The best light in which we can view its claims is that it is analogous to Russell's meaning of a sentence—"that which is common to a sentence in one language and its translation into another" (Copleston 1967: 224); it is a notion, not a criterion or a pragmatic method. This approach to the formulation of Probability has now been abandoned by many theorists.

DEFINITION 2.   *Probability* is an abstraction wholly characterized by a system of axioms. It has a certain mathematical structure (the measure-theoretic nature of which is technical) and has the following algebraic properties:

- A Probability must lie in the interval from 0 to 1 (i.e., it may be impossible or certain) or take any value in between.
- The Probability of the set must be 1. In plain words, there must always be some outcome for any Random event.
- If two outcomes of a Probabilistic experiment are mutually exclusive, the Probability that one or the other of these two outcomes will occur is the sum of the Probabilities of the individual outcomes.

From this system deductions may be made, much as the propositions of Euclid may be deduced from mathematical structures (the notions of a point, a line, a ruler, a pair of compasses, etc.) and particular assumptions about them. We do not now believe that the conclusions of the Euclidean system are precisely true in the real world, nor (as Descartes showed by recasting it in terms of algebra) is it necessary to be able to think in spatial terms to follow the reasoning of the system or to extend it.

In the same way, the axiomatic approach to Probability and its development do not depend on any capacity to translate the content of the system into terms that readily appeal to the imagination. To argue from axioms to conclusions is deduction, and is the process used in mathematics. To argue from data to axioms is inference, and is the basic process of Statistics (Murphy, Rosell, and Rosell 1982). Within this formulation, then, we may have deductions from the Probabilities of events, but not inferences about them. The latter task is delegated to the field of Statistics, which may be looked upon as a mathematical arm of empirical science. By fief, Probability is not concerned with data. Probability is prophesy; Statistics is history.

DEFINITION 3.   The *Probability of an event* is uniquely related to the odds that a rational, well-informed man would give (or accept) about the particular outcome. More precisely, if the odds such a man would give that there is no life on Mars are n to 1, then the probability that there is life on Mars would be $1 / (1 + n)$.

This formulation is an attempt to recapture the primordial nature of Probability that has been overzealously pruned by the austere detachment of the axiomatic approach. As such, the third definition has merit and is a welcome refreshment. However, the way in which the "well-informed" person arrives at an assessment is unspecified. Indeed, how a "rational, well-informed" person is to be identified is not addressed either. The definition is not intended to exclude women or even precocious children. Since, within this formulation, there would be many eligible candidates for the role, and each is to reach a Probability, the custom has grown up of referring to such an answer as *Subjective*. However, in fact, the "rational, well-informed man" is best regarded as an abstraction in the same kind of way that the law postulates the existence of the "reasonable man sitting on top of a bus";[4] that is, we do not suppose that any real person corresponds to him. By contrast, Probability in the axiomatic sense is called *Objective*.

This definition is not intended to convey any radical difference from the other two; and once it is given, the formal operation of the mathematics seems to be the same. The differences in the Statistical analogues are not nearly so readily disposed of.

This Subjective certainty would mean that the rational, well-informed man would wager anything he possesses against no gain at all that the certain outcome will occur; but it prescribes no general strategy for determining how he might conceivably reach such a state of mind.

THE NATURE OF THE STATISTICIAN'S PROBABILITY

Statisticians start—and, if true to their vocations, remain—in a world of inference and are permanently marked by that fact. It is like being a sculptor in stone who may engage in a little clandestine work in watercolors or woodcuts but is a sculptor in stone only while sculpting in stone. The task is very different from Probability theory, and the models correspondingly different.

In the first place, Statistics, insofar as it has any serious commitment to empirical evidence at all, always deals with data recorded to a finite number of decimal places. They are thus (in the technical mathematical meaning) rational data. Indeed, large tracts of the subject—denumerable variables, ranks, orders, and their multivariate counterparts—deal exclusively with integers. Example 9.5 gives an instance of a perfectly reasonable irrational Probability. But attempts to estimate it by any finite sample, however large, will always give answers that are limited to the rational numbers. The result is a domain of discourse that is not even to be called *patchy* (which connotes local continuity) but always *dotty*. What graininess a painting has may be, in principle, at a molecular level, although pointillism aims at something more massive. But the limit of the resolution of a painting on a television screen is inexorably set at a coarse level. The Statistician looks at the Probabilist's continuous theory on a television screen, the refinement of which depends on the size of the sample or the coarseness of the data. The

---

4. This reasonable man is presumably an Englishman on a double-decker bus. Lesser countries will furnish their own versions.

crudeness of the measurements may vitiate the actual resolving power of the medium; and it may be further aggravated by spurious precision (Murphy 1985, 1997). Indeed, there is a nice physiological analogue in vision, which is a map of a finite set of points corresponding to individual retinal cells from which the visual cortex constructs by confabulation a smooth continuous image, even in the neighborhood of the physiological blind spot.

A second distinction is that whereas Probability theory deals with stochastic (i.e., Random) predictions of behavior from parameters known exactly, Statistics is concerned with stochastic statements about the parameters from known values of the data. Here we must take some care about what we mean by the data being "known." The data are the realization of a process that is in itself Randomly variable, but they are perceived by methods that are subject to their own error (usually called *experimental error*) which may be further compromised by the resolving power of the system (Murphy 1997). Part of the Statistical analysis is to try to infer these various components of uncertainty, which may call for special experiments.

Third, even granted that the model proposed by the Probabilist is correct, Statistics may attempt to infer the values of the parameters *(estimation)* or to test the hypothesis about them by addressing various predictions from the model and using criteria the domain of which is Statistics, not necessarily Probability theory (e.g., sample means, variances, ranges, correlation coefficients, etc.). These numerous methods *(estimators)* enjoy special individual advantages, depending on what qualities the Statistician is looking for: simplicity, unbiasedness, efficiency, convergence qualities, robustness, and much more that we need not detail. It is scarcely surprising that on any finite set of data, different choices of estimators yield different answers, or *estimates*. Although it is easy to see how these qualities arise, nevertheless Philosophically they raise disturbing questions about the abstract theory of the ontology of Statistics. There seems to be no satisfactory general theory, although there are some well-known limits (notably lower bounds on estimates) on how even the best estimators available may operate.

Fourth, although an estimator may be based on a well-respected method and appeal to intuitively plausible reasoning, there may be no guarantee that the results so obtained will escape absurdity.

EXAMPLE 9.11. It is not uncommon, for instance, for the estimated value of a gene frequency to exceed 1, which (whatever its mathematical interest) clearly has no biological meaning at all. The same is true of occasional estimates of linkage in which the recombination ratio exceeds ½, which taken literally means that the behavior of genetic loci are more independent than independence itself.

EXAMPLE 9.12. A popular and well-tried estimator of the parameters (the method of moments) when applied to data on the ABO blood group frequencies (Bernstein 1930) yields for the several alleles estimates that do not necessarily add up to unity. Yet in other ways they have such good properties (notably simplicity and asymptotic efficiency) that it is worthwhile to use a patching-up device to correct this absurdity.

Fifth, we may note that the pentheric property (q.v.) has an important and indeed indispensable part to play for any Statistician taking responsibility for actual analysis of data. For instance, in Example 9.11 the estimator commonly gives more than one estimate, only one of which has meaning. The Statistician (with some regret but no misgivings) discards the absurd results.

COMMENT.   The reader may wonder what this discussion has to do with our main topic. Does the Statistician's model have any meaning, or does it have merely properties? Is it epistemic with no ontology at all? We await illumination on the point. Much of Statistical practice such as multiple regression analysis does not even pretend to have any ontological quality. It is not at all concerned with the inner reality of the data, but simply with how it can be summarized, described, and subjected to purely formal partitions. For instance, the usual meaning attached to *interaction* in Statistics (Murphy 1982) has no resemblance to any kind of scientific interaction and can often be made to disappear by arbitrary transformation of the data. (It is unthinkable that a chemical interaction could be changed by taking the logarithms of the concentrations of the chemicals.) Again, in a regression analysis involving three variables A, B, and C, decisions about whether A influences B will depend on the order in which the Statistician examines the data, a purely personal decision that it would seem has nothing to do with the ontology of the effects tested. But this lack of invariance that to a scientist is vitally important may seem to the Statisticians, thinking about their own inquiries in their own terms, interesting but rather unimportant (Murphy 1982). It is for precisely this reason that the scientists must preserve their own point of view in addressing the data. It is totally unreasonable to expect Statisticians to solve what are scientific problems which (if they are wise) they did not undertake to solve in the first place.

Finally, we may note the epistemic tension (Murphy 1979c) that characterizes much Statistical inquiry. Statistics has concern with two provenient properties. The one is *robustness*: the quality that minor departures from the assumptions underlying a Statistical model do not make much difference to the logic in the practical use of the model. Normal theory can be applied even to data that have a distribution far from being Gaussian ("normal"). The other quality is *power*: the quality that if the conjecture about the value of a parameter is not correct, the test has a high Probability of demonstrating that fact. Now, these two qualities are not dealing with exactly the same issues. But they are perilously close to being in open conflict. No analogous property applies in Probability theory.

THE NATURE OF THE SCIENTIST'S PROBABILITY

The scientist sees Probability under two guises that may or may not be the same.

The clearest is epistemic Probability. On the usual, largely implicit, assumptions that there exists a truth that it is the business of science to discover, and that there is yet no guarantee as to what its content may be, scientists must "live by their wits," "follow their noses," dig haphazardly in the hope of finding the meaning of clues, or of finding clues, or (at the lowest bid) of finding what might be clues, and then seeing where they may lead. One concern is to amass sound knowledge even if its implications are unclear; another is to identify what appear to be questions to answer; and all the time hoping that these two will from time to time meet and give some understanding.

· The whole formula for achievement is that there is no formula for achievement.

The best one can say is that there are some useful generalizations about how not to do science. Neither inexhaustible industry nor limitless imagination nor endless experimentation guarantees anything. The remarkable fact is not that the scientific endeavor cannot be described, but that it is even partially successful. In time, evidence accumulates, laden with ambiguities, irrelevancies, noise, low resolving power in methods; and the scientist (or, often, rival scientists) set up what are in fact models, though they are not very much like the epistemic triumphs of the Statisticians and still less like the ontological elegance of the Probabilists. There is enough global Probabilism involved in this pursuit to satisfy the most bloodthirsty. But at least there is some kind of progressive refinement in the inquiry that clarifies; and often, when the answers become clear enough, they show that the original questions were badly formulated, perhaps at odds because the theory on which they were based contained a radical flaw, perhaps even an inconsistency. But—to revive Aristotle's dilemma of the donkey that starved to death because it could not make up its mind which of two bales of hay to eat—the working scientist must decide in favor of one line of inquiry rather than another, and the guiding light will be to choose the path that seems the most Probable. But what exactly that statement means in terms of either the Probabilist's or the Statistician's meaning of the word *Probable* is obscure.

Part of this problem is the other facet of the scientist's Probability. It has been increasingly obtrusive in the last 150 years, although perhaps there are hints in classical physics as far back as Boyle's Law in the seventeenth century. It is the sense that certain of the inalienable structures of physical science exhibit Randomness in their behavior, which argues that the Randomness is not a defect in inquiry; in other words, it is not epistemic but ontological. At first, all Randomness was attributed to crudity of methods or (as in astrophysics) to the intervention of irrelevancies that were simply beyond the control of the observer. Then Clerk Maxwell in his studies of the kinetic theory of gases made bold to study the corporate behavior of enormous numbers of gas particles where there was no hope of observing any of them individually, with a kind of pious hope that the unknown multiplicity of factors concerned would (in some unspecified way) cancel each other out and make *Randomness* and *Probabilistic independence* reasonable assumptions. Obviously, this step was not taken in a heedless manner; the fact that multiple massive winds exist proves that the behaviors of air particles are not totally independent. Then Kelvin's Statistical mechanics flourished; and (an achievement neglected for forty years) Mendel not only discovered the Laws of segregation but (since the numbers involved were relatively small) felt compelled to cast them, and then illustrated them, in what were clearly Statistical terms. It is perhaps because of this last feature that they were neglected, for as fast as physics was abandoning naive Laplacian determinism, biologists—Philosophically, forever sixty or more years out of date—were trying to build a deterministic version of their own vastly more elaborate topic. Then Rutherford's work on the structure of the atom led to the discovery (now a cornerstone in nuclear Medicine) that the decay of a radioactive source follows a Poisson process, and (in the absence of a model as to how the latter could be simulated by deterministic means) that pragmatically declared it to be a Random process. The coping stone on the arch of the Random is the current view in theoretical physics that subatomic particles are in fact notionally inseparable from their distributions in space.

As we say, the biologist has been the most reluctant to accept this indeterminism and yet is unprepared to dismiss it. It is clear, in view of the unknown complexity of the biological model, that the epistemic and (perhaps) ontological components of uncertainty cannot be separated as clearly as could be wished. While some (abetted from the grave by Einstein) have dismissed all such Randomness as ignorance or faulty technique (Bohm 1957), others have been only too glad to have Randomness as an escape hatch when the modeling gets too difficult or too unmanageable. Parenthetically, we note a rather reprehensible practice among quantitative geneticists to try to account for all variation in the phenotype as due to some kind of a systematic and deterministic process, but doing so by methods (such as Fisher's F test) that expressly assume that there is a Random component (Murphy 1981b). Ultimate success for this endeavor would presumably show that the methods by which this result had been achieved were logically indefensible, a curious paradox. The Statistician stands by helpless.

CERTAINTY

In the midst of all this strife, is there any certainty? Unless the scientists are to end by pulling the carpet from under their own feet, we must suppose that there is certainty, even if it is only a certainty that ultimate matters are stochastic. Let us track down the phenomenon of certainty in the three different fields.

We start out by considering the two limits of the continuum of Probability. Indeed, a fundamental question in science (put rather technically) is, Does the scale of Probabilities include its own endpoints? The Probabilist's concept of Probability has an odd property that is often overlooked. The two endpoints or extremes of the Probability scale are the only points at which there is certainty: that the event is certain ($P = 1$), or that it is impossible and its negation is certain ($P = 0$). Curiously, these are the points at which the system is not stochastic. If the coin *always* comes up heads or *always* comes up tails, then clearly there is no Randomness in the behavior, and it is deterministic. In order to come up with a certainty, it is necessary to retreat one step up in the Chinese box: for instance, "This system is certainly Random" (although that claim might be hard to prove).

In fact, from the standpoint of modeling there are at least three ways in which certainty may be attained: tautology, decree, and exhaustion.

Certainty by Tautology

By *tautology* we mean a statement that is true either externally by definition or internally by the relations among the terms of the statement. If the right leg is longer than the left, then we can say with certainty that the left leg must be shorter than the right. If we define a tall person as anybody over six feet, then we know it is quite impossible for anybody under six feet to be classified as tall. If the tibia articulates with the femur, then it follows with certainty that the femur must articulate with the tibia. It is obvious that if these absolute statements are replaced by Probabilistic statements, and it is given that (for example) the lateral branch of the sciatic nerve usually emerges from the pelvis below the piriformis muscle, then a reciprocal statement of comparable assurance can be made that (for example) this same nerve usually does not emerge from the pelvis above the piriformis muscle. It is important to be alert to how misleading such tautologies may be, especially when they are obscured by intercurrent statements that distract from their presence.

EXAMPLE 9.13. We might document, but in the interests of diplomacy will not, studies that appear from time to time in the Medical literature designed to find what proportion of the population falls at or below the fifth percentile. Now, without any data at all, and with hardly anything that rises to the dignity of being called reasoning, we at once know the answer to that question. The fifth percentile is by definition that value on a scale of values such that 5% of values fall at or below it. So the answer is clearly 5%, or 1 in 20. Of course, that does not tell us what the actual value for the fifth percentile is in this population; but the question asked dealt not with that useful question but with a tautology.

A thinly disguised version of the same process lies in the cant for many campaigns to further some good cause. Any cause will do. Let us invent one.

EXAMPLE 9.14. The cause may start with the thought that it would be worthwhile if schoolchildren appreciated music more. A fine, if rather vague, aspiration. But appreciation of music, though no doubt in some sense quantitative, is hard to measure; and we then find it difficult to document the need that this cause is designed to remedy. So there is a campaign cry that Statistics shows that twelve million Americans are musically backward. Statistics do indeed show that, for "musically backward," which is undefined, surely means "below the fifth percentile," and twelve million is just about 5% of the American population. The number of musically backward Americans increases every year, and so long as the population is growing it will continue to do so, even if there are elaborate improvements in appreciation.

Let us take as a standard a tautology that is not intended to bamboozle.

EXAMPLE 9.15. The length of the tibia of a particular adult woman from the tip of the intercondylar eminence (A) to the tip of the medial malleolus (B) is 40 cm. Then the Probability is 1 that the distance from B to A is 40 cm. That is, it is certain; and it is certain because it is tautologous. (That is not at all to say that the *measurements* are certain to be equal, because measurements are technically fallible.) Likewise, a statement may be tautologously false. The proposition "The distance (B to A) = 30 cm" is certainly false.

Statements of that kind in science are of little interest except as corroborating statements in the face of error; or as a preliminary to purging a tautology.[5]

5. For instance, Einstein, noting that inertia and weight in physical systems always give the same information on mass, decided that this identity was a tautology and eliminated the idea of gravitation in the theory of general relativity.

Certainty by Decree

We may dispose of certainty by decree almost as easily as certainty by tautology. Scientists are always hearing from the parvenus statements to the effect that science has proved such and such an event to be impossible; that there are invariant scientific Laws that are never violated; and much more of the same. It is doubtful (Murphy 1981c) that science can give any useful meaning to the word *miracle* as it is used in the sensationalist press. But if it could, it could not be used to prove that such miracles do not occur. For if miracles do not occur, science (which is concerned with what has been observed and studied) has no part in the phenomenon any more than science can make any pronouncement about unicorns or wyverns, which belong to a different and fantastic universe. And according to the canons of science, if the phenomenon does occur, then obviously the negation is false. The final test of possibility in science is whether or not something has ever been competently reported to occur. Indeed, as every counterexample to a respected theory is uncovered, the proponents of decree close ranks and profess more fervently than ever their belief that the Laws of science are both known and inviolable.

• Nothing ever happens before the first time.

EXAMPLE 9.16. Currently there is yet another flareup of the age-old squabble about racial differences in intelligence (Herrnstein and Murray 1994). Those trenchant enough to disregard totally the dedicated endeavors of the psychometrists working in a field notoriously difficult to devise could drive a coach-and-four through the epistemology and ontology of intelligence tests, for intelligence is an extremely subtle and complicated phenomenon that quite possibly by its very nature will be forever beyond the grasp of human ingenuity.[6] There is nothing against which the intelligence tests can be validated except clinical judgment. But if that is to be the gold standard, it is difficult to see what point there is in replacing that gold standard with derivative formal tests. It seems that the test must be its own guarantee. There is a wilderness of almost intractable Statistical and epidemiological problems in defining the population of reference, the fidelity of the sampling, the choice of topics tested, the weightings that might be vigorously attacked and equally vigorously defended. All this work has to be completed and consensus attained before anything like a reputable and

---

6. This doubt is not primarily a matter of whether the mind may be in some way transcendental. Rather, it is a concern about how far the emergent properties of the mind may extend. There must be some doubt as to whether to understand the operation of the mind would require an intelligence that exceeds that of the mind. Even if the mind were totally rational, it might still be incapable of understanding itself. The problem will recur later.

scholarly approach to the racial components could even be addressed. To the scholar, there are three major flaws in the polemic—one can scarcely call it a debate.

First, intelligence tests are treated as totally privileged so as to be tacitly declared beyond question by both sides. If some sound white-box gauge of intelligence is ever available, then it will no doubt be brushed aside in the same fashion by the massive existential momentum of these tests.

Second, the issue of values has been introduced (and in a socially sensitive topic) at a stage at which the ontology has scarcely been addressed at all. We have pointed out elsewhere that a candidate may get what a Psychologist in designing the test declares the wrong answer either from being *less* intelligent than the examiner or from being *more* intelligent. As in all multiple-choice tests, in the individual case there is no redress against this judgment, since candidates are expressly forbidden to write any defense of their answers and are even apt to be penalized for doing so. This is a clear offense against phronesis and possibly the Flew principle.

Third, the current rejoinder to the claim of racial differences is to debate the claim not on its merits (if any) but on the provenience of the data, which must be faulty because the conclusion from them is condemned as politically unacceptable. Perhaps an amendment to the Constitution will put it all right by decree.

Certainty by Exhaustion

The principle of certainty by exhaustion is that if a class is finite, and some assertion has been explored in every possible case and found to be either uniformly true for all of them or uniformly false for all, then the statement is certainly proved or disproved. The most famous proof by exhaustion in recent years is that for the four-color theorem in topology (Appel and Haken 1977; Appel et al. 1977). The method was an exhaustive search by computer, and it demonstrated a conjecture made a century before to be true. There has been a firm opinion expressed that although logically sound, the demonstration does not merit the term *proof* because it does not stem from any insight into the nature of the topological relationship (Tymoczko 1979; Swart 1980). At best, the method of exhaustion is (appropriately) exhausting. In the scientific use of Probability, the result demands that all possible outcomes be codified; and in a species of even modest complexity the task is prohibitive. Hence Hume's demolition of inductive Logic (Hume 1739), and the rise of Bayes's stochastic inference (1763) (based on the studies of Pascal and Fermat) and its current virtual monopoly in the biological sciences.

CERTITUDE

So far, we have to some purpose grappled with problems of uncertainty. It is not so satisfying as classical Logic, but it has a much wider scope and is much more suited to scientific inquiry. There must be some misgiving, then, at introducing the somewhat less familiar *Certitude*.

As a reply to this misgiving, we start by explicitly denying three obvious charges: This next step is not anti-intellectual; it involves no abandonment of what has been gained by the austere standards of Probability and certainty. It is not superstitious, appealing to shapeless forms of the primitive. It is not a childish rebellion against irksome strictures.

A Definition of Certitude

To grasp what Certitude is, we need some perspective. Anybody with any scholarly discipline well knows the virtue, indeed the necessity, of both clarity and understanding, and pursues both enthusiastically. But the coin of tribute is often the sacrifice of ontology to the more showy features of shallow epistemology. It is both comfortable and easy to substitute precision for clarity and apodictic demonstration for understanding, and to try to pretend that nothing has been lost in either substitution. Judgment of paintings must be difficult if it is not to be capricious and if experts are to agree; but consensus about the sizes of their frames is easy to attain. It is vastly easier to understand the proof of a theorem than it is to explain what prompted a fruitful line of scholarly inquiry. Nothing succeeds like success. So it is not surprising that the successful, shallower, skills presume to rough-handle the deeper, more elusive ones.

There is a deeper wisdom that reserves the authority, not to overtrump the conclusions of some technical assessment, but to keep its merit in its proper standing. Some fine theory of artistic symmetry might insist that Mozart should have repeated the first bar of the *Figaro* overture, to which the discerning will say, "So much the worse for the theory of artistic symmetry." Of course, the deeper wisdom may itself be mistaken; indeed, it may be abused, and perhaps it often is. But to exercise it is not to be anti-intellectual or dishonest or regressive; it merely reminds us of the Greek myth of Antaeus, whose strength came from touching the earth; he was vanquished by Hercules, who kept him forcibly from contact with the earth. At the end of every triumph of abstraction one should hark back to the very ground of what prompted it, and test the depth of the achievement against it. The utility, diagnostic and prognostic, of intelligence tests is not on trial. But they are no safeguard of any claims that they are a wholly sufficient substitute for, indeed a replacement for, the native endowment that we call, all too glibly perhaps, *intelligence*. Here as elsewhere there is, and should be, misgiving as to whether the taproot of inquiry has been sold for the bright virtue of precision. The ultimate watchword of Statistical theory is the option, Would you rather be roughly accurate or precisely wrong? — a dilemma that bears thought.

This deeper scholarly reservation we have previously encountered in Chapter 3 in illation, in phronesis, and, at least sometimes legitimately, in the pentheric objection. We now meet it under a fourth *species* that we designate Certitude. We may define it rather informally:

DEFINITION.   *Certitude* is a state of assurance about a proposition that derives from sources other than explicit formal analysis.

Let it be noted:

1. No claim is made that Certitude in this sense lies beyond *all possible formal analysis,* for we can make nothing of statements in the natural order that the most learned scholarship can never analyze cogently.
2. Certitude is to be seen as a variable scale of assurance that, like empirical Probability, does not include the endpoints. In ordinary usage, we allow "reasonable certainty" (as indeed the law expects of a jury), although some might argue that certainty and Certitude, like uniqueness and perfection, know no degrees. Indeed, we note that Certitude uses the same scale as certainty; and like certainty it may be predicated of an ontological uncertainty such as a segregation ratio.
3. Unlike Probabilities and certainty, which may be handled quite adequately on a computer, Certitude is available exclusively to the reasoning mind. In particular, it must be clear that Subjective Probability (although its associated imagery suggests that it too is human and not formal) is quite different from Certitude.

For the time being, we are wise not to burn our boats on either side of the river: not to say either that Certitude has no place now in the paraphernalia of the scholar, or that it is guaranteed a permanent place in it.

EXAMPLE 9.17. A fair illustration of the need for this reserve is the crass identification of freedom with the physical construct of free energy. This naive equivalence led to the claim that human choice cannot be free because it would violate the principle of the conservation of energy. It seems strange now that this theory could have been so uncompromisingly upheld at a time at which there was an unparalleled concern with political freedom, a concern shared by so many intelligent people who nevertheless denied the existence of personal freedom. But even before the megaliths of Victorian physics had crumbled before the onslaught of Statistical mechanics, Gödel's (1931) incompleteness theorem, and, recently, Chaos, the sage mind obstinately held that indeed human free choice is possible, even if not often used. We may note that if the naive denial that freedom exists were true, there could be little interest, indeed little meaning, in our exploring Ethics, and none in deontology.

Empirical Certitude

Wide experience of a particular class may lead to confident statements about consequences. For instance, people do not usually die of the common cold. Now, assessment of Certitude by this approach is not really equivalent to measurement. For useful statements of this kind to be made, in general three conditions must be fulfilled.[7]

First, ontology. There must exist Things on which experience may be based. Ideally the inference should be based on a class of Things that are all exactly the same. It is doubtful that such an ideal reference population ever exists, even in inbred laboratory mice. Constructing a practical working population that conforms at least approximately to the ideal of a completely homogeneous class will, in general, involve judgments that provide a loophole through which the subjective and the nonrational may temper the processes of inference.

Second, provenience. The negotiable empirical evidence must be based on representative samples from a well-defined population. Of course, if it is possible to obtain information about the entire population, so much the better; but often, because of either the load of work or the difficulties of maintaining uniform standards, it may be prohibitive. But the sampling process at least must be representative in a fashion that itself is clearly defined.

EXAMPLE 9.18. It may be desirable to find out about the state of a patient's blood as a whole. However, arterial blood differs from venous in its oxygen content, its speed of flow, and its hemostatic qualities. Blood is, of course, ordinarily obtained from veins and so is perhaps not representative of the whole. For special purposes blood may have to be sampled from an artery or the portal circulation. Nevertheless, one cannot take all the blood out to ensure a representative sample.

Third, experience. There must be sufficient data if inferences are to be made with reasonable confidence. How to assess the uncertainty of such inferences is discussed in Statistical textbooks. If the data are Probabi-

---

7. An important distinction must be made between the *accuracy* of an estimate and the *resolving power* of a measurement, even though these two notions both imply some uncertainty, at least at a Subjective level (Murphy 1997).

listic, so are the inferences. Certainty is rarely possible and comes only from infinite or exhaustive samples. The classical Logician may not dismiss such inferences as induction under a new name, for in inductive Logic, no statement about the sample space or the sampling structure is proposed. Personal judgments based on a large, haphazard, experience of individual cases may be confidently made, but useful scientific statements can rarely be made about it. Undertakers no doubt have a much more pessimistic view of surgery than proprietors of convalescent spas. Both are confident; but the biases are clear, and the only confident statement warranted from their pooled experiences is that the operations are neither all successes nor all failures. The biases cannot be corrected by compiling more experiences of the same kind. Neither sampling nor classical induction dispels all uncertainty. However, the uncertainty left by finite sampling may be expressed by a sample standard error or by confidence or fiducial limits. The uncertainty left by induction admits of no such gauge.

Scientists recognize the tentative nature of their generalizations from experience; those using such generalizations for Ethical theory should do likewise. Uniqueness of the individual (a matter of cardinality) wars against the homogeneous class. There are well-developed Statistical techniques for dealing with factors pertinent to risk (a matter of dimensionality). Nevertheless, even these inferences involve some kind of appeal to the existence of some rather elusive assumptions that in nature orderliness exists: that risk bears a relationship to the prognostic variable that is for the most part continuous and smooth. However, that assumption cannot be proved from any finite amount of data.

Personal Certitude

Rightly or not, many clinicians believe that over and above prognostic factors that can be clearly articulated and measured, there are certain intangible qualities on the basis of which they may shade their prognosis. Confronted with a concrete problem involving an Act of some importance and immediacy, a physician might have a degree of assurance that would warrant giving infinite odds on a particular outcome, a state of mind that might not be shared by others. The grounds for attaining it may not be entirely scientific, and more will be said of this matter later. Although this Certitude resembles Subjective certainty in that both are defined in terms of odds, rather than in terms of inference from axioms and experience, there are three important distinctions.

First, the "rational, well-informed man," in terms of whom Subjective Probability is defined, is a fiction and his deliberations a *façon de parler*; from the same facts a correct computer program would give the same result. An actual deliberation is colored by explicit or implicit personal judgments (which may well modify even what data the particular clinician sees fit to collect). "Rational, well-informed" genetic counselors, for example, confronted with the same complex pedigree of hemophilia will make the same Subjective Probability statement *(S)* that a particular woman is a carrier. This is equivalent to saying, "Given the data, *S* is the correct answer to the problem." But such genetic counselors are abstractions. The actual counselor may be suspicious about some of the facts as received (e.g., about true paternity); or make errors of fact, supposing, for instance, that the patient has hemophilia (an X-linked disorder) whereas it is von Willebrand's disease (an autosomal dominant); or make errors of assumption (as in not realizing that A's assay of Factor VIII differs systematically from B's); or make a mathematical or Logical error in a complex pedigree. Nevertheless, the counselor may advise with virtually complete personal Certitude. All such suspicions and errors depend on the individual's knowledge and alertness and preconscious and unconscious functioning.

The abstraction of the "rational, well-informed man" does not take into account the physical condition of the actual observer and of the observer's instruments or equipment. Einstein's abstraction about two observers moving at different relative velocities, observing some common event and noting differences, makes no allowance for the possibility that one of them may develop a parietal lobe thrombosis and the other forget to wind his watch.

The second distinction is that the Subjective Probability statement imposes a careful constraint that Certitude does not, in that the odds are introduced symmetrically. They are the odds that the "rational, well-informed man" would give *or take* about the outcome. The argument would not tolerate an answer tainted with the aim of "being on the safe side," for such a person committed to taking bets either way would, in the long run, steadily lose money. But the person undergoing the operation, or the surgeon undertaking it in the individual case, has not that option.

Finally, Subjective Probability is a statement of grounds for intellectual conviction only; but while it may be followed by an Act, the latter is a separate matter. A computer can calculate Subjective Probabilities but is not plagued by insomnia or liable to lawsuits for malpractice. Certitude, however, implies not merely conviction, but conviction by a human mind with a commitment to act even if the Act is to do nothing. The genetic counselor having assessed the risk and communicated it to the consultands may leave what is a voluntary decision about future progeny to them. The consultation may include making a clear distinction between computing the Probabilities for the outcomes and assessing the fardels (i.e., the total burden over the lifetime) for each outcome, in accordance with standard theory (Murphy and Chase 1975). This is akin to Subjective certainty. Nevertheless, if personally confronted by the same decision, the counselor would be forced to decide whether or not to have further children, and the careful distinction between Probabilities and fardels might be difficult to preserve. Mathematics or a computer would never be in this situation.

The relevance of personal Certitude stands in sharp focus in the individual case, which is the common fare of Medical practice but unfamiliar (for example) in public health policy or in warranties on mass-produced goods. Arguably, Probabilities in the individual Ethical decision are like any other Probabilities, except that the sample is of size one. But this Oracle of Delphi policy is not amenable to critical scrutiny in so small a sample as one.

EXAMPLE 9.19. Suppose, for instance, that the failure rate from an operation is 25%. If the surgeon always promises a successful outcome, a follow-up will expose this unwarranted optimism. Likewise, a prediction that the patient has a 40% probability of dying will in time prove to be unduly pessimistic. But suppose that the surgeon gives a poor prognosis *at random,* with chances so chosen that the expected mortality rate is 25%. For instance, for each patient a card is picked at random from a thoroughly shuffled ordinary deck. If the card is a spade, the prognosis is that the patient will die, and conversely. The individual prognosis is sheer guesswork and therefore incompetent. But the predicted failure rate (25%) will be the same as if the prediction had been honestly done with ideal competence. This is a device that (like the devious Oracle of Delphi, conserving, at the expense of carefully worded ambiguities, her reputation for prophesy) is solely concerned with the surgeon's reputation and not with the patient's needs; and clearly it cannot be disproved in the individual case.

To argue uncompromisingly that each case is unique and that nothing is to be learned from experience about prognosis is merely a variant on the same theme. No doubt this could be argued both ways. The first surgeon to do a cardiac transplant, for instance, obviously had no past experience on which to base a prognosis. Nevertheless, the prudent course in most cases is to appeal to experience.

Yet at times subjective conviction may be in conflict with an objective, or at least a more nearly objective, opinion from experience. Copernicus was correct, and his fellow scientists (usually let off lightly in the Galileo affair) were wrong. Semmelweiss and Lister were correct and the surgical establishment wrong over antiseptic surgery. Harvey was correct and Galen wrong. Often such disputes may be resolved with a little goodwill and little harm to anybody. Semmelweiss merely asked obstetricians to wash their hands in a simple antiseptic solution upon leaving the dissecting room before returning to their patients.

But the conflict may be very serious indeed.

EXAMPLE 9.20. Lewis, the most respected and the most articulate of cardiac physiologists of his era, had emphatically condemned corrective operations on diseased heart valves: "Surgical attempts to relieve cases of mitral stenosis presenting failure by cutting the valve have so far failed to

give benefit. I think they will continue to fail, not only because the interference is too drastic, but because the attempt is based upon what, usually
at all events, is an erroneous idea, namely, that the valve is the chief source
of trouble" (T. Lewis 1946). How far Lewis spoke for fellow cardiologists
would be hard to say. As Brock points out (1948), the voice of surgical authority had in even more uncompromising terms condemned as unethical
all operations on the heart itself. In the face of these august opinions, Brock
in 1947 undertook to operate on patients with congenital pulmonary stenosis. Several previous surgeons had attempted it and met with uniform
failure. Thus, it might have been argued before the operation that not only
were there grave doubts that it would succeed but also, even if the operation did succeed, there were grave doubts about its benefit. In Brock's first
three attempts, two patients died, and one proved inoperable because there
was atresia of the aorta as well. How strong did Brock's conviction have
to be regarding the correctness of his empirically unsupported insight into
the pathophysiology of valvular stenosis? The Ethical decision hung in the
balance. Of course, as is now well known, he did persist, succeeded, and
started a whole new era of intracardiac surgery.

This problem is not an easy one to answer, and we shall have to explore it in considerable depth later.

A SYSTEMATIC FORMULATION OF INDETERMINACY

We now attempt a systematic formulation of indeterminacy from the
standpoint of a methodology of Medical Ethics.

Indeterminacy Due to Uncertainty

A binary process with a Probability other than the endpoints 0 or 1
implies uncertainty, which may be Objective (i.e., ontological, intrinsic to
the events themselves) or Subjective (i.e., epistemic). Perhaps (as is believed
in quantum mechanics) Objective indeterminacy in Medicine exists and is
not to be perfectly resolved by any amount of knowledge. Perhaps the contrary is so. It is not known which is true, and we can offer no satisfactory
discussion of the issue here. But assuredly, in the biological aspects of our
problem it is convenient and practical to suppose that both forms of indeterminacy exist, Objective and Subjective.

It is arguable whether from exact knowledge about the patient's physical and mental state we could predict with certainty the outcome of an
operation performed under ideal circumstances. Our knowledge is indeed
imperfect, which is the first component of the uncertainty. Also, however
precise the prognosis for the ideal, in the actual operation chance factors
in the ambiance and the surgery add a further element.

These two levels of uncertainty, ignorance (Subjective) and stochastic realization (Objective, which is irreducible), give four combinations:

1. There may be complete Objective and Subjective certainty. Most such cases are trivial ("The operation will be of finite length") or tautologous ("The operation if successful will be followed by a period of convalescence").
2. An outcome may be Objectively certain yet unknown (a matter of pure Subjective uncertainty). Thus, the sex of the fetus is fixed from conception, but the information is not ordinarily accessible until the second trimester.
3. There may be an Objective component of uncertainty without an additional component of Subjective uncertainty. Thus, some patients survive gastrectomy for cancer for five years or more. The outcome will be known with certainty in five years; but until then it remains Objectively uncertain.
4. Finally, there may be Objective and Subjective components of uncertainty. There is uncertainty about the five-year survival in a patient with mucolipidosis type IV, but the total world experience comprises no more than a handful of cases. Here the uncertainty exists both in the event in the individual patient and (a large component) in the estimate of the distribution of the length of survival as a statement about the general behavior of the class of patients.

In general, we must be prepared to accept uncertainty and, in acting, take calculated risks. But these risks must be *calculated,* wherever possible, by sound theory and sufficient empirical data of adequate quality.

Indeterminacy as Affected by Incertitude

Incertitude is an additional source of indeterminacy. In principle, it may be absent, or it may increase indeterminacy, or it may decrease it. It is clear that incertitude could increase the indeterminacy beyond that contributed by Objective and Subjective uncertainty; it is not so clear how indeterminacy could be *diminished* by taking incertitude into account. Theoretically, Objective and Subjective uncertainty may offset one another. If, for instance, there is a negative covariance between them, the combined variance may be smaller than their sum. But that is a mathematical statement; and as we pointed out earlier, theory that confronts the demands of ontology may find this supposition uncomfortably constrained, perhaps untenable. We can think of no plausible instance in which the range of ontological incertitude can be reduced systematically by further sources of uncertainty; indeed, we find it difficult to imagine how such a result could occur. On the other hand, because incertitude professes to have no explicit *rationale* (and while common sense might suggest reasonable constraints), we can make no compelling argument as to whether or not this nonrational source may offset indeterminacy from other sources.

If incertitude is taken into account together with the four combinations of Objective and Subjective uncertainty discussed above, there would be twelve possible combinations of indeterminacy. Needless to say, in many instances it has not proved possible to devise suitable illustrations. There seems to be no particular advantage in examining each entry in detail.

Reflection suggests that the contribution, if any, from incertitude may arise in various ways. Some of them are nonrational components that may reflect mood or transcendental beliefs (in the power of prayer, for one) that we cannot usefully discuss by scientific canons. Some of them may have scientific substance that nonetheless cannot be analyzed into articulate terms, although if they could be so analyzed they might be seen to have strange but quite reasonable properties.

EXAMPLE 9.21. Homeostatic, or analogous psychic, effects may damp the indeterminacy. One of the factors that contributes to the efficacy of a treatment is how well the patient adheres to the regimen: faithfully taking medication, avoiding provocations (such as alcohol in pregnancy, or smoking, or events that aggravate stress). Now, we do not suppose that a prescribed regimen is perfect or could not be improved by ever closer attention to detail. A patient's participation may be heightened to the point of promptly and constructively anticipating the Random perturbations, technical errors, and oversights that may somewhat vitiate the regimen. The effect would be not only to increase the benefits of the management but to reduce the indeterminacy in its effect. One such instance would be an awareness of the importance of prompt response to signs of placenta previa, of which the occasional unusually well informed patient would be aware. Many such illustrations could be drawn from an alert practice of preventive Medicine. Of course, in the illustration we have identified a personal factor that might, and perhaps should, be (as it were) institutionalized, made part of the regimen. And indeed, whenever we devise an overt mechanism that may be cast in rational terms, it will (and should) tend to have the same fate. But many such components may not be overt at all, cannot be institutionalized, and make up part of the inchoate mass of personal Certitude. It seems clear that such mechanisms must have Ethical implications, but it is not easy to see how they might be used to advantage.

Let us take a less rarified, nonclinical instance.

EXAMPLE 9.22. Suppose a man visits a country fair and pays the admission charge with a bill from his wallet. There is a tree-lined avenue between the entrance and the main pavilion; and after walking some distance along it, he notices that his wallet is missing. In his report to the security staff he says he thinks that the endpoint was at about tree number 7 but is not certain. He is sure, however, that it was neither further than tree number 8 (at which point he first thought to take note of the landmarks) nor nearer to the gate than tree number 5. This adds Subjective uncertainty to the point of loss. But he later has second thoughts that it was somewhere between tree number 3 and tree number 6, although he can identify no compelling reason for giving such assurance. There may be unconscious psychological reasons why he expresses himself with such Certitude, but as such they are inaccessible (for the time being, at least). Thus, there are at work Objective uncertainty (where in the interval between the starting point and the endpoint the loss occurred); Subjective uncertainty (where the endpoint is); and Certitude (which has no provenience). The latter leads to the police beginning a search between trees number 5 and 6, then going back to 3 and finally up to 8.

The Practical Assessment of Indeterminacy

In an Act there are calculated risks to be taken, preferably based on sound theory and empirical data of adequate quality. Where the latter cannot be marshaled, the ethicist will have to settle for arguments of lesser quality: perhaps by analogy with other better-studied conditions or other operations; or from experimental studies in animals; or optimal (but still perhaps inadequate) estimates from finite accumulated data. When all else fails, the ethicist is driven back to guesswork, feelings, or hunches, which may end up pointing in the right direction, despite misguided prejudice or even by lucky chance. But whatever the evidence, it seems to us that there are at least two principles involved:

1. Prediction is to be based on the efficient analysis of the totality of evidence available.
2. The uncertainty is to be cast as the appropriate unbiased estimate with, so far as possible, an estimated range of uncertainty. All should be in the open interval $(0–1)$ (i.e., not including the endpoints), for it is never wise in such estimates to exclude all possibility of failure or of success.

Granted, often neither quantity is accurate; but the very attempt to formulate these quantities will to some extent bring the Agent face to face with the nature of the decision to be made. The mature scientific mind, confronted with uncertainty, does not hold to the principle of "the equal distribution of ignorance." Even in the extreme case where there is no information at all about whether a treatment would or would not harm a patient, there is no warrant for saying that the risk is 50–50, for "50–50" (meaning, we must presume, a 50% chance of failure and 50% chance of success) is a statement for which, it has already been admitted, there is no basis whatsoever. But in fact it is unthinkable that any responsible clinician would undertake a procedure about which nothing whatsoever is known. Even the most radical always plead some kind of a case for trying it; and then although the estimated risks and benefits from the outcome may be very imprecise, it is implausible that the point estimate is 50%.

COMMENT. It must be understood that the intent of the previous paragraph is neither Moral nor deontological. It is not a prescription for how the clinician or the ethicist should behave in making decisions. Rather, the goal is to identify what good scientific practice accepts as sound methods of making inferences in the face of uncertainty.

On the other hand, a retreat into the heuristics in vogue before Pascal and Fermat is deplorable. There is still too commonly a practice of talking about moral certainty. Those in a position to make decisions are commonly advised to evaluate the facts, to resolve the uncertainties of the problem as best they can, and then to act only in "moral certainty." As usual, we shall not attempt to decide on whether or not the proposed Ethics is sound. Our ontological concern is twofold.

First, what exactly is meant by *moral certainty*? Does it mean that the Probability of success is 0.5? 0.9? 0.99? 0.999? Or if it is a matter not of assurance about the outcome but of the accuracy of the estimate of the outcome, then some kind of a confidence statement would help. If the issue is how much effort has gone into the analysis, no doubt suitable measures could be devised. If it means anything more than that, it probably is beyond the point at which science has any contribution to make. As Medical scientists, we are not even sure that what is meant by *moral certainty* can be expressed in the conceptual terms we have formulated.

The second concern is why an explicit statement of risk—always supposing that it is known—should be forsaken for something that is gratuitously vague. If a Moral judgment is made under the auspices of some discipline totally removed from the reputable practice and science of Medicine, then we withdraw from the discussion on grounds of incompetence. To people brought up to think like scientists, failing to reduce Ethical decisions to such terms seems regressive. We do not intend this complaint as a variant of the earlier criticism of billiard-ball Ethics. To go from a concern with precise risks to crass categorical assessments seems to involve, not tolerating, but advocating vagueness.

It is a fair generalization that in Medicine any Act (starting with small sips of cool sterile water by mouth) that can do nontrivial good may conceivably do nontrivial harm. Furthermore, many activities have uncertain outcomes. If some Medical Acts are (in some undefined sense) good and others bad, then probably most will be intermediate. The notion of representing this infinitely fine gradation as a two-valued function surely seems to conform to nothing in the experience of scientists, most of whose effort is devoted to measuring things on a continuous scale rather than arbitrarily putting them into categories.

Expected and Actual Values

Whatever system is used, results will vary and preclude easy judgments. There is an analogy here that we would like to keep in mind. Healing the devastation left by Hume's (1739) demolition of inductive proof was set in motion by Bayes (1763) and his stochastic proof. Since the outcome from an Ethical decision is not uniform, what can we substitute for the naive putting of Acts into the binary good-bad patterns, when the best we have to go on is a guess based on possible but not certain effects? The fact that we may not be able to arrive at certainties does not mean that we cannot, in the face of uncertainty, devise any counterpart of the simple, certain event. Stochastic outcomes for Acts offer a multiplicity of candidates.

EXAMPLE 9.23. One possibility is to use the average (i.e., the mean or expected) damage. By this gauge, subjecting two people to a 50% chance of death may result in neither one, only one, or both dying, the average being one death. It could be argued that this average outcome is equal to, and Ethically strictly equivalent to, one certain death. That concrete proposal will, and should, be disputed. To subject a very large number of people, say, ten thousand, to a risk of 10% of dying causes on average one thousand deaths; and here equating it with exposing one thousand to 100% risk is much easier to defend. In view of the much larger sample size, it is virtually certain that there will be more than, say, six hundred deaths. Insofar as a person is to be responsible for a particular Act, it does not seem to change the moral weight of the Act whether or not, so far as the chance aspects of the Act are concerned, the result turns out to be favorable. On the other hand, an overstrict interpretation of responsibility does not really seem to make much sense. Submitting a man to a 1 in 10 chance of dying and submitting one hundred men to a 1 in 1,000 chance of dying is a quantitative difference only. It may be the case that a quantitative change on a continuous scale does produce some qualitative difference in the significance of the Act, but we do not see how this can be demonstrated; and thus, our attitude toward this proposal must be one of agnosticism.

The average is, of course, only one proposed solution. We shall have something more to say about such assessments toward the end of Chapter 10. In the last half-century, Statistical decision theory has proposed several criteria for the making of decisions where there is uncertainty. They take into consideration loss, gain, and the Probabilities associated with them. One strategy is to attempt to maximize the average gain; another, to minimize the average loss; a third, to minimize the maximum loss or maximize the minimum gain. Almost any therapeutic or diagnostic procedure carries risk—sometimes a serious risk—and as well there will be some demands, in time, in discomfort, and, of course, in financial cost. None of these factors, although often trivial, can be dismissed as Ethically altogether neutral. However, benefit accrues from a well-thought-out procedure: the cure or prevention of seriously incapacitating conditions; or the allaying of anxiety; or the ultimate, less personal, advantages to others, such as the promotion of public health or the advancement of Medical science. At times the loss may be certain. A venipuncture is going to involve (at least) blood loss for the patient. A fifteen-dollar test costs money. But often there may be some uncertainty about either the benefit or the disadvantage. In everyday life, in our balancing of possible loss and gain (e.g., in crossing the street), we accept risk as at least implicitly negotiable.

The ideas we have been discussing are of concern to some thinkers. They seem to imply that a rate of exchange can be struck between money, on the one hand, and the delivery of care to the sick and the preservation of human life, on the other. To many people this detailed, even cold-blooded approach is repugnant. But it seems to us that it is a false judgment of decisions in practical cases to say that it is repugnant to formulate this policy explicitly but to accept the implication when it is merely shrouded in vagueness.

EXAMPLE 9.24. Consider a group of patients with massive cerebral hemorrhages. If the policy is to spare no expense or trouble or care in keeping these people alive, no doubt the results could be better than they now are. Yet even those with the tenderest consciences would accept that there are reasonable limits to keeping those particular people alive as long as possible. Surely nobody would feel, for example, that the entire nursing and doctoring resources of the hospital should be diverted to looking after such people to the detriment of other patients. And evidently implicit in this judgment is the notion that the expected gain is very small. Such people have a poor chance of surviving with even the best possible care, and even if they did, it is likely that they would be so severely incapacitated that neither they nor society would derive much evident benefit from prolonging life. Now, there are those who believe it more compassionate to retreat from a hard analysis into vague impressions. All may tolerate the notion of an inarticulate judgment because often no more precise way exists in which to handle the matter. We do not insist that every conscientious judgment should be relentlessly overridden by a quantitatively precise analysis; both must be allowed a say. But we have little sympathy for the practice of replacing a Probability already calculated at 0.92 with the statement that the "patient will be all right," any more than we tolerate the statement that a patient's blood pressure is high, which might mean any-thing from 145/95 (a minor matter, especially in the elderly) to 390/260 (which is a dire Medical emergency at any age). Without trespassing on Moral Philosophy, we see little to be said for gratuitous vagueness, a kind of metaphorical coin-tossing in the mind.

EXAMPLE 9.25. There can be no doubt that the number of road acci-dents could be reduced, for instance, by constructing barriers so that pedes-trians could have no access to streets. But there would be a price to pay, notably in constructing the barriers and the means by which pedestrians could cross a street without meeting the traffic at all. And the necessary de-mands on taxation would certainly excite protest. This would demonstrate, if demonstration were necessary, that some voters, at least, imply that there is a de facto equivalence between money and life, however squeamish they may feel about saying so. If human life were indeed believed to be price-less, any such economy would be unthinkable.

But if a cost-and-benefit formulation is to underlie policy, then the Probabilistic approach in the many individual cases is equivalent to the as-sessment of averages over many people. If we adopt this criterion, it follows from the Statistical principle of sufficiency that the assessment will be the same regardless of how the total cost or the total benefit is arrived at. To expose one person to a risk of 100% would be equivalent to exposing two people to a risk of 50% or four people to a risk of 25%. A series of gratu-itous small risks spread over a large number of people on this scale would involve just as much expected damage as one risk of large size inflicted on one person. This conclusion is inescapable from the terms on which our decision principle is based. There are those who may protest that this is unreasonable—which can only mean that they would deny the principles from which our inferences have been drawn.

At the least it may be said that this approach using expected damage and injury is formulated clearly enough that it can be disputed. To say that persons must follow their individual consciences may be a very lofty senti-ment, but it does not help in the slightest in deciding how to act in concrete situations. It must be recalled again that the uncertainty underlying a diag-nosis or prognosis may be either Objective or Subjective. Matters of this kind commonly occur in genetic counseling.

EXAMPLE 9.26. Because her father is affected, a woman is known to be a carrier for an X-linked disorder. The Probability that her next child will be affected is, then, 1 in 4. This uncertainty is merely a matter of what appears to be Objective indeterminacy about the outcome of the next preg-nancy (which has not started yet). But there may be uncertainty as to what this risk actually is. Suppose that the woman's daughter is the consultand.

This daughter is at a risk of 50% of being a carrier. If she is a carrier, the risk for her first son is 1 in 4; if she is not, the only risk of her son being affected is the minute risk of new mutation. So the black-box risk should be computed as follows: there is a 50% risk of a risk of 1 in 2, and a 50% risk of a risk of virtually zero, in all, 1 in 4. This answer will be modified in the light of subsequent data (Murphy and Chase 1975). Although from a strict mathematical or Philosophical standpoint there is a confusion of two Logical principles here, this seems to create no particular difficulty from an Ethical standpoint.

An interesting question arises as to how far the expectations can be identified with existence itself. Would it be possible to argue that, insofar as human life is to be used as a value for the basis of such a system of Ethics as we have been discussing, the value lies in the expectation of life—that is, not only the quality of the life but its expected duration? This large topic is deferred to Chapter 11.

10 On Making Decisions

The fundamental concern of Minor Ethics is the making of decisions: wherever no decisions can be made or where the decisions lack impact, no pragmatic Ethical problem can exist. To make a decision one must be presented with a concrete problem and particular abstract principles to the point. Nevertheless, it seems possible and profitable to explore in their own right the principles whereby an Ethical decision is made; and it is with this subject that the present chapter is concerned. It will be necessary to define and expound certain basic ideas; we shall not be put off from doing so explicitly because of any concern over their obviousness or the rhetorical perils of laboring the trivial, for it is often in the ideas that seem to be beneath our dignity that the seeds of confusion and disagreement germinate.

THE ONTOLOGY OF DECISION

The words *decide* and *decision* come from the Latin word *caedere* (to cut), from which come a great crop of words: *incise* and *incision, precise* and *precision, Caesar* (the man born by incision),[1] *concise* (trimmed of details). The literal meaning is so powerfully taken over by a metaphorical sense that the two may lie side by side with no incongruity except a clash to the ear; so we might wonder whether decisions about decisions are decisive, or incisions are precise. The image that most readily comes to mind is that of a sharp butcher's knife and the edge as the knife goes through the meat, clean-cut, not ragged. The romantic image conjured up of the great leader—who does not procrastinate, does not do things by halves, is never at a loss, never in torment with his conscience, can make bold actions to gain big ends—has led to adulation of the decisive. The great leaders are not those who are right but those who are sure. And this idea of fierce neatness has been taken over unchanged into Ethics. It lies at the very heart of billiard-ball Ethics, its imagery, its methods, its uncluttered lines, and its indecomposable Acts.

1. Thus, the common term in obstetrics *Caesarian section* is redundant.

Now, there is no doubt that there are real examples to sustain this sense of *decision*.

EXAMPLE 10.1. The practice of surgery before anesthesia: "If it were done when 'tis done, then 'twere well / It were done quickly" (Shakespeare, *Macbeth*, I.7.1–2; Harbage 1969). For a competent surgeon, it should take no more than minutes, even seconds, to amputate a leg on a conscious patient; and that left little time for arguments about niceties, still less for endless decomposition into steps.

To treat all, or even most, modern Ethical decisions in this fashion is at best ludicrous and at worst tragic. Indeed, it is so incongruous that we wonder whether we should retreat from this severe, sharp-edged, Latinate idea of *decision* to the much more temperate and appropriate Anglo-Saxon equivalents: "making up one's mind," "weighing the matter," "thinking the thing out," above all being ready "to hold to a steady course," "to wait and see," much the better part of the wise and the tried. If we are to stick to the Latin, at least we must sound a warning about the persistent misunderstanding of how all this bears on Ethics. In fact, leaving aside a considerable class of cases that for one reason or another are straightforward, decision is in general a complicated process, a negotiated path, a course navigated, not an instantaneous choice made once for all, "at one fell swoop" (Shakespeare, *Macbeth*, IV.3.218; Harbage 1969). We shall take some pains to discuss the components in detail. Of course, our decomposition is artificial and made for purposes of exposition only: in practice, all will be interlocking and operating simultaneously. Unfortunately, it is not possible to express everything at the same time; and we ask the reader's patience if the speculative parts at times seem exasperatingly labored and far from the concrete whole.

In the first place, a decision encompasses three main components:

1. *Facts:* Assembly of appropriate particulars about the specific case and the general theory and knowledge needed to put it in context, to make a diagnosis, to make a prognosis.
2. *Implications:* Consideration of not only the semantic meanings of these data but their implicative meanings; the issues of policy; the possible courses of action and their consequences.
3. *Execution:* Implementation of what is considered the appropriate course.

Facts

We should perhaps be using some more solemn term here than *facts*. In using it, we must pay some attention to vocabulary. Carnap (1966) makes an important distinction, vital in symbolic Logic, between *fact* denoting the truth of a general proposition (e.g., "It is a fact that in human ontogeny six branchial arches develop") and *fact* denoting a particular item of information that, with some reservations, we equate with a datum ("It snowed this morning"). What are loosely called facts embrace a wide diversity of phenomena.

Clinical facts, for instance, cover an assortment of gleanings by the clinician from interviewing the patient: unsolicited, unprocessed stimuli (visual, auditory, olfactory); a preliminary sorting out of those that are worthy of attention, a process that converts *sensations* into *perceptions;* edited, telescoped, and often unconsciously made inferences from these perceptions that we dignify by the term *data;* a more sophisticated process of sorting them out into data that are of interest to the problem in hand. There is no doubt that this account is sketchy, and the processing is being quite artificially disarticulated. A fair account of the clinical interchange would be a much more elaborate affair, permeated at all stages by revision; by a continued flow of fresh stimuli and perceptions; by a perpetual readiness to accept that a datum noted previously but dismissed as beside the point is after all germane to the whole problem; and by the occurrence of intermediate states of relevancy that lead the clinician to make notes about them but perhaps not make any larger inferences from them. Our point here is not to describe the diagnostic process with anything approaching fidelity but to warn the nonclinical reader that what are glibly referred to as facts ("Just give me the facts!") are not a tidy collection of unit parts like coins that can be treated as homogeneous and interchangeable lumps of evidence.

Fact further comprises that whole set of information and perspective contained in the history and the physical examination of the patient; the various tests and special diagnostic procedures; the diagnosis and prognosis.

Fact also embraces the unbounded mass of knowledge on the etiology, pathogenesis, natural history, prevention, treatment, and transmission of disease, what emerges as the disease runs its course; everything, indeed, wherein the responsibilities and concerns of Medicine reside.

Needless to say, we have no ambitions to discuss this vast topic even in outline. The brevity of our comment is due notice that the topic is huge. We must warn those unaccustomed to Medical practice against any attempt or even supposition that it can all be compressed into a simple sentence on which without more to do the Ethical process may neatly operate. Whatever Medicine is, it is not a set of one-liners.

Implicative Meaning

When all the facts and scientific knowledge have been assembled, there will normally be a more or less careful deliberation over the possible courses of action. It would again be a monumental task to expound this topic in adequate detail. There may be several possible courses of action in each of which it will be necessary to appeal to the various benefits and disadvantages, both in the short term and in the long term: the benefits and disadvantages to length of life, to quality of life, and to disability, physical, psychological, and social. Persons other than the patient (relatives, colleagues, professional help) as well as the more abstract demands on society may have to be considered. The technical issues of making decisions in the light of implicative meaning will be discussed in general later.

Execution

The component of execution is much more complicated than it may at first appear. More than fact and meaning, it is of the very substance of Medical Ethics. We have to recognize two main topics here: what the process comprises, and (in the broadest possible terms) how it is to be paid for.

The process: compact decisions. Sometimes the fulfillment is simple and clean and brief in the execution.

EXAMPLE 10.2. An amputation may be done sometimes for local and purely cosmetic purposes (e.g., removal of a sixth finger) or enhancement of the body image. At other times (e.g., excision of adipose tissue) the goal is less clear and may have some concern with general health, such as the effects of excessive strain on the weight-bearing joints.

EXAMPLE 10.3. Amputation of a leg may be regarded as an Act that is ontologically dense and virtually irreversible. We shall suppose that the part excised is a danger to health or even life (e.g., from a cancer or a severe infection); or that there is no prospect of healing (as in frostbite, an arteriosclerotic gangrene, or an indolent ulcer) and there would be no reason to consider restoring it to the body even were this course of action technically possible.

EXAMPLE 10.4. Sometimes, of course, amputations are inadvertent— for example, as a result of an industrial accident, or through deplorable surgical error whereby the healthy member of a paired structure (arm, leg, breast) is removed in mistake for the affected one. In such cases the amputation may be reversible, and skill in this area continues to improve.

EXAMPLE 10.5. Some procedures are done that it may be desirable to reverse and are carried out in the first place with this in mind. Instances include an "-otomy" or an "-ostomy" rather than an "-ectomy." Such procedures include closing a temporary colostomy or (more precariously) undoing a tubal ligation originally done as a means of birth control.

EXAMPLE 10.6. The diseased organ may subsequently be replaced by a graft (e.g., a kidney or the liver), although the grafting of the replacement is usually done during the same operation as the excision.

EXAMPLE 10.7. Serial operations that have meaning only when taken as a whole may nevertheless be Legally distinguishable.[2] For instance, atlanto-occipital fusion (an operation on the upper cervical vertebrae) may involve a preliminary operation to fit a halo-cast to ensure that when the fusion is done the parts will be kept immobile until the consolidation is complete and firm. It is possible that the patient, having agreed to undergo the two-stage operation, will after the first stage decide to go no further in the process. For the surgeon to operate at this stage against the patient's wishes would be at the least assault and battery. The same revocation may occur where there is a whole series of operations (e.g., in an elaborate plastic reconstruction).

The process: protracted decisions. Many instances, however, may be of a quite different character. The decision is a much more diffuse matter: it may not be quite so urgent, and it is not accomplished anything like so quickly.

EXAMPLE 10.8. The decision about appropriate action may be reached promptly, but the carrying out of the decision may last a considerable time: days, as in management of severe diabetic ketosis, or weeks, as in treating tuberculosis. During that time the treatment may be stopped either on the judgment of the clinician or at the demands of a dissatisfied patient. It may subsequently be resumed, but perhaps with some loss of benefit through delay because the patient's condition has deteriorated, or because through mutation the infecting organisms have become resistant to treatment.

EXAMPLE 10.9. The treatment may be just as important to life and health but involve a change of regimen rather than therapy. The conduct of the later parts of the treatment may be changed in the light of the results of the earlier part. Dietary treatment of obesity, diabetes, heart failure, and the like may be just as important in the long run.

Such a regimen differs from the previous types in that it depends vitally on not merely the complaisant consent of the patient but also the patient's active, continued cooperation. As such, it involves two components. The first component is a resolution to change habits, or at least a disposition to have them changed—a *metanoia*. We need a definition:

2. We have already addressed the Ethical issue in connection with the principle of double effect in Example 6.3.

DEFINITION.   *Metanoia* is a radical change of attitude, a resetting of patterns of behavior strongly affirmed with the intention of persisting. It thus involves a more serious exercise of freedom than simply acceding (or not) on a single occasion.

The classic example from literature is Ebenezer Scrooge.

The second component in the change of regimen is *perseverance,* the day-to-day realization of the metanoia. The traditional "New Year's resolutions" are commonly moderate as to metanoia and feeble as to perseverance.

EXAMPLE 10.10. The most striking instances here are diet and exercise to lose weight; group and social therapy to handle alcoholism, especially in those already having disease of the liver; withdrawal of drug addiction; and management of antisocial behavior. But it will be clear that the patient's broad good intentions are not enough. It is necessary for the patient to cooperate continuously and repeatedly: in taking medicines, in avoiding some undesirable factor (alcohol, sodium, dietary excesses, etc.). It may be noted that there have been Ethical disputes over how far the clinician may, or should, override the patient's reluctance.

EXAMPLE 10.11. In engaging the patient's metanoia, the clinician is in a delicate balance. On the one hand, it is important to make sure that the patient has really grasped what the advice consists of, and that is not usually easy to judge even when the patient claims full understanding. Even more difficult is how far the clinician may go and what instruments of persuasion are appropriate to excite a metanoia. Theoretically, the fact that the patient has consulted the physician is a kind of implicit permission for the clinician not only to recommend treatment but to urge it. Of course, the patient is free to break off the professional relationship at any stage (except where the competence of the patient is impaired). But short of that stage the intemperate urging of advice may still be overt harassment.

EXAMPLE 10.12. As to invasion of perseverance, the tactical management of drug addiction may be distressing. Aversion therapy (i.e., the use of drugs that in the presence of the addicting substance may produce acute distress, with the object of reinforcing the patient's purpose) is more controversial. Opinions differ as to how far this strategy is an abrogation of the patient's freedom at a lower level (to indulge the harmful habit), and how far it is a help at a higher level of freedom (to avoid the ill effects of the bad habit).

The Payment and the Day of Reckoning

No decision would be necessary if there were not some benefit, or at least perceived benefit. But almost as regularly, there is a price to be paid, even if it is only the trouble of attending to medication or other recommendations. We have seen many of the commoner examples, and they need no further illustration. However, just as the substance of the treatment is by no means limited to a brief, almost instantaneous treatment, so also with the price paid.

EXAMPLE 10.13. There may be an immediate and overt price: not merely money and the discomforts of convalescence but also disabilities that are permanent (e.g., after amputation of a limb or lung or kidney, residual blindness, etc.). There may be the day-to-day stresses and deprivation of pleasant but harmful habits. We may note also that after some major surgical event, there may be further action that is to complement it but is nevertheless quite distinct from it. For instance, after amputation of a leg the usual course may be to fit a prosthesis, which will involve some further trouble, discomfort, and the demands (including occasional falls and injuries) of learning to use it. Some elderly or neurologically disabled patients may decide not to go through this further ordeal.

Moreover, there is a day of reckoning that must be taken seriously when diverse options exist; and sometimes they are complicated by intricate Probabilistic components.

EXAMPLE 10.14. The disorder or groups of disorders known as hereditary polyposis of the colon (HPC) are autosomal dominant traits in which there is extensive multiple polyposis of the colon and sometimes of the small intestine or the bile duct as well, each of which may give rise to various troubles of its own (McKusick 1994: entries *174900–175510). However, the main concern is that there is a high rate of bowel cancer among those affected; in several forms of the condition it seems to be ultimately certain, but it occurs on average perhaps twenty years or so after the polyposis appears (Veale 1965; Bussey 1975; Morales, Murphy, and Krush 1984). Options, then, may be exercised in various ways. A major issue is the hereditary nature of HPC. Setting aside nice issues of ascertainment, the risk of having the disorder is high in all close relatives. There are increasingly refined methods of detecting the latent state of the gene (Smith-Ravin et al. 1994; Nugent et al. 1994; Caspari et al. 1994; Giardiello et al. 1994; Wallis et al. 1994), but in fact the mean age of onset of overt polyposis is probably about twelve years (Morales, Murphy, and Krush 1984). When polyposis is diagnosed, the patient may want to have the colon removed without waiting for any signs of malignancy, and in any case to have it done even at a stage at which there are very few polyps and presumably a relatively low immediate risk of cancer. It is a reasonable supposition that the earlier the colectomy, the lower the lifetime risk of cancer, but the longer the time with what disability there is from colectomy; and conversely. But there is a day of reckoning that makes indefinite postponement unacceptable in the present state of our knowledge.

In this formulation of the day of reckoning, there is a maximum penalty of loss of one genetic human life (i.e., extinction of one genetic line). However, with its attendant morbidity and other troubles, the reckoning may be unbounded.

EXAMPLE 10.15. Where Mendelian disorders are concerned, the reckoning may go on indefinitely. A person with a dominant Mendelian disorder may decide to have children, each of whom will be at a 50% risk of inheriting the disease; the consequences to them (depending on whether they in turn have children) may include passing it on to yet another generation, and so on indefinitely. Traditional deterministic theory of genetic dynamics under certain reasonable but nonetheless precarious assumptions predicts that eventually these impaired traits are certain to become extinct.[3] A more realistic stochastic theory tells another story. The direct Probability of extinction (Murphy, Krush, et al. 1980) leads to an estimate that in one form of HPC (namely, Gardner's syndrome), if the distribution of family sizes remain unchanged, the Probability is 0.28 that the line of descent from a person bearing the gene will never die out. On the face of it, this means that the average number of affected descendants has no upper bound.

If this theory of perpetuation of a disability (which is certainly mathematically sound) seems rather fanciful, we do well to remember a famous example that is surely not unique.

EXAMPLE 10.16. Most, perhaps all, human beings need vitamin C in the diet and would sicken and die of scurvy if deprived of it. The reason is that they are descendants of a mutant stock that as a result of mutation lost the capacity to make their own vitamin C. Thus, scurvy, which from an evolutionary standpoint is a genetic deficiency, has come to be regarded and treated as a deficiency disease. It has proved a great boon to the citrus industry.

COMMENT.   We may note here results of empirical but informal observations on those seeking genetic counseling. Consultands vary consider-

3. The assumptions are that genetic disorders reduce fertility; that there is a hard upper bound on the world population; that this must lead by hook or by crook to constraint on reproduction; and (a very precarious assumption) that this constraint, when it occurs, will be strictly proportional to unconstrained fertility.

ably in the range of their concerns in the face of a diagnosis. Some are concerned about their own phenotypes. This concern is particularly sharp about traits like HPC that are age-dependent in their manifestations and their dangers (as opposed to static traits like color-blindness or blood group). Such persons may be concerned about how much burden they may come to impose on others, notably in dementias such as Alzheimer's disease; severe neurological incapacitations such as Huntington's disease or Joseph-Machado syndrome (McKusick 1994: entry *109150; Livingstone and Sequeiros 1984); or progressive physical disablements.

Another group of consultands shift their anxiety to the next generation, most strikingly those who are proved carriers of traits but are not themselves affected. This is, of course, the classic substance of genetic counseling (A. C. Stevenson, Davison, and Oakes 1970; Murphy and Chase 1975; T. E. Kelly 1986).

Yet other consultands have spouses who are not carriers, and they are concerned not that their children may be affected but that they too may be carriers: their concern is really with the third generation. A concrete instance is the woman who is the carrier of an X-linked trait. For every son this woman has, there is the 50% risk that he will be affected; but for every daughter, there is the 50% risk that she will be a carrier and will have to endure a repetition of the mother's burden. Still others may push this problem a stage further to embrace what they may or may not contribute genetically to the future of the human race. This last concern is more akin to eugenics than to traditional genetic counseling: the view that it is not enough to have carrier children and tell them not to marry other carriers. In this connection we may cite the Muller-Haldane principle (Murphy and Chase 1975): the total number of genetic deaths ascribable to a new deleterious mutation depends only on the pattern of inheritance, and not on the severity of the disorder. Roughly speaking, this principle depends on the idea that in a very severe disorder—one incompatible with postnatal survival, or leading to early death or sterility—the day of reckoning is prompt: the person affected will have no progeny. In mild mutations, such as color-blindness, the gene has a low, perhaps extremely low, risk of being lethal. Fertility is then little impaired, and the mutant is apt to become widespread. There result many individuals at a low risk of lethality; and the total risk for the mutation risk will amount to the same number of deaths as for the severely detrimental traits.

A REPRISE OF TERMS

To approach a working model of the decision process, we call attention to particular principles and terms explored earlier.

Tautology

The term *tautology* is addressed in Chapter 9, where the emphasis is on tautology as a source of certainty, or perhaps an arid source of illusory certainty. We understand the word *tautology* in the usual sense, as a statement of an intrinsic, rather than an extrinsic, truth. "*A* is greater than *B*" is an extrinsic truth; there is no problem in constructing particular examples for which such a claim would be false. But the statement "*A* is greater than *B* if and only if *B* is less than *A*" is a tautology, since it is universally true and ultimately it follows from the notions of "greater than" and "less than." No counterexamples are imaginable. It seems, then, that a tautology is merely a rearrangement of terms; as such, it is epistemically trivial, though it may have value in clarifying the mind confused by complexity or by the opacity of style in which a proposition has been stated.

However, here we find a rather more constructive interpretation. There is another facet to tautology, a quality that suggests it is by no means empty. In general, deductive Logic and axiomatic mathematics are entirely concerned with statements that are, at least in principle, tautologous. The structure of such a system is prescribed a priori, implicitly, and the system already contains all the legitimate inferences of which it admits: the ideal mind would at once discern all these inferences without explication. However, there is a well-known and disturbing theorem due to Gödel (1931; Penrose 1989) showing that under quite general and reasonable conditions, no finite set of axioms can ensure that there is a solution to every well-formed problem in that system; sooner or later there will be encountered cases that cannot be solved except by adding supplementary axioms. Perhaps that takes some of the gilt off the tautologous gingerbread.

These instances of tautologies have their counterparts in Ethics. Many methods of resolving Ethical issues are reducible to the trivially tautologous.

EXAMPLE 10.17. To say, "Ethics requires that patient A be kept alive" is at once to imply, "Ethics requires that patient A be not left to die." Despite the serious substance of that proposition, it is rather difficult to think of this jump as containing any useful insight.

There are other instances in which the jump is scarcely less trivial but in which, because of obscurity, rhetorical distraction, and the like, many people have difficulty in seeing the connection between two statements. When all semantic confusion has been cleared away, the appropriate decision may then be obvious. That is perhaps a foretaste of the confrontational version of Ethics: the stance that when all the facts and their implications, and the implications of the consequences of the decisions, have been clearly and explicitly laid out, no further formal apparatus of adjudication is necessary.

Nevertheless, it is misleading to imply that all Ethical problems are purely semantic. It may be, at the opposite extreme, that many of them cannot be resolved by any degree of analysis whatsoever, and the most that can be hoped for is that analysis will lead to an unambiguous comparison of the activity in question and its consequences (which we shall have to treat as a cardinal feature of consistential Ethics).

There remain the cases that lie between the extremes of the patently tautologous and the unresolvable, where the strategic objectives are clear enough but the tactical details are not. It is such cases that concern us here. We might hold the reduction of the total suffering of a patient to be a strategic objective; but the means of doing so may be another matter, to determine which may present formidable problems.

We consider, then, that Ethical decisions in general are not trivial, and that therefore we must equip ourselves with the machinery necessary for making decisions.

Uncertainty

Most nontrivial Ethical decisions involve uncertainty. We use the term in the various technical senses defined and discussed in detail in Chapter 9. There are undoubtedly cases, exemplified later, where no decisions whatsoever can be made without some risk of error. Thus, one might say that over a sufficient number of such individual decisions, it is to be expected that errors will be made, perhaps serious errors, perhaps even lethal ones.

It is vain to demand petulantly that no step should be taken until certainty is attained. To embrace the policy "No step should be taken" is itself to take a step. Awaiting certainty may be the very course that destroys all hope of doing any good whatsoever; and the amount of damage or risk may increase as the delay in making a decision is prolonged. Decisions may be required, not from all eternity and in generality, but *abruptly, unhesitatingly, and uniquely.*

Uncertainty (as we have seen) may be Objective or Subjective; it may be difficult to distinguish from incertitude. In scope it may be within the domain of fact, of reasoning, of values. There may be no grounds whatsoever for resolving it; there may be no means of ensuring that the problem about which the decision has to be made is not illusory.[4] It seems, then, that there must be a wide range of Ethical confrontations in which uncer-

---

4. An ambiguous component of Certitude is the appeal to the proverb. McHugh and Slavney (1983) have pointed out that proverbs, comforting forms of assurance, evocative of mellowed experience and ripe wisdom, nevertheless commonly come in contradictory pairs. "Many hands make light work," but "Too many cooks spoil the broth." "Look after the pence and the pounds will look after themselves," but "Penny wise, pound foolish." "Faint heart never won fair lady," but "Marry in haste, repent at leisure." Turning to a proverb for guidance will involve a choice between conflicting advice; and it may amount to little more than a rationalization.

tainty of some order is important; and where uncertainties adhere to all conceivable courses of action, the question must arise as to how a course is to be chosen that is, in some acceptable sense, best.

Integrity

As the proverb says, "There is no point in keeping a dog and barking yourself." If Ethics is to have coherence and not be merely a matter of caprice, then the solution to a problem invokes an agreed system of argument from a set of accepted facts, aims, and principles. Two things follow. First, insofar as one may rely on the system, its directives will relieve much of the burden of conscience involved in making a decision. Second, the price for this relief is a certain binding force on the ethicist. The connection between the two is really a tautology, for, of course, if the Ethical principles involved impose respect, why, they have to be respected.[5]

Nevertheless, we make the point with some diffidence, since this principle of respect can itself be, and too often has been, abused. In Chapter 1, indeed, it was proposed that principles and conclusions should be mutually correcting. No set of principles that cannot transcend the limited and commonly distorted observations on which they are based should ever be allowed to tyrannize the making of the Ethical decision. On the other hand, in conduct no less than in science, the greater the true momentum that a principle has attained, the more reluctantly should that principle be set aside, overridden, or abandoned. Two hundred years of demonstrable success from Newtonian mechanics did not save it from the inroads of relativity mechanics. But the iconoclast's fervor generated from this example (and others) may be tempered by two aspects of the replacement. First, the scientists abandoned Newtonian mechanics only after a serious and determined struggle to accommodate the dissident facts inside the older system. Second, the new system turned out to be not so very different and, indeed, could be shown in limiting cases to give the same rules as the old. There was no arrogant discarding of the fruits of the older scheme just because it had imperfections, and in fact it is still widely used three-quarters of a century and more later in cases where exquisite refinement is not germane to description or prediction.

However, in the appeal to the momentum that a principle has acquired from experience, only authentic experience should be respected. The vivisections of Procrustes were not authentic experience and did nothing to alter the fact that the height of the human species has a variance. No number of ruthless applications of a policy, apt or inept, can establish it as a principle. Hard cases make bad law, indeed; and a law that generates hard cases is not a good law. If a law leads to repellent decisions, we escape it

---

5. One useful purpose for a tautology!

first by phronesis and illation. Then, more formally, in accord with the Flew principle, we may conclude that it is inadequate and arguably incompetent.

In demanding integrity in ethicists—that is, in demanding that they abide by, or at the least have the gravest respect for, the conclusions of their arguments—it is necessary to beware of three major pitfalls.

The first is inadequate formulation. A principle can hardly be worthy of the name if it is so vague or so ambiguous that it cannot be applied without confusion. Some of the terms commonly used are shrouded in vagueness that it has been the goal of this book to dissipate. Several have been dealt with earlier: *normality* and *disease; Acts* and *Things*. In other instances the ideas may be based on false phenomenology: the principle of "double effect" ("the act of two effects"; see Chapter 6, under the heading "Complex Action") if used in reference to Medicine may be an example of such a principle.

The second pitfall is lack of cogency of the proof. There is always peril that a line of argument is fallacious at a Logical, a semantic, or a scientific level. It is vital to keep alert to tautology. In the real world, proof (like reflex action) has both afferent and efferent pathways. From sound scientific facts fallible particular inferences about action are made: error in the efferent pathway. But also, "facts" are put forward from (fallible) inferences depending on observation: error in the afferent pathway. Moreover, the two may reinforce each other. It is a common failing of the more pragmatic to gloss over these weak points in the reasoning; and the conclusions, while roughly true, are often more precarious and less binding. Popper (1959) has sagaciously pointed out that every application of a principle is commonly taken as a further corroboration of that principle. In 1963 M. Campbell advanced a persuasive theory that the apparently meteoric increase in coronary disease in the twentieth century is an artifact generated by the mounting awareness of the existence of this disorder, which made physicians more likely to diagnose it; and the more fashionable the diagnosis, the greater the reinforcement of that trend. Of course, the converse applies to a principle or a diagnosis under suspicion. As a result, the estimate of Probability for a rare event is of the order of the square of the true Probability (Murphy 1981c: Appendix).

The third danger is imperfect relevancy. The perils of substituting mere knowledge for scholarship are admirably illustrated in the learned professions, which give us terms to belittle those who do it: *textbook doctor, sea lawyer, cookbook statistician*. These false experts may know answers to classic cases but without any grasp of the principles by which they were reached or how a new case is to be solved. The temptation among them is to try to force the new case into a classic mold willy-nilly.[6]

---

6. Compare the classic schedule of the railway conductor on the charges for transporting family pets in the luggage car: "Dogs is pigs and cats is sheep, but tortoises is insects and travels for nothing."

It is regrettable that so many who practice a profession or have a scholarly training have recourse to stereotypes. Scholarship is rare and painfully acquired; and yet anything less must cause injustice and unnecessary pain, and eventually—since clients may be well-informed critics—discredit and scandal for some honorable profession. The closer the field of interest to human affairs, the worse the indignation. Incompetent weather-forecasters are figures of fun, at worst contemptible: who ever sued one for incompetence? But incompetent Medicine, professional law, Ethics, and Morals are beyond laughter.

No doubt Ethical argument and analysis may be at times grossly incompetent. That is scarcely a matter for us authors to judge or amend. Inside some systems of belief, inadequacies are readily enough recognized and condemned. We are sure, however, that inept Ethical decisions may be due to incompetent Medical and scientific formulation. The respectable of the last century may be quite unacceptable now. That is not mere cant, nor just one more instance of "chronological snobbery" (C. S. Lewis 1955: 26): the attitude that any statement made long enough in the past has been disproved simply by the passage of time. In the mid-nineteenth century little was known about the unconscious mind, about semantics, symbolic Logic, genetics, the pharmacology of behavior, Statistical inference; and nothing about DNA, quantum mechanics, the ontological ambiguities of viral disease, hormones, and countless other fields in science, Philosophy, and the arts. These fundamental developments are not to be squeezed into nineteenth-century Ethics as extra, nonpaying, passengers with just a little reshuffling of baggage. No doubt most Ethical solutions then were distorted by underdimensioning, just as a two-dimensional map of the world is distorted even if over a small region the distortion is so minor as to leave its threatening presence unsuspected.

But in practice, most ethicists, like most judges, apply their conclusions with leniency by binding, but (to extend the metaphor) binding with some "slack." While in most real-time decisions there may be no other recourse, it is, in our opinion, simple laziness and incompetence to rest content with discretion or clemency as a formal institution for redressing any gratuitous inequities of incompetent Ethics. Vagueness and imprecision are defects, not virtues. However, finding better answers calls for hard work. A simple analogy may help.

EXAMPLE 10.18. A man wants a suit made to measure. He writes to tailor A, who asks for two data, his height and his waistline. From them the tailor makes a poorly fitting suit, which the customer nevertheless believes modish because tailor-made. Next time he is persuaded to telephone tailor B, who asks for six measurements. Lacking detail, B does not risk a close fit and produces a loosely fitting suit, comfortable but hardly fashionable. The man's third attempt is with tailor C, who insists on seeing him in person, takes a multitude of measurements, and produces a well-tailored suit that will retain its shape for years. In the Ethical or Legal analogy, A is like the village headman, who can grapple with only a few facts and coarse-grained arguments. B is the common judge or ethicist with some finesse who, lacking the insight to scrutinize his limited professional knowledge and makeshift arguments, ascribes (with perhaps some vanity) the vagueness entirely to the nature of things, and believes that incongruities may be dealt with by padding and shrinking. C is the Solomon, the ideal maker of decisions. Perhaps, however, there is a yet finer type D beyond our ken. Certainly at none of these levels of sophistication is there room for complacency.

Epistemic Symmetry

When a proposition has been proved beyond any shadow of doubt to be true, and the only admissible Ethical course of action can be rigorously deduced from it, there is no dilemma, and further speculation is fruitless. Our concern here is not with such cases but with those in which two or more solutions, all more or less plausible, exist. Then we appeal to a deep-rooted, if not very well articulated, principle that what is sauce for the goose is sauce for the gander. The elements of a system of Ethics are to be treated strictly on their merits: no part of the system is to be treated as privileged or is in itself to furnish a criterion of judgment. This latter demand is in accord with the principle of conterminality. There is excellent support for this stand from Philosophy, mathematics, Psychology, and historical politics. This principle means that where there is no authentic certainty, no hypothesis is "in possession," though it may be favored a priori. No part of the system is privileged; and none may be given the status of inalienable principle to make or break other parts. This evenhandedness we shall refer to as *epistemic symmetry*.

EXAMPLE 10.19. A nice illustration is provided by the contrast in Anglo-Saxon law between trial at criminal court and trial at civil court. In all trials, of course, we take it for granted that the judge is privileged by delegated power. Beyond that, we recognize that criminal trials are not symmetrical. Always the hypothesis "not guilty" is in possession. There is no requirement for the accused's defense to be argued. Onus of proof rests always with the prosecution, and should the prosecutors fail to make any case or should the judge (or jury) consider the case inadequate, the hypothesis of not guilty prevails by default. (Note that the very terms of the verdict reflect proof by default: the accused is not said to be "innocent" but rather "not guilty." The verdict is a description not of the merits of the accused but of the case presented by the prosecution. Something more like symmetry is attained at Scottish law, where there are three verdicts possible: "innocent," "not proven," and "guilty." But disposition remains asymmetrical. Only the third verdict leads to punishment.)

At civil law, on the other hand, where two parties are disputing a claim—say, a wallet found in the street—symmetry is preserved. It is true that "possession is nine-tenths of the law"; but this is not an asymmetrical relationship, rather a strong balance of evidence a priori for one party. (A nice point arises in the sequelae of the trial. While two parties may dispute in good faith, in many cases it is evident that one of the parties must be lying. But subsequent trial for perjury of the party who loses the case takes place only where there is other evidence of perjury. Even in such instances, the conclusions of the civil case, disposed of symmetrically, have no necessary impact on the asymmetry with which a trial for perjury would be conducted).

In the Ethical context, we cannot accept that a mass of opinion, even of sound and independently operating minds, can ever extinguish the possibility, however remote, that some alternative hypothesis may yet prove to be true.

- No truth was ever established by a majority vote.

However, it is conceivable that at times truth may be attained by consensus. Of course, the majority opinion may dictate the behavior of the reasonable person; but decisiveness in action, as we shall see, is not at all the same thing as decisiveness of conviction.

Asymmetrical arguments are characteristically used where the force of the prior evidence has not been, or may not be, adequately assessed. Thus, in criminal trials, while it seems evident that a previous conviction for a similar crime makes it more likely that the accused is guilty, such evidence is not admissible until after conviction, when the severity of the sentence is being decided. In civil law, prior evidence is used. Possession is strong evidence of ownership; the evidence of a written contract is stronger evidence than claims for a verbal agreement. Where all else fails, the law will treat the claims a priori as equally strong; but even this is implicitly an a priori stance and, as such, falls into the class of decisions known in the theory of Statistics as Bayesian (or symmetrical) hypothesis testing, distinguishable from the Neyman-Pearson or Fisherian (or asymmetrical) systems.

True and Approximate Isolation

The term *isolation* is used in a wide variety of ways. In the present context we use it to characterize the relationship between components of a system such that one component has no impact on any other component.

EXAMPLE 10.20. For definiteness, consider the common Ethical principle "I may do what I please provided it does no harm to anyone else." We shall not attempt to adjudicate on the content of this principle, but it will be of value to explore its form. Is any Act a person performs completely free of impact on somebody else? The answer is by no means obvious; and recent theory of Chaos (Gleick 1987; Devaney 1989) has reinforced doubts in particular cases at least, though there are dissident opinions (J. Cohen and Stewart 1994).

It may help to consider a simple example.

EXAMPLE 10.21. Three men live in the Sahara Desert hundreds of miles from each other. One man sings loudly; one practices karate; one does not believe in washing. All consume oxygen. It is difficult to believe that their individual peculiarities disturb each other. But suppose, now, that their dispersion is a few miles, or a few hundreds yards. Imagine them, finally, confined within a single telephone booth. In the last instance it is quite obvious that their behaviors are not mutually isolated; it is fatuous for any one of them to suppose he may indulge his practices because he is not harming any one else. Yet it is difficult to see at what stage of physical separation the line is to be drawn between such so-called isolation and nonisolation. A pragmatic lawyer would no doubt solve the problem by arbitration, which would do well enough in practice, though there would surely be borderline cases. However, there seem to be two clear consequences of such a pragmatic approach.

First, the isolation even under the most remote separation is, strictly, an illusion. Without doubt, as matters stand, the relationships among the three men are well enough *approximated* by supposing them isolated for all practical judgments. But as the distances gradually shrink, these departures from true isolation gradually become more obtrusive and eventually can no longer be ignored. It is worthy of comment that a stimulus may have an effect without entering the conscious or even the preconscious mind (see Appendix 1); it is not to be supposed that unless there are overt symptoms demanding Medical attention, a person at interest can suffer no harm.

Second, it is difficult, perhaps impossible, to state a principle that depends on an approximation of unspecified accuracy. Such a statement may be a reasonable working rule, but as such it is always too brittle to be a principle. What is a trivial distinction in practice may be only accidentally, not essentially, trivial. In principle, the right (in the sense of "Let right be done"), unlike the law, must always be concerned with trifles. One might even say *especially* with trifles, for one litigant's trifle is often another's grievance. It is difficult to imagine that any poacher has ever been charged with stealing water for having drunk from a lake while trespassing on somebody else's property. But it is not difficult to think of circumstances in which drinking from a precious store of water would be a serious crime. A Legal principle that stated that stealing water to drink is not a crime would founder readily enough on extreme cases.

———

Lest our treatment of isolation seem too theoretical, we quote examples of two kinds of cases over which there has been much soul-searching. They illustrate that in an Ethical problem, as in a chemical one, the pattern may be dominated by the "rate-limiting step," and where that changes there may be a fundamental change of decision. We expressly make it clear that we are withholding our personal opinions in what follows. First, we have a set of three problems focused on a single issue.

EXAMPLE 10.22. Consider the question of whether a child with serious mental defect and atresia (i.e., total blockage) of the duodenum should have the latter defect relieved by operation so that normal feeding may be instituted and the child kept alive. While there is a range of opinion, there is little doubt that many believe the only ethical course is to operate. But in the situation envisaged there is only an approximate, not a true, isolation between the fate of the child and that of other children.

Let us suppose, first, that the setting of the Ethical problem is one of those African nations—Somalia, Eritrea, Rwanda—that have been in the news in recent years, where, as a result of famine, the risk for any child taken at random dying of starvation is perhaps 30%. We may infer, then, that whatever happens, children will die in such numbers as to equalize the food supply and the number of children to be fed. It might then seem foolish to keep alive by extraordinary means a defective child and thus decrease the chances of survival for some "structurally normal" child. No doubt many would still advocate operating; but there seems little doubt that the center of gravity of opinion will be shifted away from operating. The point of the example is, of course, that the first-order simplification—that abundance of food is totally irrelevant to the operation—no longer even comes close to true isolation; the serious limitation on food has ensured a most intimate interdependence.

EXAMPLE 10.23. Now suppose that the number of surgeons sufficiently skilled to perform the operation is small. It would again be argued that where a conflict exists, they should give priority to "normal" babies rather than those with mental defect. In this instance, where the rate limitation is imposed by the number of surgeons, the nonisolation of the fates of the babies is so gross that even the most slovenly Ethics could not ignore it.

EXAMPLE 10.24. Suppose, finally, that the question is whether enough surgeons should be trained to deal with all babies affected, mentally impaired or not. Where resources are unlimited, expense involves no constraints, and there is an inexhaustible supply of suitable pediatric surgeons who have no other demands on their energies, many would favor providing for operations on all in whom they would be effective. But again, in undeveloped countries, such straits do exist. Even in the richest, most developed, countries, it is mere cant to pretend that no expense should be spared to allow optimal health, a fact we are slowly and painfully learning.

Consider now a second, very different topic: the appropriate birth rate.

EXAMPLE 10.25. It might well be argued that in a world almost empty of human beings, ensuring the survival of the species is a sufficient good to make unrestrained reproduction not merely permissible but a benefit, even a duty. The limitation on the size of the family is mainly imposed by the number of children too young to look after themselves that the parents can provide for. Later, as the population expands, the need to reproduce to keep the population from extinction is less urgent, but the right to do so is strenuously asserted. Later still, the right is still asserted, but the demands of a complex civilization and the limits to natural abundance make it financially exacting. Still later, severe restrictions such as that recently in force in mainland China may be imposed. At the present era there is an awakening of a sense that limits do exist and that sooner or later having large families will imperil survival. At some time in the future the right to have an unlimited number of children may be legally revoked. This shift in position reflects the transition from the scale of the stewardship of parents, as the limiting factor in determining family size, to abundance; in other words, there is progressive obtrusiveness of nonisolation of families as the population steadily increases in a finite economy.

The Incommensurate and the Incommensurable

Two terms that arise in this area of decision making, and indeed wherever there is any attempt to balance qualities, require a brief analysis at this stage.

Commensurate has something of the sense of *proportional,* although that is rather too narrow a statement. We expect that removing a thorn from the skin will be a smaller task than removing a brain tumor; it will require less staff, less support, much less of the operator's time, and much less skill. There will be less liability. Time is, of course, not charged by the minute or bandages by the square centimeter. But we expect that the surgical fees should be correspondingly smaller for removing the thorn, fees commensurate with the task. No doubt a completely rational scale of charges might be devised. But underlying any scheme of Medical care is the idea that there is some equitable correspondence between the charge and the time, strain, elaborateness, and so on of the treatment.

Commensurable is a more subtle term to be predicated of more than multiplicity. It supposes that there is an intrinsic, natural, rate of exchange between two things that are associated but not the same. Strictly, two qualities are commensurable if they are capable of being expressed in the same units. The height of Mount Everest and the width of the Amazon can be expressed in a common linear measure, say, meters. The color of a ruby and the tragedy of *King Lear* are incommensurable because they have no common descriptor; one could not, for example, declare apodictically which is the greater. The commensurable units may be real enough, but they may not really get to the heart of what is being measured. Food and paintings can both be weighed. But one buys sugar at so much the kilogram; one does not buy old masters at so much the kilogram. They are commensurable as to weight, but weight is not the point of the painting. There is a commercial perspective that says that a painting is strictly equivalent to its commercial value and hence to so much sugar; other opinions would condemn that belief.

There are special cases in which apparently incommensurable *qualities* can in fact be compared by *quantity*.

EXAMPLE 10.26. The color of a ruby and the pitch of a note, though at first consideration incommensurable because they affect different sensory modalities, nevertheless can be expressed as wavelengths or as frequencies per second. The flaw is that the frequency of sound is expressed in a longitudinal compression wave in gas, and that of color in lateral electromagnetic waves. It is a nice point as to whether wavelength should be accepted as an exact equivalent of color or of sound (each according to its proper medium). Observers may reject the notion that because they derive more pleasure from crimson than from middle C played on an organ pipe the difference is ascribable to the shorter wavelength, and that therefore they should prefer ultramarine to both, because it has a still shorter wavelength, and that X-rays should make them ecstatic. Nevertheless, at least some aspects of the two qualities are commensurable. Indeed, it is one of the achievements of Galileo to have recognized that all physical measurements may be reduced to some combination of three scales (time, mass, and linear extension).

Now, while it may not be possible to set up demonstrable rates of exchange between quantities, it may be necessary in the real world to do so artificially.

EXAMPLE 10.27. Superficially, the Portuguese escudo and the German mark are commensurable at one level, if the premise be accepted that they are equivalent to so much gold. In fact this equivalence is economically naive. What determines their gold equivalents is somewhat artificially controlled. Inasmuch as the one is an agricultural/fishing/tourist economy and the other industrial, it seems doubtful that they are sensitive to the same factors. But at least in theory the coins are indices of credit, and it can be argued that at any specified instant of time they are commensurable.

There are a great many instances in which no pretense of commensurability can be maintained.

EXAMPLE 10.28. A painter may sell a painting to buy food. As we remarked earlier, in a narrow, commercial sense one might argue that this makes paintings and food commensurable because they are both reducible to money. But food decays and loses its virtue, whereas certain paintings do not, so that the rate of exchange may change enormously with time; and this very fluctuation suggests that the commensurability is a fiction.

We take note of another, nobler but also more romantic, view of the commercial transaction.

EXAMPLE 10.29. The contempt in which prostitution is held is that it is an attempt to equate two things (love and money) that are incommensurable. By analogy, a man is said to be prostituting his art if he believes in the commensurability of art and money so firmly that he measures his achievement by how much money his art will buy. This prostitution applies not only to the finer arts but to the professions and the skilled trades as well. Simony is held sinful, and dishonest workmanship the hallmark of lack of pride in one's trade. A less demeaning, though no doubt impractical, viewpoint is that an artist does not work to obtain an income but has an income in order to pursue a vocation. Certainly it is absurd to suppose that (however much or little one might respect their views) missionaries working in a leper colony can be said in any simple economic sense to be paid adequately for their services.

But not all incommensurable transactions are meretricious.

EXAMPLE 10.30. In speculating as to what career young people should be encouraged to pursue, society might have to decide between promoting, say, teaching or Medicine. If they become teachers, they will contribute (one hopes) to the cultivation of the mind but not to the restoration of health, and conversely; the better supplied the one profession, the worse supplied the other. This is a real decision that has nothing to do with money. Even in a society without money or property, it seems to be a perfectly real problem of promotions. It involves no degrading surrenders, since both professions are honorable and useful. Yet ultimately there is some kind of implied equivalence between things of the body and things of the mind. How much of studying of Shakespeare is it proper to sacrifice to keep children free of colds? We do not condemn out of hand anybody who feels that society must also pay major attention to material well-being. The individual person may, of course, make a choice. But society is an aggregate of nonisolated beings. Society is, in a word, social; and it is necessary that it should have some policy about the relative importance of various goods.

Optimization

If it be agreed that many choices are to be made in the face of some indeterminacy, and that in time some errors must occur that cannot be avoided by any strategy, then we must address how best to apportion the errors. *Best* here is an undefined term to be dealt with only after a system of values or other criteria may be introduced, a step we have resolutely avoided in this book. Nor do we propose to address it now. Nevertheless, we shall take for granted the following somewhat contentious rules, which, however much dispute there might be about details, and however unpalatable in principle, are nonetheless implicit in the fact that people do make decisions in the face of uncertainty and where incommensurable quantities are at stake:

1. All elements that enter a decision—death, life, pain, embarrassment, money, time, disfigurement (anatomical or physiological), resources available, competing demands, and so forth—all these elements are capable of being expressed on a single common quantitative or at least ordered rating scale.
2. Negative ratings denote the undesirable, positive ratings the desirable, and in strict proportion to their magnitudes or ranks.
3. The best strategy for making decisions is that which in the long run may be expected to yield the highest rating for the outcome; that is, it will maximize the good effects of correct decisions and minimize the bad effects of erroneous ones. To any such statement of variable courses of action is added the general cautionary phrase "other things being equal."

Lest there be misgivings as to what these rules commit us to, we make the following comments.

First, the first axiom may seem distasteful, although fully in accord with the *P* (for *practice*) coding given in Chapter 2. We construe Ethics to reflect, among other matters, actual behavior of societies; and there can be no doubt that implicitly such equivalences do exist.

EXAMPLE 10.31. Human life is everywhere treated as having equivalents. Road deaths could be reduced, at a large expense, by ensuring that pedestrians have no access to roads containing vehicles; at some inconvenience and economic strain, by lowering speed limits (as was done during the 1970s in response to the oil crisis, apparently with considerable reduction in mortality) and enforcing them strictly, perhaps by mandating the installation of governors on engines; by setting more stringent standards in driving tests; by narrowing the age range at which driving is permitted; by promoting public transport; and by a dozen other measures. Now, all these methods could be used without themselves leading to loss of life. If it were indeed true that in principle life is beyond price, there would be no choice but to take all steps possible and necessary. Most people would regard this as an excessive price to pay for the benefit obtained. Thus, whatever the orators may profess to believe and the public applaud, there is certainly no common enthusiasm for this policy to promote safety. It seems inescapable, then, to infer that most people implicitly accept a rate of exchange between human life and money. This is the result we are concerned to establish: our argument must not be construed as an attack on the appropriateness (or otherwise) of public policies about protecting life.

Second, the system can be made to accommodate inviolable principles by the simple device of attaching a positively infinite rating to make sure that they are observed and a negatively infinite rating to prevent them from being violated. However, ethicists at their peril set up a policy as an absolute principle. For instance, how are they to adjudicate between two principles, both declared absolute, when they are in conflict? To be sure, the matter can be dealt with by invoking different orders of infinity; but apart from being cumbersome, such an approach involves the problem of ranking absolutes, which is arguably a contradiction in terms and at the least will present formidable difficulties. Furthermore, it is experientially doubtful that any society has ever consistently behaved as if there were any absolute principles.

Third, the terms in the argument are expressed in mathematical expectations—that is, averages—regardless of how arrived at. By this reckoning, a gross neglect that causes the unnecessary death of one person is neither more nor less culpable than a gratuitously neglectful policy applied to a hundred persons that raises a possible mortality rate of 5% to an actual mortality rate of 6%. This will be an unpopular conclusion, because much of the indignation that crime generates lies in the suddenness and the disruptive nature of the criminal Act. But it is difficult to see the justification for this counterargument, and we suspect that such a matter of sentiment rather than cold Logic has no weight.

EXAMPLE 10.32. There are those who would insist that raising the mortality rate by 1% in one hundred persons is less culpable than letting a particular person die unnecessarily. They would surely not countenance a pharmaceutical company randomly making vials of morphine of which, on average, every hundredth contained a lethal quantity (although the difference in the mortality rate is still 1%). We may have to accept it as a limitation of the power of arguments from expected costs that such distinctions are in fact made. Constructing an Ethics means, in effect, showing people what the effects of their activities will be; that is, it is as much a matter of confrontation and evaluation as it is of decision and prohibition. As we have previously argued at length, in our treatment of Probability and certainty (Chapter 9), the broad outcome must be in terms of averages; indeed, we concluded that for the purpose of introducing numerical values into Ethical arguments, the average value could be treated as equivalent to the actual one.

TYPES OF ETHICAL DECISIONS IN MEDICINE

We may state at the outset that there is a major existential problem in what follows. The traditional stance of the clinician is that each patient is an isolated universe: it is the understanding and the duty of the clinician to act from the point of view of that patient as if the solitary occupant of a personal universe. This involves giving whatever care and treatment may be personally appropriate. Further, the ineluctable competition more and more may extend to diagnostic procedures as well. Where this duty means a competition for scarce medications or treatments, the clinician should plead the patient's cause by all methods short of deceit.

But some clinicians also have some commitment to public health and perceive that they are bound to consider other issues. Notably, they must recognize that the unbridled advocacy of the patient may not square with what public health perceives to be the most advantageous policy to society as a whole. The false isolation in their experiences of inner, smaller, matters leaves many unprepared to modify their intransigent principle of unwavering duty to their patient's individual interests. These competing loyalties are not totally disparate; but neither are they matters of minor adjustment. For this reason we are obliged to deal with several types of cases, realizing that the preferences, the demands, even the urgent necessities of the individual patient can less and less reach the stage of being an absolute principle of good.

Decisions about One Person: Only Trivial Outside Considerations

There may exist many dilemmas in which the only issue is the welfare of the patient—there are no competing issues—and they cannot be resolved with certainty by any expenditure whatsoever outside the patient. Even so, the best policy may not be straightforward. Two classic illustrations may be given.

EXAMPLE 10.33. Acute left ventricular failure (pulmonary edema or cardiac asthma) may be difficult to distinguish from bronchial asthma, especially where certain special tests are not available. For acute pulmonary edema, among other measures, morphine is a drug of choice, while epinephrine is strongly contraindicated. For bronchial asthma, epinephrine and similar compounds are valuable drugs; morphine is to be avoided at all costs. Both drugs cost a little money. Here that consideration and the risk of depriving others in need of them are usually trivial. However, there is an Ethical conflict concerning the patient alone. The physician must decide which diagnosis is probably correct and treat accordingly; but in dealing with this kind of problem there will be some errors; and there is no coin in which this uncertainty may be bought off.

EXAMPLE 10.34. Acute abdominal pain may be due to (among other causes) a perforated peptic ulcer, which should be operated on promptly; or to acute pancreatitis, in which a surgical operation increases the mortality. Even in the best of hands and circumstances, they may be confused and the wrong decision made.

Decisions about One Person: Outside Considerations

The person may be thought, on very slight evidence perhaps, to be suffering from a dangerous disease that calls for treatment. Further investigations, expensive, time-consuming, and uncomfortable but involving no danger, may resolve the doubts. The physician must decide how far these further investigations should be pursued before being reassured.

Unlike the last kind of problem, this Ethical decision involves setting an equivalence between two quantities not intrinsically commensurable: dangerous disease on the one hand and discomfort, expense, and so forth on the other. We may take it that special investigations rarely settle such matters with complete certainty, and that the stopping point will leave some, usually small, residual uncertainty.

Decisions about Two Persons

There are many instances where making the decision involves danger to two persons, especially where the flow of benefit is, or appears to be, in one direction only.

EXAMPLE 10.35. An operation for the transplant of a kidney (or, even more so, of a heart) is an example. The procedure is equivocal because the "books cannot be balanced": a decision to imperil a person's life that confers no benefit is, prima facie, unacceptable. The balance might be restored, however, by introducing the donor's personal love and anxiety for the survival of the recipient, or by introducing that larger love known as altruism. (Of course, the origins and Moral force of these issues lie beyond our present scope; we have not as yet any Medical means of evaluating them.) The problem here is to strike an equivalence between one person's life and another's principles of benevolence. There are other, more mundane, possible equivalences:

1. The donor is rewarded financially (e.g., in blood transfusion) or by remission of a prison sentence or the like.
2. The decision is the outcome of a pact for mutual assistance agreed on beforehand.
3. An element of duty is involved, as for the clinician who must look after a patient with a disease that is serious and readily communicated.

Decisions about Three or More Persons

A decision concerning three or more persons is a case worth treating separately from the last one because of the relevance of real and approximate isolation (discussed earlier in this chapter). The Ethical burden imposed by the needs of a patient might be intolerable for any one donor.

EXAMPLE 10.36. A patient undergoing an aortic replacement may need ten pints of blood. That would put an impossible burden on one donor, but it would exact less and less from each as the number of donors involved was increased. If it could be argued that a patient needs two kidneys, there would be two Ethically different cases where the kidneys were derived from one person and from two.

Decisions Involving More Than One Person Indirectly

Wherever the benefit of medical care is equated with a value in money —even if this is merely for purely administrative purposes, as in setting one service equal to another—there is usually, perhaps invariably, some degree of nonisolation involved. The more expense, labor, or medication is made available for one person, the less there is for another. This constraint arises from the finiteness of the commodities; and while often the treatment may be cheap and simple (e.g., dosage with ferrous sulfate available), in other cases (notably renal dialysis, the "artificial kidney") there will be concern with priorities, and some will have to be denied and may die. In principle the demand could be met by expanding the supply; but the lack of money may reflect the implicit policy of society. Medicine is, of course, an art of the possible; and however much clinicians may deplore scarcities, they must be prepared to make the decisions where they have no other recourse.

THE MAKING OF A CLINICAL DECISION

A clinical decision is commonly a matter of the diagnosis or the treatment, and often both. We shall therefore concentrate our efforts in this field. The theory is laid out in various texts (e.g., Murphy 1997). Although some features (e.g., ascertainment) may seem a little strange, they are all factors that bear on the sample space from which the patient may have been drawn. The process comprises two ideal steps: first, describing the problem in formal terms; and then optimizing the decision.

Description

In general, the following considerations will be involved in the process of describing the problem: prior Probabilities, ascertainment bias, conditional Probabilities, and cost.

Prior probabilities. The first consideration is the prior Probabilities associated with the competing states (e.g., hypotheses) among which a decision is to be made. In the diagnostic process this is mainly a matter of the prevalence of the disease; but its clinical impact is something like the readiness of the clinician to make the particular diagnosis. Paragonimiasis occurs in Baltimore, but not often; and the mind-set of the diagnostician is one of reluctance to diagnose some exotic condition and readiness to diagnose the commonplace. In choosing between a perforated peptic ulcer and an acute pancreatitis as the explanation for the abdominal pain, the surgeon will take into consideration the relative frequencies of these conditions. Other things being equal, the commoner diagnosis should be chosen; but that stark course would be appropriate only in the excessively rare contingency where no other evidence was available. (Of course, as we shall see, it is rare that other things are equal; nevertheless, prior Probability will still carry some weight, which in special cases may be overwhelming.)

Ascertainment bias. It is not enough that a physician should accept the Probabilities for the world in general. The patient is a member of a diagnostic sample space, and part of sound Diagnosis is discerning what that population is.

EXAMPLE 10.37. Even the wisest and most experienced clinicians in Kansas or Wyoming would have little experience of erysipeloid. But those who see patients in a fishing port would be familiar with it.

It is not difficult to think of many such factors that radically change features in a naively stated space: occupation, sex, and diet, as well as the reason for referral.

EXAMPLE 10.38. A classic example is the rather uncommon disease thromboangiitis obliterans, originally described in 1908 by Buerger (1908). He recorded that most of his patients were Polish and Russian Jews. That preponderance has not been sustained. McKusick and Harris (1961) reported that the disease is very common in the Orient. Although it earns a brief note among possible recessive diseases (McKusick 1994: entry 211480), the genetic evidence is of the feeblest. It seems likely that Buerger's original note on racial distribution was an artifact of ascertainment to be expected in view of the high concentration of Russian and Polish Jews among his patients in general.

EXAMPLE 10.39. When a patient presents with severe central chest pain, coronary disease will be uppermost in the minds of internists—but not in the minds of pediatricians, who in the scope of their practice see patients of a type in which this disorder rarely occurs.

EXAMPLE 10.40. The physician with a practice that is largely composed of Ashkenazi Jews will be on the alert for Tay-Sachs to a somewhat greater degree than the physician who sees mainly African-Americans; and conversely for sickle-cell disease.

As to the characteristic signs and symptoms ascribed to a disease, the cases of disseminated lupus erythematosus (a notoriously pleomorphic disorder) seen by the dermatologist and the gastroenterologist or *referred from them in consultation* will have different symptoms and different diagnostic criteria. There are many such disorders.

EXAMPLE 10.41. Inbreeding may be an important telltale sign in, for instance, familial Mediterranean fever (FMF), an autosomal recessive condition in which there are commonly attacks of abdominal pain that may simulate the acute abdominal emergency. Yet a clinician catering to a population (e.g., the Amish) in which there is an almost universally high rate of inbreeding will need to modify the results; diagnostically, all patients from that population are likely to have an inbred ancestry. Epidemiologically, FMF is rare in that community.

Conditional probabilities. The physician must also consider the conditional Probabilities of the signs and symptoms under the various diagnoses.

EXAMPLE 10.42. Wilson's disease is less common than alcoholic cirrhosis, and if the decision rested on prior Probabilities alone, Wilson's disease would never be diagnosed at all. But the prior Probabilities are really attributes of the population at large. Examination of the individual patient might discover a Keyser-Fleischer ring and a low serum ceruloplasmin level, characteristic findings in Wilson's disease but rare in the general population. Hence, the priors and the conditionals tend to offset each other. The existential choice, then, may lie between supposing rare manifestations in a common state or common manifestations in a rare state. It is not difficult to imagine instances in which these two conjunctions balance each other and render the competing hypotheses about equally plausible.

Cost. The term *cost* must be understood in the widest possible sense. It is probably unnecessary to repeat a list of the factors subsumed under the terms, and it would not be easy to be sure that the list was exhaustive. While the three other factors given above are (in principle, at least) easily determined by empirical means, converting well-being, pain, disability, and so on into an acceptable common metric presents all the thorny problems of commensurability. But it is easy enough to see that, for example, stringency of proof should be relaxed more for diseases that if neglected are disabling, dangerous, and easily communicated, and for which treatment is highly effective, especially if given promptly in the early stages. Conversely, for those disorders in which early diagnosis has no other effect than possibly precipitating a prolonged period of mental suffering, given the prospect of ultimate disability or death, the standards of Diagnosis should be stringent.

Optimization

It is a fairly straightforward, if technical, procedure to optimize decisions once the problem has been formally described. The matter is dealt with in textbooks that address decision theory (Blackwell and Girshick 1954; Raiffa and Schlaifer 1962; DeGroot 1970; Murphy 1997), and details would be out of place here. As to the gold standard for optimization, we mentioned one earlier in this chapter: to maximize the average benefit. Others should be considered: to maximize the benefit for the individual case, or to minimize the harm, for instance. Inasmuch as the physician applies decision-making procedures to a great many cases, we think that the best criterion is the maximization of the total good, which is equivalent in any individual case to maximizing the expected gain. But that is a Diagnostic principle, not an Ethical discussion.

III Involvement of the Person

So far we have kept our analysis at the level of formal discourse, no doubt much of it debatable, but at least operating in a well-defined area and by methods well known and familiar to the scientist. Something deeper is needed, however, that is not nearly so easy to define but is vital if the peculiar character of the ontology of Medical Ethics is not to be lost entirely. As nearly as we can state it, this element arises from the fact that Ethics addresses human beings both as discussants and as subjects for discussion. We want to take heed of these two senses and of the considerable difficulties of integrating them without confusing them. Yet we want to keep faithful to our principle of not proposing any particular Ethics or intruding (in particular) any specification of values or how they might be broached.

However, the default position—the impression left if we said nothing at all—is by no means a neutral one; and an active process of purging inept and undisciplined systems of values is important. In Chapter 11, for instance, we point out that an adequate representation of life must be more than a simple binary classification (live or dead); and, indeed, unexamined and poorly comprehended use of mean survival may grossly distort judgments. Likewise, in Chapter 12 we try to purge shallow rhetoric and misplaced compassion from the discussion of pain and suffering. To alert our readers to these misdirections by analyzing in depth is not at all like prescribing answers about how these intricate topics are to be managed. The analysis is something like a cautionary tale; but the goal is not to show how inadequate current notions should be improved, but rather to implant in the reader's mind the question, Have the notions that you have taken for granted in the Ethical analysis been seriously examined?

Chapters 13–15 deal with progressively more intricate topics in which the full weight is felt of analyzing notions (like respect, intention, and responsibility) when the analysts themselves are an inextricable part of the very system they are analyzing.

Chapter 16 is an attempt to pick up the not wholly reconciled outcomes of these analyses and to try to safeguard the integrity of each for future inquiry and application.

11 Duration and Quality of Life

L
ife is as sensitive a topic in Ethics as it is in many other branches of learning. Emotions may run high, and ethicists adopt diverse attitudes, some appealing to absolute principles of the sanctity of life, some to existential judgments; some rely on common sense; some elaborate an Ethics of exceptions, which they may or may not attempt to codify. Here, we start with no such theory and have no aims to reach prescriptive or proscriptive conclusions.

We are, however, impressed by the contrast in treatment of human Ethics between the subtlety, imaginativeness, and intricacy of the Ethical arguments, on the one hand, and, on the other, the wanton lack of attention to the ontological aspects of what is being discussed, aspects that would be regarded as commonplace to the scientist and the clinician. There is a temptation for us to make a catalogue of errors and misadventures that have resulted from such neglect, and to illustrate them by citing examples. We shall resist this temptation firmly. For one thing, it would beggar the tact of a diplomat to do so without gratuitously irritating many readers. The examples we would give may be very much to our point. But it is to be remembered that to other authors and the points *they* were trying to make, our criticism may be quite irrelevant and may be mistaken for mere carping. But even if, throwing all caution to the winds, we were to take that outspoken course, it is doubtful that it would do much good. Vivid examples might point up the need for better perceptions of particular points. But one cannot coherently deal with how a process should work by relentlessly citing examples of how it has not worked. We shall try, instead, to give a systematic exposition. If occasional examples used here seem trivial, even absurd, they are not for that reason to be supposed supercilious rhetoric. To the contrary, they are one way of cultivating solid ground for agreement by capitalizing on what we hope is beyond dispute.

There is need for the usual exercise of identifying and defining terms. Once it is conceded that life is more than a black box and has features by which it might with genuine discernment be described and evaluated, we are obliged not only to explore these features but also to try to examine what aspects of life they address and ponder whether these aspects are such as appeal to the discussants. The pattern is now a familiar one. We can look for no benefit from summarizing the topic; there is already too much syncopation at work. To the contrary, we must unpack it, tease it out at length so that no major aspect remains unexplored.

LIFE AS A BINARY VARIABLE

Primary Cells

In Table 3.1, we gave a range of levels of ontological density, with examples stretching from those that are perfectly dense or close to it, at the one extreme, to those that are so ill formed as to appear as if arbitrarily carved out of a homogeneous and featureless empirical landscape, at the other. Some writers seem to treat life as ontologically dense with respect to features that are already partly known, as if there is at least enough homogeneity within what is living to make it amenable to common principles that can be of use in ontological and Ethical discourse. Now, as a first approximation, that may not be wholly false or even useless. For instance, even without digging any deeper, it is possible to devise effective epistemic uses for that claim.

EXAMPLE 11.1. There is a field of nonparametric, or distribution-free, statistics, that uses methods concerning so-called *order statistics,* devised for analyzing variables that may exhibit ordering of magnitudes without being representable on a quantitative scale. For instance, there are better and worse pianists whom we may rank in a competition even though we cannot give them grades on which all would agree. But order statistics may also be used, and commonly are used, to analyze variables that exhibit more than order alone and can be scored on a strict quantitative scale. They may be used because the scale is unknown, or when for one reason or another (such as that the distribution function is unknown, or known but unfamiliar, or the distribution is not conveniently tabulated) the Statistician chooses to ignore the existence of a scale. Theorists even explore such topics as power. One instance is how applying the Mann-Whitney nonparametric U statistic to data that are known to follow the Gaussian ("normal") distribution compares with the preferred parametric method (the t statistic). In particular, converting a continuously distributed variable into a binary variable according as its value lies above or below some arbitrary cut point is a well-accepted procedure, even if (to the disgruntlement of the investigator who collected the data) some loss of Statistical power or efficiency results.

Nevertheless, this *binomialization* of a continuous variable may at times be something more than a makeshift or a quick approximation. In populations of simple cells, it is not difficult to think of examples in which the primitive perception may be of fundamental scientific interest. The question is, then, whether the cell is alive or dead, not how alive it is.

EXAMPLE 11.2. It is not many years since an expedition to Mars was mounted to answer (among other matters) the question, Is there life on Mars? The burden of the argument was that if there is any kind of life at all on Mars, it is liable to be diverse. The radical question was whether on Mars there might be an independent repetition of evolution of life such as is supposed to have occurred on Earth.

EXAMPLE 11.3. A technical challenge, of rather less basic character but of major clinical and scientific importance, is to prepare a system freed from foreign living matter to a specifiable degree. At one extreme is the completely germ-free environment, in which experimental studies have been done in raising children affected with various congenital immunological defects in their ordinary means of resisting infections. There is also the maintenance of the very strict standards of sterilization in aseptic surgery. There are other instances where the aim is not extermination of all life but where only certain organisms are to be eliminated or at least reduced to a sufficiently low concentration to avoid some danger (e.g., in the pasteurization of milk or the delivery of acceptable but not necessarily sterile drinking water).

EXAMPLE 11.4. The most exquisite operations of all are those in which the goal is to deliver a nicely calculated dose of some attenuated form of a harmful organism that will generate active immunization without undue risk that the infection in the recipient will get out of hand.

This last instance is the first hint of a state of living in which we address a feature of life other than the pure primordial fact of life (or its absence), even if it is only a Probabilistic attribute. To describe the process, we need something more searching than the two categories living and dead.

Populations of Unicellular and Multicellular Organisms

Without unduly laboring the point, it is clear that from time to time it is necessary in society to decree some control of higher animals, either because (like venomous snakes) they are dangerous in themselves, or because they are reservoirs of infections that they may transmit themselves (e.g., rabies in foxes) or through insect vectors (trypanosomiasis in cattle). These topics have a *point d'appui* in Ethics from standpoints like public health, ecology, management of national parks, and the like.

Extension to Human Beings

In extending this line of thought to human beings, we must proceed carefully and deliberately.

EXAMPLE 11.5. We do well to recall that, from the standpoint of organization, the sponge is an ambivalent structure, being a facultative assembly of organisms each consisting of a single cell. For certain purposes and at certain times these cells may band together to form a kind of primitive society that acts in unity. It is, indeed, the typical example of the evolution of the multicellular organism. The importance of such a relationship to the human species is pertinent at a highly theoretical level, neither fanciful nor farfetched. An unsparing view of the biology sees the phenomenon of the human being as an assembly of individual cells participating in a hierarchy of functions. Acting as a whole, it is under the illuminating control of a unifying principle. At the present time, at least, that unifying principle is beyond the understanding of the organization itself. However intellectually unsatisfying these uncomprehended and unresolved ontological and epistemic questions may be, we know of no responsible and intelligible opinions that dispute these main facts.

We are treading here on the preserves of the Philosopher, and we promise to get back to biological science and Medicine promptly. But if the arguments are to be concise enough to be intelligible or at least expressible, there is need of some vocabulary and some notional framework. We cannot argue concisely if we have to repeat some wordy periphrasis every time we refer to the principle of unification in the process of organization of the human being as a whole. The appropriate Greek word *psyche* has come to refer exclusively to the mind. As the result of semantic overload, the concise and earthy Anglo-Saxon word *soul* threatens us with an incursion into more recondite and arcane fields, even if it is only to fight a battle of disengagement from them. The best compromise seems to be the word *individual*.

DEFINITION.   An *individual* is a system of components that cannot be divided without loss of its identity.[1]

---

1. It is noteworthy that *individual* is the Latin translation of the Greek word *atomic* (unsplittable), although traditionally it has come to designate unsplittableness at a much higher, more elaborate, and more subtle level of organization. In this sense we are getting into problems of levels of language. It seems to be evident that if any disruption of the whole threatens this identity, then no part of the system can grasp, analyze, or adjudicate upon the whole. The individual, then, cannot grasp the working of his own brain. This argument seems suspiciously easy, and no doubt there will be those who for that reason will declare the whole structure of individuality meaningless. As clinicians, we are unintimidated but dismayed by the prospect of that sanction, which seems ominously close to intellectual excommunication.

——

Inquiry into the scientific nature of this individual, a responsibility that we authors undertake, must be approached with care. Its integrity is not (to appeal to a cognate Greek word) anatomical. The individual will survive many and vast structural abridgments: amputations, "-ostomies," and "-ectomies." It survives many and vast functional abridgments also: failure of endocrine glands, metabolic processes, the special organs of sense, processes of ingestion and excretion. In a sense (admittedly one much harder to grasp), it survives much brain damage, even when accompanied by gross impairment of brain function, including sense of reality, even sense of identity. The conventional usage (and we see no need to quarrel with it) is that, however battered or distorted, the individual is the substantive of which the words *living* and *dead* are predicated. Without probing too deeply into the Philosophical problems (notably the ontological and epistemic issues of death) we may say that in writing a death certificate, the clinician is not making a statement about gangrene of one foot, or loss of speech, or hepatic failure, but is declaring that the individual no longer exists: the minimum principle of organization of the whole has radically and irrevocably disintegrated. That coarse statement is, of course, no fundamental product of exquisite argument and inference. To the contrary, it is an unrefined but inescapable, crassly empirical, datum. It is, if you please, the starting point of an analysis, not a finely processed concept; a discovery, not an invention. All the more so, it is not some clever intellectual device to be outmaneuvered by nothing more than a yet higher level of cleverness. The epidemiologist advisedly calls it a *hard endpoint*. The cogent test that interaction of the Ethical analysis and the domains of science and Medicine has been fruitful is that their joint verdict must without evasion accommodate that uncompromising datum. Nevertheless, the crass fact is capable of refinement. And our own goal here is to explore that refinement from the Medical and scientific side.

STRATEGIES FOR THE ANALYSIS OF COMPLEXITY

The word *analysis* seems to us to have acquired a bewildering diversity of precise technical meanings. The chemist's analysis breaks a mixture or a substance down into its components. A mathematician denotes by *analysis* (more obscurely) that class of problems that make use of the calculus. There is endless confusion between forays into breaking down problems and questions, on the one hand, and breaking down solutions and answers, on the other.

Some Definitions

We wish to introduce some terminology appropriate for those examinations of topics of discussion that may involve changes in complexity. We shall impart no very technical meaning to the word *complexity* (although for those interested we provide a definition in the Glossary) but appeal to it in a broad intuitive sense. It is then customary to recognize distinct patterns of direction that may be applied to the various disciplines of discussion (ontology, epistemology, Logic, Ethics, science, etc.).

Parsing (top-down inquiry). The gist of the top-down strategy is the successive conceptual breakdown of the organization of the system into simpler and more fundamental components. The archetypal pattern is the inquisitive small boy taking a watch apart because he wants to understand, literally, what makes it tick.

Syntaxis (bottom-up inquiry). To extend the illustration, the great watchmakers have been at their task long before the boy even starts on the search. They have been engaged in an activity that would be much more happily called *synthesis,* a putting together. They have analyzed what it is they want to do and the properties of the parts with which they want to do it; and by trial and error they have built up the watch, which is one way of keeping track of the time, subject to certain constraints of size and weight. (Evolutionary theory proposes the same kind of pattern, except that it would be a misrepresentation to talk about invention in the watchmaker's sense. But the analysis will be unchanged by that fact.)

We may think of the two ways as being opposite in direction. The watchmaker is *inventing* the workings of the watch; the small boy is *discovering* them. The top-down strategy is like a mountaineer finding a path down the cliff face, and the bottom-up strategy is like one finding a path up it. The primary objective in neither strategy is to get to the top or the bottom of the cliff; a helicopter or a roundabout road would be a much quicker and safer solution. The objective, rather, is to ascertain whether or not a path on the cliff face connecting the bottom with the top *exists*. In the analogy as applied to the ontological analysis, the objective is to see whether there is more needed in the system (in some sense) to account for the complexity at the top of the cliff in terms of the raw materials at the bottom.

Paraphrasis (the transversal). The image of the crag prompts a third strategy (Murphy 1987) of a somewhat more subtle flavor, yet no less important for that. It involves no vertical shift; that is, it is making for neither higher nor lower levels of complexity. Instead, it translates a more or less complicated level of organization to one that is just as complicated, but with the hope that the recast pattern will in some sense be easier to grasp.

A simple domestic instance may help to make paraphrasis clear. This example is ontological.

EXAMPLE 11.6. Consider a new bar of soap in the form of an ellipsoid. Its length, breadth, and thickness are all mutually unequal quantities, so that even when wet and slippery the soap can still be easily rotated or held in any particular position. Now, the shape of this bar is a property that ignores spatial orientation, a useful property when orientation is irrelevant. When the statistical theorists (in rather forbidding terms) prove the theorem "The eigenvalues of the variance matrix of a quadratic form are invariant under orthogonal transformation," what they are saying is something like, "The shape of a bar of soap does not change however it may be rotated." The equivalence of those two statements is a twofold transversal. First, shape is the same whatever the coordinate axes, but the representation of the bar of soap in a coordinate system is not. From the perspective of form, shape is thus much easier to grapple with than a set of typical coordinates from an arbitrarily oriented figure. Second, a bar of soap is a much simpler system to deal with intuitively than the formal definition of a quadratic form. Yet in neither instance is there any change in the complexity involved in the system, only in our way of looking at it. We are neither better nor worse equipped with information about the bar of soap or how we might dexterously use it to work up a lather.

The Strategy of Ontological Parsing

To revert to our ontological analysis of that multicellular individual the human being, we have noted that there are large parts that are present in the normal[2] person that may nevertheless be impaired, even totally missing, without evidently compromising the individuality. This activity is more or less top-down analysis in the sense that it is bent on determining how much of the phenomenon of the human may be dispensable. (To say it is ontologically dispensable is not, of course, to say it is unimportant.)

For that matter, we might appeal to the computer, though not as a model but strictly as an analogy.

EXAMPLE 11.7. The hardware of the computer is something like the essence of the individual. If it ceases to function, then the computer might be regarded as dead. But from the other side, the fact that the hardware is intact does not guarantee very much. The merit of the computer lies in the remarkable things it can do when given sophisticated software. Yet hand-

---

2. After the strictures of Chapter 8 we crave the reader's indulgence for this slovenly use of the term, even though it is a very rough substitute that will do well enough for our purposes here.

some as it is, the software (like the stag's antlers in Aesop) avails nothing without sound hardware.

It is hard to say whether or not this finding should cause surprise at how much damage and curtailment the individual can survive. But we are habituated to the reality of this survival. Our bias is perhaps that the seat of individuality is the mind (whatever that may mean in biological terms); but the sheet anchor of our current scientific-Medical analysis will lie in the elusive area between the empirical facts we know and common terms of discourse about personhood.

Unfortunately, because of the coarseness of our methods of experimental disruption of the individual and (where human beings are concerned) the Legal, Ethical, and Moral constraints on experimentation, it is not easy to go far with top-down analysis, at the present time, at least. For instance, is it possible that there might exist a damage, operating diffusely, cell by cell, throughout the body, that without in any other way interfering with the operation of the separate cells would abolish the coherence that distinguishes a multicellular organism from a large colony of unicellular organisms? We know of no such evidence. But that may be a technical and temporary setback. Yet, as we shall see, there is some bottom-up evidence on the point.

The Strategy of Ontological Syntaxis

There is no doubt that certain physiological functions can operate adequately in a foreign environment and in a host organism.

EXAMPLE 11.8. There is close to a century of experience in the transfer of erythrocytes (red blood cells) from a donor to a recipient. The key to success was the remarkable insight of Landsteiner (1901) in recognizing the existence of different immunological types of blood groups; and while there has been a vast and probably inexhaustible elaboration of this central idea of immunological types in the technology of blood transfusion, there is every reason to believe that the fate of the red cells is little affected by the disturbance involved in transfusion, if they are given to an immunologically compatible recipient. Any criticisms there are of this argument are not such as to undermine that latter claim in any way, but they do urge decent caution in generalizing from it. The erythrocytes are very peculiar cells. They are biologically almost inert. With a limited metabolic equipment, they exercise the solitary biological function of transporting oxygen and carbon dioxide, a function so primitive as to be little more than a mechanical chemical device. They do little else. They have no nuclei, so they cannot reproduce their kind; they have no means of repairing injuries done to them; they cannot regenerate enzymes. For various technical reasons—their abundance in the body, their free mobility and mixing, the ease with which radioactive labeling studies can be carried out—more has been learned about their natural history in the bloodstream than about any other bodily structure. Life span can be measured accurately and is known to be about 120 days in most ordinary states. There is a well-developed theory stemming ultimately from Schiødt (1938) and Mills (1946), and first coherently laid out in generality by Dornhorst (1951), about computing the survival of cells; and it does not seem to be appreciably changed upon transfusion into a compatible host. Part of the cause of this success is that erythrocytes are not treated as foreign bodies and are not attacked by scavenger mechanisms (such as phagocytosis). In all these respects, erythrocytes seem to be strikingly different from other bodily cells, and there has been little success in finding another cell type that is so readily and simply enabled to function in a host.

EXAMPLE 11.9. The ambition of genetic engineering is to restore a normal mechanism at an even more fundamental level. Bodily cells that function well in all respects, except for a flaw in a single gene that governs a single enzyme or structural protein, may be repaired by introducing into every cell (by means of a vector such as a virus) a functioning version of the gene that had been flawed. This procedure, which is still in the stages of careful and circumspect development, is a matter of effectively manipulating the function of a single simple structure. As such, it is akin to chemically pure replacement therapy in an endocrine disorder such as diabetes or thyroid deficiency rather than to the great diversity involved in a full-thickness skin graft.

The great impediment to effective transfer of extraneous tissues seems to be immunological; and to offset this incompatibility the main devices are careful immunological typing and the use of drugs that suppress the (ordinarily beneficial) immunological responses. Details, which are many and highly technical, need not concern us here. Sometimes (as in skin grafting) the extraneous material is intended in the first place only as a temporary structure to be replaced in time as ordinary bodily means of repair fulfill their functions.

EXAMPLE 11.10. A more ambitious undertaking (e.g., when the recipient's marrow has been infiltrated beyond repair by leukemic cells) is total removal of the population of the marrow and replacement, not by red cells alone, but by a full complement of healthy extraneous marrow components. This procedure provides not only a supplement of blood cells but also the apparatus for generating a steady supply of cells. As is well known, with exquisite care in subsequent management, these methods will work well. Thus, it seems that not merely mature cells but simple bodily processes may survive transfer into the body of the host or (equivalently) transfer outside the body of the donor; and (obviously) they do so without depriving the donor of the biological necessities. There is thus both top-down and bottom-up evidence involved in this system.

EXAMPLE 11.11. But we can do better still. Under much the same carefully regulated conditions, it has proved possible to transfer a whole heart from a donor to a recipient who, to judge by a steadily mounting experience of actual operations, may survive a long time thereafter. This is an example of the transfer, not of a gene or a cell or a tissue, but of all these things that taken together and on a massive coordinated scale perform an elaborate function that is large-scale. Here there can be no longer a question of the resemblance of a *restitutio ad integrum*.[3] The method of the replacement is not at all like the recapitulation of the explicit process by which the normal heart developed in a fetus. There is a very real sense in which, however long the heart functions, it will always belong to the donor. *Belong*, here, is used not in the sense of legal possession ("This car belongs to me") but in the colloquial American middle-voice sense of being at home ("This is where I belong").

There are two further considerations from this last example. The first is that even though a functioning heart is vital to ordinary survival of the human being, it may be adequately replaced by an extraneous heart or its equivalent. The former is illustrated by the transplant of the heart, the latter by the mechanical heart, which, while cumbersome, is effective. Although the cardiac role is an essential feature of the individual, the heart is not. This view would have seemed strange in earlier ages in which the heart was seen as the seat of certain qualities of the individual, like love and courage. Frankenstein's creature in the famous story by Mary Shelley (1818) could be declared a monster because it lacked the quality of humanity. Now, humanity implies no precise anatomical commitments. What concerns us here is a very different belief: the idea that the heart, qua and ubi heart, has a nonabstract quality something more than a metaphor, a belief that some are still reluctant to abandon. Brock (1948), embarking on intracardiac surgery, remarked on the false mysticism with which the eminent surgeons had condemned as grossly unethical an operative intrusion on the heart, as if it were a profanation. The idea of a man having not a heart but a metallic contrivance instead would do war against a vigorous tradition of romantic poetry, still a key point in *The Wizard of Oz* (Baum 1900), and still treated

3. This term, roughly to be translated as the therapeutic "restoration to the whole state," refers to the tissues as they stood intact before the disease occurred. It is typified by the perfect resolution of pneumonia in the intact lung tissue; however, the tissue destroyed in an abscess complicating the pneumonia is not restored but is replaced by simple scar tissue that fills the space left by the destruction of lung tissue.

as a literary vehicle of Philosophic criticism taken seriously within the last half-century in *That Hideous Strength* (C. S. Lewis 1946).

The other reflection is that the heart has certain autonomous characteristics. It is an inherently rhythmical organ, the beat of which is modified by the autonomic nervous system but not dependent on it. In this respect, for instance, the heart is quite different from the lungs or the special senses. In its autonomy the heart remains a kind of physiological republic working under treaty with the rest of the body. It is therefore all the more remarkable that the heartbeat should be taken not merely as a sensitive sign of the bodily metabolism as a whole but traditionally as a vital sign, the word *vital* being taken in both of its senses: as essential and as living. This autonomy is paralleled in the kidney, another complex system that operates on its own resources. It too is susceptible to the influence of the individual, mainly though physical factors (e.g., perfusion pressure, osmosis, etc.) and, in more refined terms, by endocrine messages from antidiuretic hormone, parathyroid hormone, cortical steroids, and the like.

Ontological Syntaxis and the Analysis of Autonomous Survival

Such multiplication of cases may soon lead to darkened counsels if we do not here pause to tidy up. We have noted that extraneous devices at various levels of complexity and organization, from erythrocytes (which are biologically almost inert) to kidney function, may be used to sustain the individual. In a rough analogy we might see the individual as like a manufacturing company, at times fortuitously benefiting from migrant workers, at other times subcontracting necessary functions to sophisticated providers. Although the individual is ordinarily provided with its own full complement of necessary services and substances, perhaps by supplements from outside, both are extraneous to the main core of the individual. These facts raise the reciprocal question of the self-sufficiency of the extraneous resources. Can the heart, the kidney, and the separate body cells survive without attachment to the organizing genius of an individual? The general answer seems to be a qualified yes. The heart may, in a warm and chemically favorable environment, continue to beat for some time after total isolation from the body. The success is greater with the small and easily perfused heart of the frog. In the larger and more intricate mammalian heart, the muscle of the heart itself needs its own blood supply (the coronary vessels), which, in the intact individual, the heart by its circulatory function itself perfuses. Again, in a favorable environment separate cells will grow and reproduce effectively as tissue culture; typically the culture will survive for only a relatively short time, but certain cancerous cells have been maintained in culture almost indefinitely. (The HeLa line of epithelial cells has been maintained in culture for over eighty years so far.) The great enemy to autonomous survival is the lack of an organizing system; in laboratory culture we might say that the careful handling and provisioning by the scientist is a vicarious form of organization by the individual. Left to fend entirely for themselves, the cultured cells would stand a negligible chance of survival.

On balance, we are led to believe that the individual is more important to the components, subcontractors and all, than the components are to the individual. Still, we should be careful in interpreting the oblique meaning of this relationship. The individual may transcend the components, but we should not for that reason make shallow inferences about independence. The real strength of the whole probably lies in the *relationship* between the individual and the essential services. On the other hand, we seem to have reached the conclusion that it is the (admittedly elusive) individual that is the unique and essential feature, whereas the general services are more or less nonspecific, and substitute means of providing them are possible.

That is about as far as we can take the ontological syntax at present. No doubt in due course the prospect of brain transplant, total or (much more likely) partial, will furnish more bottom-up evidence on the nature of the individual. At the present time the best we have are the highly capricious flights of science fiction.[4] Most of it is loaded with the idea that the "fierce light which beats upon a throne" of consciousness—what we might envision as the cursor on a computer screen—resides in the highest levels of cognition and is located in the cortex. The neurological facts seem to be at variance with this supposition and suggest that consciousness is a diffuse function of the whole neurological assembly. There is an assumption (almost always implicit) that no part of the body other than the brain harbors consciousness (or individuality, for that matter). We do not know of the scientific evidence for the supposition that this is universally true.

The Strategy of Ontological Paraphrasis

In a fashion that is comfortably familiar to the clinician but that the narrow scientist may be slow to grasp, paraphrasis may be the most profitable strategy of the three for exploring the ontology of the individual. At present there is some insight at the bottom and some at the top. But there is little hard scientific information connecting them. That there must be a path on the cliff face seems likely, and some would regard the degree of certainty of that belief as overwhelming. But the decorum of due scientific process will not allow that unbridled confidence to pass unchallenged. No doubt physicists are committed in the same way to the belief that an unbroken chain must exist from particle physics through solid-state physics to

---

4. Heinlein's *I Shall Fear No Evil* (1970) is a typical example of the exercise of literary rather than scientific imagination in the face of a negligible supply of facts.

cosmology, or biologists an unbroken chain from chemistry through bio-chemistry and molecular biology to histochemistry and classical pathology. But any sober critic armed with decent skepsis[5] will perceive that all these claims are devoid of evidence and are in fact pure acts of faith.

Transversal analysis may, in a way, be more accessible to us, for the inquirer narrowly driven by epistemic issues commonly overlooks the fact that exquisite criteria of proof tell us nothing whatsoever about the nature of scientific discovery. The important discoveries are made not by science in all its abstract majesty but by scientists. While, at the one extreme, romantic histories commonly make much of the moment of inspiration— Archimedes in his bath, Newton's apple, Watt and the boiling kettle, Flem-ing and his contaminated petri dish—it is more and more clear that, at the other extreme, discovery of new ideas is not a systematic manufacture by formula but a product of some uncanny operation that we wot not of. Popper, the arch-epistemologist, discussed at length the peculiar, the sin-gular, phenomenon of how scientific theories and formulations are devised, but with no satisfactory conclusions (Popper 1963: esp. chap. 3); and he is to be honored for that frankness. No doubt the richest epistemic results come from the bottom-up and top-down studies. But their chief virtue is that they are of an objective character and a strict discipline that conduce to proof; nevertheless, by this very fact they deprive us of the peculiar per-ceptiveness of the subjective approach. Furthermore, epistemology is an objective discipline, but epistemologists and their operating medium are at least colored by the subjective. It is one thing to prove the theorem of Ex-ample 11.6. But how did it come about that anybody sought the method of proving it? It is a subtle experience of mathematics that the discovery of a proof is wonderfully promoted by knowing that a conjecture is true (e.g., because it is reputably stated that there is a sound proof even though no details have been furnished).

Just how such insights, inspirations, and encouragements come about is unclear. Polya (1954) offers a vivid account of how he himself pursues patterns consciously and, in a sense, systematically. It is in some sense a *rationale;* but it is not clear how successful other mathematicians would be with it.

EXAMPLE 11.12. One classic instance is that of R. A. Fisher, who be-cause of poor eyesight in his youth was advised to spare his eyes as much as possible. He developed much of his inspired Statistical theory (notably in the partition of variance) by manipulating geometrical images in his mind

---

5. There is a sharp and useful distinction to be preserved between *skepsis*, the sober intellectually calculated *un*belief of the careful scholar for whom all the dross must be purged from lucid scholarship, and *skepticism*, the rhetorical and often highly emotional *dis*belief of the partisan or the reluctance to make any commitment to belief (Murphy 1981c).

until he had grasped what he wanted to prove and then translated the results into algebra.

We noted above that in the adept, at least, some problems are solved outside the ordinary operation of the conscious mind. We have no particular wish to endow the unconscious mind with uncanny properties (which would in any case do nothing to advance our understanding of the ontology of discovery). But it may be that a large part of such discovery is a matter of patient searching and even exhaustive search after the manner of the proof of the four-color problem (Appel and Haken 1977; Appel, Haken, and Koch 1977; Tymoczko 1979; Swart 1980). We have to allow for the possibility that this mental activity outside of the conscious mind may contain some element of ontological parsing. That is, in the conduct of a paraphrasis, the investigator's recognition that a perspective *A* is equivalent to a perspective *B* is an operation at a somewhat more complex level than either *A* or *B* and therefore strictly involves an element of ontological parsing. This supervisory activity (at least to the point of making intelligent judgments that enhance the efficiency of the search or other routine activities) may, without invoking the uncanny, also be supposed part of the unconscious contribution.

There have, however, been many uncanny thinkers, and the texts by Koestler (1960) and Miller (1987) make healthy reading for those besotted by the epistemic at the expense of the ontological insight. Indeed, the distinguished mathematicians Poincaré (1913) and Hadamard (1954) had remarkable experiences in becoming instantaneously aware of the solutions to complicated problems, which in some unconscious fashion they had discovered while consciously engaged in thinking wholly about something else. They do not give enough detail to warrant any sophisticated Psychological analysis of the facts. Such a skill, though not unique, is much less commonplace.

Now, just as in the natural perception that the sighted have of the physical world, eye level (which also happens to be at much the same level as the visual cortex) is given a preferred status, so (by analogy) our natural and comfortable perception of ourselves is pitched at the same level of elaborateness as that at which we ourselves work. To appeal to our metaphor of climbing, it is much easier to see what is at eye level than what is far above or far below. That is perhaps why clinicians in thinking about Ethics hanker after authentic attention to what it is they actually see rather than the ingenious abstract purifications of the theorist. It is almost inescapable that the level of complexity of our thoughts about our thoughts is much the same as that of the thoughts themselves. Indeed, it is difficult to imagine otherwise, which in itself is perhaps a self-referent statement. So perhaps transversal strategies are the most typical and the most useful. Whatever opinions the scientist may express pro forma (on the basis of doctrinaire assumption from ontological syntaxis that the mind must operate like a computer), it is very difficult to believe intuitively that that is so. It is still less easy to devise an assumption from ontological parsing that the mind is a system that can enable us to cultivate intuitions of how it works, including the mechanism of developing the intuitions themselves. By comparison, it is easy to grasp how intuitions of reasonableness can be converted transversally into Logic, or Logic into set theory, or set theory into symbolic Logic, which are all about the same level of complexity.

Our ability to see these equivalences rests on the possibility of higher levels in the Chinese box (q.v.), which we take up again in Chapter 15.

LIFE AS A CONTINUOUS VARIABLE: DURATION

So far we have supposed nothing about life other than that in any particular instance it does, or does not, exist. An Ethics that had nothing else to draw on could only make statements of the kind that curtailment of life—regardless of whether by ten seconds or by seventy years—is, or is not, deplorable. This model underlies the spirit of much of absolutist Ethics and Morals, the law, and the more demonstrative perceptions of preventive Medicine. We pass no Ethical judgment on it. But ontologically it is restrictive, unreal, and often misleading, even occasionally by any standard ridiculous.

EXAMPLE 11.13. There is an increasing prevalence of periodontal disease in the population, and no doubt that calls for improvement in preventive dentistry. But that is not to say that the increase is in itself any cause for alarm, for there is a false premise in the enthymeme involved. To say that periodontal disease is increasing is a marginal Probability statement that disregards the change in the composition of the population. A major cause at work is that dental caries is more and more successfully prevented, so that more teeth are surviving long enough to permit the predations of periodontal disease. The same might be said about atherosclerosis, Alzheimer's disease, and many other instances. They may be showing an absolute increase because a larger proportion of the population is living to an age at which these conditions are common.

Statements of the kind "As a result of one campaign to discourage smoking, two thousand fewer people died of lung cancer" have little meaning and, without further careful commentary, are of no scientific importance. For instance, if the subjects were all centenarians, the triumph would be hollow. If we accept that life is of finite length and always will be, then if fewer people die of some particular disease, more of them must die of something else; so if preventing death is the only consideration, why, the total mortality is always going to be 100% and the whole endeavor is (tautologously) hopeless. There simply cannot be a decrease in total lifetime mortality in all diseases. That is not to deny that constantly delaying the age of death is worthwhile. But unqualified statements about mortality are simply not a useful gauge of what is happening.

To rescue the discussion from absurdity, we have to address issues other than mere mortality: change in length of life, the quality of life, the quality of death, freedom, perhaps other yet subtler, deeper, or personally significant changes.

Now, this subject is not, as may at first be supposed, at all so easy to deal with. We shall have to lay out a little detail, some of it technical but not particularly elusive, that dogs the merely rhetorical use of such terms. As might be readily imagined, it is much easier to state the principles than it is to supply the details. There are many reasons why this should be so: lack of sufficient explicit, empirical, data; lack of agreed values or means of interpreting them; the general neglect of even the most rudimentary Philosophical analysis. Our strategy will be to start with the most colorless topics and end with the general systems that allow the impact of values to be introduced, without preempting what particular systems of values there are to be intruded. In brief, the goal is again to identify and present the issues rather than to make prescriptive statements or to solve any particular Ethical problems.

CHANGE IN THE LENGTH OF LIFE

Life is lived dynamically. The lures of quietism, the tranquil, contemplative habit, the disdain for the material notwithstanding, duration is of the essence of life. It is very different from a certain kind of static art. In Keats's "Ode on a Grecian Urn" (1819), "For ever wilt thou love and she be fair" is a beautiful line. But it is the statement of a poet, and one ill and doomed to an early death, meditating on an abstraction about life rather than about life itself. The spirit of the line is the poet's total detachment from *time* as having *duration*. "For ever" does not mean "for an infinite period of time" but rather indicates that, of its nature, the work of art is outside of time. It is wholly at war with what might be called the *metabolic quiddity* of life, the fact that maintaining life in even the most economical circumstances involves minimal consumption of energy, minimal wear and tear, a minimal rate of irreversible aging.

Not only is there a finite duration to life, but this duration varies widely. Length of life is considered a variable that may be displayed on a continuous scale calibrated on the conventional time scale of physics. It is not at all wholly obvious that the physical scale is appropriate. Indeed, it is a common, albeit grossly subjective, conviction that in comparison with the measurements of the clock, time passes more quickly at some times than at others. There is no prior warrant for the view that this judgment is inferior or less relevant than physical time simply because it is subjective. But this personal component invokes a conceptual luxury that we can scarcely afford in the fragile borderland between the Probabilist's (highly individualistic) representation of Probability and the Statistician's (essentially generalized) representation. In any case, its highly subjective quality is perhaps better delegated to the discussion of the quality of life.

On these terms we must insist that duration is an inalienable part of life. Obvious, even trivial, as this claim may be, it seems to be commonly overlooked. (In the following example it must be clearly understood that we are prescinding from all Ethical issues. We are concerned only about the ontological implications.)

EXAMPLE 11.14. An argument ardently put forward against capital punishment is that it is an irreversible curtailment of life by an amount that may reasonably be equated with the expectation of life for the condemned individual — for definiteness, let us say thirty years in a particular instance. Should the executed individual subsequently be shown to be innocent, no recompense in kind can be made. The criticism is to the point, and the injustice must be regarded as a reproach to the judicial system. But if the punishment is commuted to imprisonment and the prisoner's innocence is established just as he is dying thirty years later, there is still an injustice, every bit as irremediable and every bit as much a reproach to the judicial system. Of course, it will be argued quite reasonably that total loss of life is a greater loss than loss of liberty and of those other benefits owed to a law-abiding citizen. But that is merely a matter of degree, and the force of the argument — which is purely about the impossibility of restitution — is just as strong in principle. And if the period of unjust imprisonment is five years rather than thirty, it is still wholly irremediable in kind. The gravamen of the complaint may be smaller, but the principle is just as strong.

There must be a reasonably strong presumption that the law has operated throughout competently and without malice; and that the conviction of the innocent from time to time is a sad but inevitable consequence of the limitations of knowledge and Legal inference. There must be a machinery for amending such mishaps as well as possible, a machinery that we must perhaps leave to the dictates of Legal Ethics and the practices of the law. It is in that domain that rates of exchange between the incommensurable must be negotiated. But ontologically, to equate a million dollars of recompense with five years' loss of civil liberty is obscene commercialism.

The Characterization of Length of Life

The full treatment of length of life is as a continuous Random variable that can be cast in terms of a distribution. For our most immediate and practical purposes, it does not really matter why it varies, how far it is Random, how far due to a Random generation of phenotype and how far depending on environmental and other factors. It suffices that it varies, and that attempts to predict its duration in any individual are very far from perfect. It varies and has a conventional interpretation with which we live and which in some existential sense we claim to understand. One such understanding is the criterion of the expectation of life: the simple perception that there is a difference between an expectation of seventy years and one of seventy-five years and that, other things being equal, this increase is to be applauded. With this existential understanding we shall not tamper. Expectation of life and similar gauges are ambiguous properties used differently by the Probabilist and the Statistician, and the nonspecialist cannot reasonably be expected to understand the difference. But at least we may try to exhibit the notion that the brute existential fact that the expectation has increased may make for misleading interpretations. To clarify this issue, we shall have to lay out a little theory in terms that are somewhat unusual but are designed to lead to a ready grasp.

Three Ways of Displaying Length of Life

When seen as a distribution, length of life may be displayed in three forms (Figure 11.1).

The probability density function. We are used to seeing the histogram of a series of measurements on some such variable as height. If based on indefinitely large samples and finely scaled, the histogram would be somewhat like the Probability density function (PDF) illustrated in the top panel of the figure. Age at death (or, indeed, any time-dependent variable such as the age of red cells) might be displayed in this fashion. However, in demography it is rather unusual to do so. We may take a cohort of newborn babies and present on the vertical scale the rate at which its members will be dying at any particular time in the future. That rate will be small at age five because most are healthy at that age. It will be small at age ninety-five because there will not be many members of the original population who have not already died. The rate will be at its highest at some intermediate point, termed the *mode*.

The (cumulative) distribution function. The (cumulative) distribution function (DF) illustrated in the middle panel of the figure shows the proportion of the original live-born group who will have died by any particular future age. Clearly—indeed, tautologously in a live-born population—this proportion will be zero at birth, and as age increases the proportion dead also increases. If over some interval no deaths occur, the level of the DF will remain flat; but at no point and over no interval can the DF fall with increasing age, because that could only mean that some dead people were coming

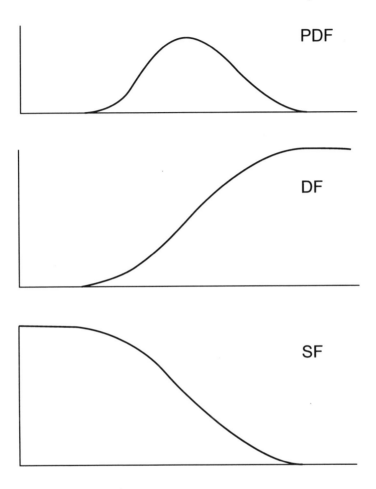

Figure 11.1   Three representations of survivorship of a cohort of subjects. *Top:* The instantaneous rate of death as a function of age (Probability density function, PDF). *Middle:* The cumulative proportion dead as a function of age (distribution function, DF). *Bottom:* The proportion surviving (survivorship function, SF), which is the mirror image of the DF.

back to life. Leaving a wide margin, we may confidently state that by age 150 all will be dead and the DF will have attained the value 1 (i.e., 100%).

The survivorship function. The survivorship function (SF) illustrated in the bottom panel of the figure shows the proportion of the original group who are still alive at any particular future age. Since all who are not dead are alive, it is clear that at any age *t,*

$$DF(t) + SF(t) = 1 = 100\%$$

That is, SF is the complement of DF. This SF is the typical "decay curve" for populations of labeled cells, enzyme activities, or the like. Many of its main properties follow at once from the DF. That is, in any region, the curve may fall or be quite flat (the latter indicating no deaths); but it cannot rise at any point or over any interval, because death is irreversible. However, the SF has an interesting further property that will greatly help understanding. The property is not difficult to prove (Murphy 1979b: 138–40) to the satisfaction of any but the strict mathematician.

• *The principle of the mean survival:* The area enclosed between SF and the two coordinate axes ("the area under the curve") is equal to the mean survival.

It follows at once that any change in mean survival will be reflected by a change in that area. So if the mean survival is increased by five years, then the area under the curve increases by five units. We shall make extensive use of these facts because they furnish a simple and vivid impression of what changes in the mean may tell us and how they may be achieved.

Note that this principle of the mean survival depends on one and only one assumption: that the mean in fact exists; and that property is assured for any individual biological system that has a finite life span.[6] Beyond that it does not matter whether the risks of dying are continuous, or intermittent, or a mixture of the two, or whether they are homogeneous in time or in space. Indeed, in real life none of these further (and unnecessary) assumptions may be safely made.

A Brief Note on Some Simple Models of Survivorship

Let us start with the simplest model of survivorship.

EXAMPLE 11.15. For soldiers in battle doing the same task, the risk of being hit by a bomb or a bullet is no respecter of age. If the rate of bombardment is constant, the risk of being hit will follow the exponential curve (familiar from radioactive decay curves).

The *model of homogeneous risk of death in continuous time*, or *exponential model*, that we have just used may be generalized in various ways. Death may occur after and only after a succession of such hits that are indepen-

---

6. Since there are still animals (including human beings) that continue to exist, the whole story is not available, and it is not at all clear that survivorship of the animal kingdom as a whole is finite.

dent and identically distributed. This is the *gamma process*. The folk belief that an English cat has nine lives means that its survivorship should follow a gamma process of order nine. (The Spanish cat has seven lives.) If the risks are not necessarily homogeneous, then we speak more generally of a *nine-hit process* (or the international version, a *multiple-hit process*). Unlike the simple exponential process, multiple-hit processes of all kinds "have a memory" (i.e., the past history of the animal still alive influences the distribution of its further survival). If the past history depends solely or partly on imperceptible wear and tear—old cats may, for example, become less agile—we may use the yet more general term *Erlangian process*. If there are two or more processes of which at least two are more complicated than exponential, and death ensues when any one of them is completed, we have a *bingo process*. If, for example, death results after the heart has sustained eight episodes at homogeneous risk or the brain four such episodes or the kidney twenty, then survivorship is a *gamma-bingo process* (i.e., death results from whichever of several independent gamma processes is completed first). Such models may be endlessly elaborated. There is good reason to think that human survivorship exhibits these various features.

EXAMPLE 11.16. The survivorship of blood platelets in acute thrombophlebitis, which is very harmful to them, conforms to the exponential distribution (Abrahamsen 1968); and we reasonably infer that they are destroyed indiscriminately of their ages or past encounters. However, when the thrombophlebitis has subsided, the pattern of decay is more like that expected when cumulative wear and tear bear on future chances, the kind of pattern due to cumulative effects of multiple insults (multiple-hit or, more generally, Erlangian processes). It is general experience that the Erlangian pattern is the usual one exhibited by platelets in ordinary functioning (Murphy and Francis 1971; Belcher et al. 1977; Hill-Zobel et al. 1982).

EXAMPLE 11.17. It is an evident, even commonsense, view of human life that aging leads to death and is itself caused by repeated insults from the wear and tear of living. The pattern, however, is analytically rather more complex, for again common, primitive, experience tells us that the patients "die from what kills them." Sometimes it is the heart that reaches the end of its tether first; sometimes the kidneys, or the liver, or the nervous system, or the lungs, or the blood. All of them are perpetually under some kind of attack. The length of life, then, is the time it takes until the first of many separate and competing processes fails. As we noted above, this constitutes the so-called bingo model (Murphy, Trojak, et al. 1981).

Indeed, it is difficult to imagine a rational biological model of survival that cannot be classed under some version or another of this model. The properties of this model explain much of the enigmatic detail encountered in human survival patterns. Its details are rather complicated to expound and would be quite out of place here. In any case, what follows requires nothing more complicated than the principle of the mean survival. Parenthetically we remind the reader that the bingo model, unlike noncompeting Erlangian processes, may be negatively skewed (see Example 4.7).

The mean survival. While the mean survival enjoys some popularity, we may anticipate by saying that it is of limited use as a descriptor, and indeed may frankly mislead.

EXAMPLE 11.18. Consider, for instance, robust and healthy men and women of twenty who learn that in the last thirty years the mean length of life has increased by five years. They commonly perceive this information as meaning that instead of dying at, say, seventy-two, they will die at seventy-seven. They see that increase as five more years of disability and imperfect health, and they view it with little enthusiasm. If the meaning were as stated, they might have a point (even though those now aged seventy-two would perhaps not wholly agree). But in fact the meaning that they are attaching to it is highly misleading, as we shall try to make clear. To do so, however, we shall have to elucidate a few points.

The principle of the mean survival is based on the convention that the initial value of the SF (i.e., the value at birth) is 1, or unity, or 100%. If we were to express it as 100 percentile units, the number of units of area would be 100 times as many; and to find the mean number of years, we should then have to divide the area by 100. In general, if the initial value were set at B units (instead of 1) and the area under the curve were A units, the mean survival would be A/B. Now, suppose we set B at 5,000, the number in a cohort of babies; the mean survival would be $A/5,000$. If we change B by excluding the number (e.g., 200) of stillborn babies (who would obviously contribute nothing to the area under the curve), then the mean survival in *live-born* babies would be $A/4,800$, which would obviously be greater by about 4%. If we excluded babies born with congenital defects from which they are likely to die early, we would have to decrease both A and B; but since the contribution of the babies eliminated to the area under the curve is much smaller than average, the mean survival would again be increased. By an extension of this idea, at any age we could determine the *mean further survival* by dividing the remaining area under the curve by the number of people surviving to that age, and it may be clear that the greater the age at which we do that calculation, the smaller B will be and the greater the mean total survival (i.e., age lived so far plus the mean number of years of further survival).

Now, consider survivorship in live-born children. The typical pattern of the SF (Figure 11.2) shows the following features. There is a moder-

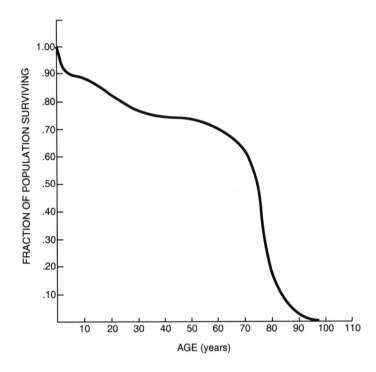

Figure 11.2   A schematic representation of the SF in an advanced society, not drawn to scale. Details vary. There is a fairly abrupt fall in the first year—indeed, mainly in the first few months—due to disorders (e.g., infections) and anomalies that allow the infant to exist only precariously, if at all, outside the mother's body. There is a second fall in adolescence, which is here exaggerated for clarity, and then fairly steady survival until the sixties, when vital organs that have been repeatedly insulted begin to fail. The death rate at any age depends on both personal hazards and the numbers at risk; hence the flattening out of the curve at the older ages. The logarithm of the SF plotted against time would show that the hazard increases for all ages over sixty.

ate, but fairly sharp, drop in the first year of life, which largely reflects the deaths of infants who manage to survive in utero but are ill equipped to survive outside after birth. The abrupt mortality at birth reflects not so much the harshness of the world outside as the fact that certain patterns of physiology—mainly nutrition and oxygenation—change over within seconds at birth from one system (the umbilical cord) to direct provision by the alimentary and respiratory tracts. There are also striking changes in the operation of the cardiovascular system. This abrupt fall reduces SF sharply with little loss in area. As a result, there is the anomalous fact that the mean *further* survival at age one is higher than the mean total survival at birth.

Beyond the first year, the decay in SF is slow. It is true that there are deaths from genetic disorders in infancy such as fibrocystic disease or Tay-Sachs disease; but in a general unselected population, such disorders are rare enough to have little impact on the whole. In adolescence there is something of a further drop, due to car accidents and trauma generally, suicide, homicide, and (increasingly) AIDS. Although this drop must not be exaggerated, it is generally held that these deaths are in principle preventable. The further decay of SF is comparatively slow, but the age-specific death rate increases rather sharply and steeply after age sixty-five, more so in men than in women. The actual decay flattens out eventually, but that is because while the age-specific death rate goes up, its absolute impact is reduced simply because the number of people at risk is also decreasing.

Now, against this background consider some of the many ways in which the mean survival in, say, live-born children might show an increase (or decrease) of five years. Any possible change requires two conditions to be fulfilled: first, that the total area under the curve be increased or decreased by five years; and second, that SF cannot increase at any point or have a positive slope, although it may remain unchanged.

EXAMPLE 11.19. It is theoretically possible for the mean to be increased five years by the SF being moved bodily from the origin five years to the right (Figure 11.3A). This would mean that there were no deaths and no deterioration between ages zero and five. Given that the starting value of SF is 1, the increase in area (represented in the figure as shaded) will equal that of a rectangle of sides 1 and 5. This theoretical Sleeping Beauty change is, of course, quite unreasonable unless the ill effects of genetic disorders and birth defects could be suspended for five years, and the occurrence of wear and tear be arrested for the same time and correspondingly delayed throughout life. But the illustration shows in principle how misleading it is to suppose (as the healthy young in Example 11.18 did) that the extra years are merely added only in old age.

Let us take a rather less fanciful scenario.

EXAMPLE 11.20. It is possible that preventive measures increase mean survival by five years because of improved survival in adolescents and young adults. The SF is displaced upward between ages ten and forty (Figure 11.3B). At the end of that time there will be more people at risk from the other causes, so the total mortality from them is higher, and at a later age the new survivorship coincides with the old one. So what has been gained in the population is an increased enjoyment of the years of youth and middle age, presumably what the healthy young appreciate.

EXAMPLE 11.21. Another pattern would be one in which the measures have no impact on the mortality in the young, but morbidity in them is

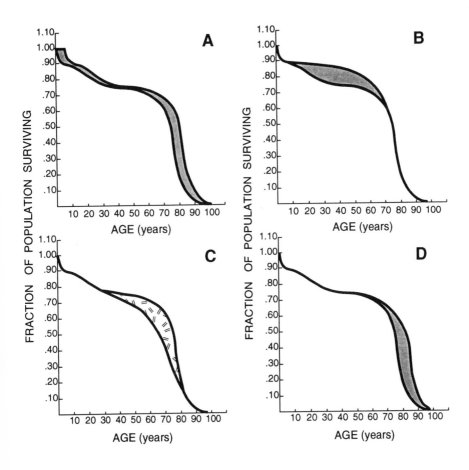

Figure 11.3   Some patterns in which a five-year change in mean survival might occur. In each diagram the control SF and the changed SF are plotted. A shaded area signifies an increase in survivorship relative to the control SF; a stippled area signifies a decreased expectation of life. *A:* The changed SF has the same shape as the standard SF but is displaced bodily from it by five years in the positive direction. No death occurs in the first five years. *B:* The changed SF results from a decreased mortality rate between the ages of ten and forty, and thereafter an increased mortality, so that the two curves fuse again by age seventy. *C:* There is a loss in survivorship of five years in late middle life. *D:* There is no change in survival until age sixty, after which expectation of life is increased.

increased and leads to aggravation of the mortality in diseases that have a long latent period. Such diseases include cancers, diabetes, coronary atherosclerosis, and hypertension. Perhaps the "high living" that leads to high vitality in youth is a threat to old age. One thinks of those who play serious football in college but run to fat in middle life. The result is an average loss of five years' survivorship in late middle life (Figure 11.3C).

———

The main benefit may be in forestalling diseases that occur still later in life.

EXAMPLE 11.22. Recent retrospective studies by Breitner and his associates (1994) in twins have shown that the use of anti-inflammatory drugs for other purposes delays and decreases the lifetime risk of Alzheimer's disease, especially in women. The typical age group for this disorder is sixty or older. Figure 11.3D shows a five-year increase in mean survival distributed from age sixty onward.

The variance. Examples 11.18 to 11.22 have (rather insidiously) introduced quality of life, though simply as a means of stressing that there is more to consider in interpreting survivorship than black-box statements about mean survival. But even ignoring quality of life, there remains the question of where an extra five years might be spent; and the diversity of the possible answers is not reflected in the mean. There are all manner of other measurements, each with its own implications and meanings. One of these measurements is the variance or (in more general terms) the distribution in the length of life.

EXAMPLE 11.23. The scatter could be abolished altogether: all subjects might die at exactly the same age. The form of the SF is then rectangular, the upper limit of which is exactly the mean survival (Figure 11.4). We ourselves regard this as quite unreal, implying as it does that death is a totally deterministic process at absolutely zero risk at any age below the mean, and at that point at infinite risk. Death is something like an alarm clock going off. However, we must record that there are some gerontologists who believe this pattern to be an ideal that can at least be aimed at (Fries 1980).[7] Gavrilov and Gavrilova (1986: 112 ff.) critically evaluate both the theoretical issues and the empirical information. They explicitly note that the changes in survivorship in recent years, far from tending toward the extreme "rectangular" pattern shown in Figure 11.4, are showing a progressive "derectangularization," in that the upper (higher age) tail of the curve is becoming more extended than ever.

7. The only possible interpretation of such a SF would be that all subjects lived to exactly the same age. It turn, that could mean one of three things: (1) All are impervious to genetic and environmental factors. (2) These factors act in such a way (by regeneration, homeostasis, etc.) as to cancel each other's effects. For instance, there might be accidental injuries, which would be perfectly corrected by reparative mechanisms, but there would be neither permanent injuries nor deaths due to accidents. (3) Because of sheer multiplicity of effects, asymptotic convergence to all pertinent parameters is guaranteed. For instance, if survival were the composite effect of multiple gamma processes, the order of gamma would be so large that the coefficient of variation for each would be virtually zero. Though technically possible, these imaginative assumptions do not commend themselves to serious scholarship.

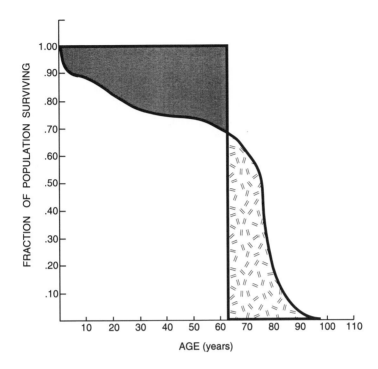

Figure 11.4   The relationship of the mean to the SF. The standard SF is shown, and superimposed is a rectangle drawn such that the shaded and stippled areas (see Figure 11.3) are equal. The rectangle corresponds to the survival curve, with the same mean as the standard SF but with no variance in the age at death.

Further and more sophisticated parameters. It should be noted, however, that in any real population no matter how carefully studied, to know the mean and the variance exactly is, in general, insufficient to reconstruct the form of the curve. The unarticulated assumption that the mean and the variance are sufficient information is a legacy of the slavish use of the well-known Gaussian ("normal") distribution. Other explicit models call for information on the specifications (the *parameters*), or the use of equivalent forms, well known to the theorist, such as generating functions and other transforms.

The hazard function. The specifying device of the hazard function provides a formula, as a function of time, for the instantaneous risk in the fraction of the population not previously destroyed. It is approximated by the epidemiologist's notion of the age-dependent mortality rate. The exponential function, for instance, has an unvarying hazard, so that if at any age the function is rescaled to 100% (unity), the future pattern of survival is exactly the same for old individuals that have survived so far as for totally new individuals.

There have been attempts to describe the empirical survival curve in human beings by ingenious devices like the hazard function of Makeham (1860), which proves fairly accurate. However, the biologist will object that this function is merely a clever actuarial trick that is purely descriptive and has no heuristic value whatsoever. That is, it leads to no insights as to how the causal components might be interpreted, explored, evaluated, or modified. It is like having a beautifully carved box that is jet black. Any attempt to translate this conjectural hazard function into literal biological assumptions seems to lead to absurdity.

Authentic modeling. The preferred method of describing the SF is to devise a tractable model that aims to capture the known biology of the system and translate it, term by term, into a mathematical form while preserving the qualities of at least approximate interpretation. The bingo-gamma model (i.e., survivorship determined by the time to completion of the first of several independently operating multiple-hit models at constant risk) gives a pattern very similar to human survivorship. In that sense it is a success. But paradoxically that outcome is epistemically perhaps even more dismaying, for the bingo model is founded on biologically plausible, even compelling, but minimal assumptions; and we reasonably suppose that the actual individual components are of a much more complex pattern. Yet the fit is already so good that we can hardly hope for any much better fit from a fuller and more explicit model. The model, taken as a whole, works too well and is Statistically not powerful enough to allow the individual components to be explored and tested. It illustrates well the epistemic tension. However, too much should not be made of this shortcoming. As in the faithful exploration of any complicated pattern, the remedy is to break up the problem into manageably small parts and study, for instance, the survival patterns in each of the organ systems separately. This strategy is permitted here by the nature of the model (which is already shown to be compatible with the data); but it is not workable in Makeham's clever, but purely actuarial, device.

LIFE AS A CONTINUOUS VARIABLE: QUALITY

Apart from hints here and there, we have so far ignored the fact that life is a state that has value. Moreover, that quality varies from time to time, has vastly heterogeneous components, and exhibits systematic and Random variation. No reputable Ethical analysis can ignore that authentic feature, even if some writers in some cases attach overwhelming weight to naive and unconditional issues of choice. Again, we make our strong affirmation that we are not proposing any Ethical solutions or even evaluations.

Our examples are intended not as recommendations or even as hints of our own preferences, but rather as explorations in unearthing and introducing quality in particular cases.

EXAMPLE 11.24. How is life in the deaf to be evaluated? Deafness is perceived as a disability that seems usually to be accepted as the price for continued existence. But there are some few people who are, in a sense, protected from distractions by deafness. For instance, Beethoven's deafness was no impediment to the almost apocalyptic quality of his later compositions (notably the last group of string quartets). It might be argued that had his experiential knowledge included developments in the physics of the piano as a musical instrument, it might have inhibited the boldness of his writing; instead, his compositions stimulated the piano manufacturers to greater feats of design. Likewise, one thinks of the remarkable blind organists in the Parisian tradition who in some way not readily perceived by the sighted seem to have capitalized on their disability in their remarkable skill in improvisation. Or again, there is a long tradition of blind poets, not those such as Milton to whom it was incidental, but those like Homer to whom it was perhaps of the essence because of the demands it made on his memory. These instances are merely some of the many in which shallow appraisal of values may be profoundly misleading. It is a not uncommon criticism of scholars that they read too much while they savor and reflect too little.

To presume to express this perplexing issue of value under the slick term *quality of life* experienced moment by moment only is to miss much of the point.

EXAMPLE 11.25. A great part of the satisfaction lies in the detailed carrying out of long-term strategy. Enjoyment of excellence in some intensely physical sport is something that may take ten or fifteen years to achieve, years of denial and effort that contrast with the slovenly ease of those who seek only instant satisfaction. Yet the champion figure-skater, the tennis player, the swimmer, the sprinter, may be past the peak by age thirty and may expect thereafter nothing but decline. All know of athletes who, at high risk of lethal damage to the liver as well as to professional honor, have been prepared to take anabolic steroids, trading one hour of glorious fame for an age without a name. Again, there is mounting evidence of the risk, especially in women, of the athlete, or more generally the professional celebrity, intensely preoccupied about surplus weight, ultimately losing control and succumbing to anorexia nervosa and premature death.

The serious academic scholar reckons maturity to be something attained much later,[8] at the age of perhaps fifty, with a decline in the seven-

8. Mathematicians seem to be a notable exception.

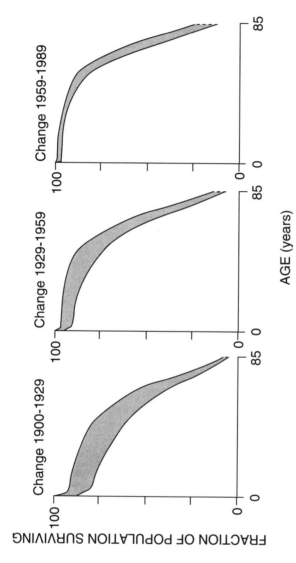

Figure 11.5   Changes in survival pattern in white males in the twentieth century. In each diagram the upper limit is the curve for survivorship at the end of the era indicated, and the lower limit that at the beginning (which, in turn, is the upper limit for the previous period). It is evident that gains in early and middle life dominated the improvements early in the century but that the recent gains have been greatest in middle and later life.

ties. This goal represents mortgage of a much greater part of one's life, and a greater irrecoverable forfeit of life seen by those concerned, yet judged by them a fair price to pay. A year or so of one's youth lost in some blind alley, which the scholar might genially "chalk up to experience," would to the athlete seem a major setback.

How may we view this set of values in terms of survival? Those who cash their survivorship bonuses at once take none of the risks of investment and live only for the present. Those seeking physical prowess accept the risks of failure and live with their prospect of reaching maturity as athletes, musicians, or craftsmen in mind. Those pursuing academic careers perceive that, to stand any chance of scholarly achievement, years of patient and perhaps even physically dangerous toil and deprivation are needed, and they will not merely curtail immediate pleasure, rich rewards, even health, but will carefully husband the remnants of life thereafter when they are mellowed and respected scholars. The extra five years between seventy-two and seventy-seven (which the physical and healthy young view with contempt, even apprehension) may be treasure beyond price to the late-maturing.

Dr. Helen Abbey pointed out to us two matters that bear on survivorship and excellence (Figure 11.5). In the past, the toll on the young was severe, because of the poor quality of hygiene: diet, ignorance, malnutrition, infection, inadequate warmth and clothing, abuse, industrial labor, and the like. These deficiencies were largely remediable, and between the start of the Industrial Revolution and perhaps 1940, the SF in childhood and young adult life was greatly enhanced. But the most striking change was effected by the introduction of antibiotics, which for the first time greatly improved survivorship in the elderly. At present, Dr. Abbey pointed out, if all mortality below the age of thirty were eliminated, the increase in expectation of total life would be not more than two to three years. Clearly there is limited scope for improvement there.

For the rest, we apologize for making so much of these commonplace notions. However, they show that people have various ambitions, and that to achieve them they adopt quite diverse strategies in life, including their patterns for husbanding health and even survival. Arguably, given the choice of how to appropriate some fixed expectation of life, the various kinds of people might make very different choices. To counterbalance the policy of instant gratification, there is the shift in how age is perceived. In 1300, Dante, then aged thirty-five, began his *Divine Comedy* by identifying himself as middle-aged.[9] In the American Constitution the age qualification for being a senator—that is, a (wise) old man—is still thirty-five. In 1912, E. C. Bentley could refer to Mr. Cupples, "nearly sixty years old," as "wiry and active for his age . . . a retired banker"—in fact, a picture of arrested

9. "Nel mezzo del cammin di nostra vita" (In the middle of the road of our life) (Dante 1300: *Inferno* 1.1.).

decrepitude. Dixon McCunn, the elderly hero of John Buchan's *House of Four Winds* (1935), was a retired grocer, aged sixty. The point is that most people do not form their images of "middle-aged," "elderly," and so forth from vital statistics, but from what they have experienced socially. An abstract Ethical point of view directed to promoting survival as an absolute, homogeneous value, without due attention to the choices of individual persons, is a travesty. For the ethicist to arrogate the moral power to prescribe this disposable expectation according to the goals of the individual would be a slight improvement, but not much. While we may agree that there are values involved and even that, in principle at least, there must ultimately be a way of measuring them, it would be idle to suppose either that most people have a single ambition without compromise or that, given multiple, even conflicting, ambitions, it is a simple matter for the external evaluator to set a rate of exchange among the values.

The Domain of Freedom in Survival

It seems likely to us that catering to the perceived need of the individual is a personal choice to be evaluated and exercised in the domain of freedom. In this book so far we have not put much stress on freedom. We perceive that it is an issue of major, even overwhelming, importance that we shall have to return to later. At the same time, we have ontological concerns, first as to how the term is to be defined, how it may operate, what the conditions of its operation may be; and beyond those concerns, the much more intricate epistemic problem of how far we might gauge freedom to be involved in any decision. We shall present a brief discussion of how it may be guarded from abuse.

First, freedom operates in the domain of truth. This principle, though sound enough, is dangerous and open to gross abuses. However (to pinpoint one item), it seems to us to be the principal warrant for compulsory education. Granted that freedom is not merely a rich and treasured luxury characteristic of humanity, but also a matter that in some degree has been demanded by the needs of every society, it has loomed large in the general theory of rights. The latter topic has little bearing on this book (see Appendix 3). The idea of education (or, to be more precise, de facto education) is something that is resented and resisted by most children. The claim is made that by compelling children to be educated, one is promoting freedom, the main putative purpose of education. This principle is so profoundly paradoxical as to leave us perplexed unless we accept the claim that knowledge and disciplined understanding are a great part of freedom itself, although they clearly cannot be all of it. But as we discussed earlier and at length (Chapter 7), effective freedom is constrained by truth, and that relationship cannot be tampered with.

Second, truth is discovered, not invented. We do not say or imply that it is easy to discover or that what is discovered empirically is ever altogether secure. Yet however cautious we are about the claim, there is reasonable assurance that on the whole our existential grasp of truth makes progress. There is a danger that a pretentious concern with safeguarding the truth may be used as an excuse for making authentic freedom of choice inaccessible to the individual. That strategy puts an impossible load on the quality and fidelity of the perceived truth. Much, far too much, of tragedy in human history has been due to the pushing of truth or (more significantly) what purports to be truth; and the custodians have abused their limited powers too often to encourage us to have much trust in them. It seems to us that however grievous these abuses in the past, the risk is currently as great as ever, or greater, for the current abuses are based on two specious assumptions masquerading as truth themselves: that the confines of empirical science set the limits on all truth, which, if a mistaken view, is at least honest; and the much more insidious, because manifestly unwarranted, claim that the truths pertinent to empirical science are adequately known. The first assumption ruthlessly excludes much that has long been tested and applauded, in the fields of art and esthetics, law, Morals, politics, sentiment, religious belief, and much more. The second assumption is related to what purports to be truth in the conclusions reached from limited data and vulnerable inference from empirical science. The assumption is that these propositions are in no way answerable to criticisms that may be leveled against them even by serious scientists—that any persons who take issue with them can only be on the side of obscuration. As a result, it opens the door to shallow merchandising of the most precarious speculations by the bigot. The explicit criticisms by Feynman (1989), a distinguished physicist,[10] of the abuse and misuse of the syllabus of education, as decreed by those in power, should foster some serious doubts in those who can bring themselves to examine his complaints.

Third, there is a tension between the individual and society in the apprehension of truth. On the one hand, it is well argued that in making free decisions, the individual is obliged to pay attention to relevant truth. Society has some right to give the individual access to that truth and is itself under obligation to discover and discern what that truth is. We can accord no respect to educational policy that substitutes for honest scholarship devious propaganda advanced for meretricious purposes.

On the other hand, ultimately personal freedom can operate only within that part of the domain of truth that may be existentially appropriated by the individual acting. The limitations of human understanding of truth may be wider than the power of individuals to understand the truth and its relevance to their own lives. What purports to be truth must also leave room for the operation of the illative sense and for phronesis (qq.v).

---

10. On his own admission, not without his blind spots and his prejudices.

A Note on Expectation and Realization

Before we leave the topic of survivorship we must clarify a distinction that has been glossed over in the foregoing sections. If the exact outcome were known in advance, the individual might choose to change the grand strategy.

EXAMPLE 11.26. If a girl of fifteen with both physical prowess at skating and intellectual talent for Philosophy knew that because of some latent genetic disorder, she would never reach thirty years of age, she might decide to make the most of the skating; and conversely if survival to age seventy were assured. But usually that prescience does not exist, there are inescapable uncertainties, and then the decision must in effect be a wager. Of course, it is not a totally blind guess but one that will make the most of what information is available. There will be different outlooks for different combinations of familial, environmental, and other conditions. The gymnast or the swimmer might aim for the pattern shown in Figure 11.3B. The ambition to attain deep scholarship will require a prolonged training, so naturally it calls for a fair chance of attaining that age. Thus, for a given mean length of life, it would be appropriate to forgo much of the increased Probability of surviving to the age of fifty enjoyed in the population of Figure 11.3B, and to enjoy an enhanced Probability of surviving to age eighty as in the population of Figure 11.3D. The golfer, an athlete with a long career through middle age, may elect an intermediate pattern.

We need hardly labor the point that *the option is exercised in the plan only, not in the outcome.* If would-be Philosophers die young, then they have lost the bet, but of course some will survive and may go on to great things. But those who pursue a career in professional boxing may live a life of prosperity, but because of repeated head injuries they would be seriously reducing all prospects of ever being serious scholars. (We say nothing of their other possible disabilities.) At the present time, these, or elaborations of them to include variance and whatnot, are the only terms in which we can grapple with the problem of choice.

Now, of course, in any particular case the outcome is a success or a failure; and the question of what the three Brontë sisters or Evariste Galois or Schubert or Keats might have achieved if they had lived to the age of seventy is a matter of historical sentiment only, for in fact they all died early—all of them, perhaps, because of careless and avoidable risks. Now, on the principle that the outcome in any one individual is what it is, and that there are unaccountable differences between any two individuals, it is easy to slip into irresolvable nihilism. On the other hand, if we force all individuals into one class, subject to what the crass call inalienable principles, then we trample all over personal sovereignty and turn our backs on anything that distinguishes one individual from another. If we go to the other extreme of fanatical obsession with individuality, then negotiating on these terms, tautologously, we have no fund of experience on which to base reasonable predictions, and hence no wisdom to offer the individual in counseling. Nevertheless, we can salvage these Probabilistic structures for Ethical discourse, if in using them we are prepared to forgo the extremes. That is equivalent to supposing that the fates for many individuals, in prospect as in retrospect, are not totally disparate. The ethicists are engaged not in fortunetelling but in promulgating carefully husbanded collective wisdom for ready uses in many cases. They are to do so in such a way that the individual's personal characteristics are taken seriously into consideration; that is, they have to grapple with a problem of innumerable individual cases inside a system of secure and parsimonious dimensionality.

Finally, we may note that Ethics is operating on its own terms but using the best scientific information that is available. Setting aside the question of how far Ethics is mutable and subject to change, there is no doubt that what purports to be the best scientific information is a moving target, for science of its very nature is tentative and perpetually subject to amendment. Even the most practical Ethics, then, should not be so structured as to make amending it (in the light of improvement of knowledge as a result of perceptive iteration between theory and data) impossible, or even cumbersome. No doubt it would be an impertinence for us to presume to instruct ethicists on that obvious point. However, our audience for that statement is not ethicists but the "sea lawyers" who, having once heard an ethicist's judgment in a particular case, imagine that it is a final and irreformable opinion about an unspecified class of similar cases.

With that preliminary discussion we may make bold to address our last topic, by far the most subtle, the most readily suspected of casuistical deviousness, and the most difficult to apply in any practical decision. It should not be necessary to say yet once again that what follows is not an attempt to make any kind of Ethical prescription. But we insist that *insofar as Ethics makes an authentic appeal to any aspect of life other than life's primordial existence or nonexistence, it cannot convincingly escape the elements that follow.*

THE OPTIMIZATION OF EXISTENCE

Life has not only order but also duration, to which we may for convenience assign the conventional designation of physical time, t. The number of the issues to be taken into consideration is, in principle, infinitely divisible. For simplicity we start by supposing them twofold: value of life as seen by the individual concerned, and that as seen by others. Then we may suppose that there are two functions of t denoting time (or age): namely, $p(t)$, the personal perception of value of the life, and $s(t)$, the outside or ex-

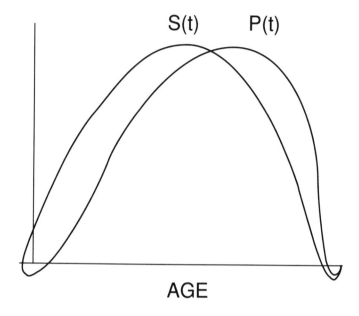

Figure 11.6   A schematic display of the quality of common enjoyment of life; *p(t)* is the personal viewpoint of the subject, *s(t)* that of associates. In our view, society sees pregnancy and birth as occasions of joy but the baby's escape from warm squalor into a cold world as unpleasant. Society sees most members as peaking rather earlier than the members themselves do and feels the burden of care of them rather earlier. The assessment is, of course, arbitrary and disputable. What matters is that the pattern is age-dependent, and that there are internal and external views, both of which need to be taken into consideration in Ethical evaluations.

ternal or social value of the life. They may be represented as functions of age (Figure 11.6).

Clearly the mathematical values of these functions may be positive or negative. Positive values would be largely a matter of well-being and the sense of usefulness, negative ones the patient's view that "life is not worth living" and the external view that the patient would be "better off out of it all." Neither catch phrase is to be taken as having any serious Ethical weight. The attitude may, for instance, be a matter of mood or the run of environmental experiences and pressures. For instance, there may be some stage at which a patient is undergoing a surgical procedure that is uncomfortable, debilitating, and incapacitating, and in which the sole merit is the hope for serious improvement in the future. But the long-term outcome might be excellent.

There will in general be a pervading agreement in the order of the numerical values for the two functions, but they are certainly not identical. At the outset, there is no clear evidence one way or the other whether the fetus derives any satisfaction. Probably there is none to the parents. The newborn baby will so far have derived nothing but discomfort from the birth and will not share the delight of the parents at a successful outcome. Even for the parents, a major gratification is the prospect of years of pleasure from the child. We may reasonably represent $p(0)$ as negative and $s(0)$ as positive. Both will increase in a diverse and complicated fashion. A decrepit old age may again yield negative values, perhaps rather earlier in $s(t)$. And at death, time d, the (earthly) account for the individual will be closed, and aside from an expected bereavement, $s(t)$ will also become zero. So the starting and the finishing values will be the same, zero, for both functions.

The adaptation of these ideas to Ethical inquiry would not be an easy matter. We would accept readily enough that both the individual and society are parties at interest. Society may reasonably lavish more care on individuals of widespread importance than on others, although we recognize that the details of that argument would be a hornet's nest of controversy. The converse of it would be to give the criminal less consideration than the law-abiding. An orderly system of judgment would, of course, be to construct an Ethical function $E(t)$ by taking both lines of argument into consideration in some superfunction $H\{\cdot\}$:

$$E(t) = H\{p(t), s(t)\}$$

However, it is not at all clear what an appropriate superfunction would be. Obvious simple suggestions would be to act on their weighted sum

$$E(t) = m \cdot p(t) + n \cdot s(t)$$

(where m and n are arbitrary constants), or their product, or some such relationship. A better case might be

$$E(t) = \int_t^\infty H[p(t), s(t)] \, dt$$

where the limits of integration are set by the present time and any time after the patient is dead.

Commentary

These final issues fall squarely in the domain of Ethics and outside our self-appointed domain of discourse, namely, the contribution that Medicine and science can make to coherent Ethical analysis. That terse dismissal leaves us open to the charge that we break the backs of the ethicists by first devising a horrendous challenge and then leaving all the hard work for them to do. We acknowledge the force of the rejoinder and sympathize. However, we are moved to three comments.

First, Medical Ethics will gain nothing in either depth or respect if the elusive sensibilities of some Medical ethicists are responsible to nothing but the elusive subtleties of other Medical ethicists; and if all incisive dialogue with science and Medicine is cut short, as if it were in the nature of things that black-box Ethical analysis is preferable to white. Above all, this strategy would in the long run do nothing to cement the relationships between Medicine and Medical Ethics.

Second, Medical ethicists, we freely recognize and sustain, have a grievance if scientists and clinicians should arrogate to themselves the right either to propose an arbitrary system of values of their own or (what is perhaps worse) to impose some measurement (e.g., the numbers of days spent in hospital per year, or the amount of productive work done by the individual), the main epistemic value of which is the fact that it is measurable, without serious thought about its meaning, implications, and so forth. For this reason we back off from the analysis at what is the farthest point we can go without introducing prescribed explicit values. The main motive is not faintheartedness but respect for the ethicists' professional perceptions.

Finally, we express in principle our readiness to try to bridge the hiatus and to collaborate with Medical ethicists in a fruitful dialogue. Moreover, as reassurance, we recall an earlier passage in which we explained what we mean by *dialogue*. (A fuller and more explicit statement of terms is given in Chapter 16, footnote 1.) The terms of not only the arguments but the method of argumentation must be acceptable to both sides. The scope for the dialogue does not have to be that given above, which is used by some decision theorists. However, if there are to be radical changes, it seems evident that to attain the dignity of a formal component, the notion of values will demand a much more detailed and explicit ontological analysis than we have given so far.

12 Pain and Suffering

No serious Ethical analysis may ignore pain and suffering. In our role as Medical and scientific caterers to Medical Ethics, we may not neglect them either. But it must be admitted at the outset that the task is a difficult one, almost uniquely difficult. Before we get seriously to work, we must first deal with impediments that, although not really of the essence, nonetheless befog any articulate approach to it.

THE TABOOS ON PAIN AND SUFFERING

In these days of frank and explicit portrayal in the theater and kindred arts, it is usually forgotten that originally the word *obscene (ob-scene)* meant not fit to be portrayed on the stage. Thus, strictly, an "obscene play" is a contradiction in terms. In this aboriginal sense both pain and suffering are also obscene topics. They are certainly part of the authentic reality of life. Monumental industries thrive on offering relief from them. We may take for granted that all our readers have personal knowledge of them. The cry of the infant is a call for rescue from need, discomfort, pain; and the cries cause anything from discomfort to distress in the nearby adult. Such experiences are indeed so matter-of-course that none will recall their first encounters with either pain or suffering. Yet this familiarity does not help us to address them; quite the contrary. At the outset, our attempts are so festooned with emotion as to make rational discussion precarious and to undermine any useful approach to austere evaluation.

But there are greater difficulties. Pain is distressing, as grief, bereavement, and disability, physical or mental, are. Long before any conscious experiences of any of them, and long before any notion about the nature of compassion and sympathy, social pressures arm the superego with taboos against these topics. Jokes about them, for instance, offend. A curious exception is the jokes told by the sufferers about themselves, for humor is part of a general device of protection against distress, and jokes against oneself are often taken as a sign of a carefree bravery (Maugham 1938: 42 ff.). Thus, Saint Lawrence during his martyrdom by roasting on a gridiron is applauded for his sally that it was time they turned him over and did his other side; or Charles II could apologize for being "an unconscionably long time a-dying"; or Oscar Wilde, solaced in his last hours with a glass of champagne, could remark that he was dying beyond his means. But for anybody else to have made such jokes would be deplorable.

This disapproval is reinforced, in the case of pain, by the shadow of vice. Inflicting pain was the most unseemly of the sexual perversions of de Sade and, for all we know, of many of those attending the festive events of the Roman Colosseum. There is a common belief, of what provenance we cannot say, that inflicting pain is a vice among professional torturers and among those who are morbidly attracted by details of torture.

But beyond all these gross perversions there lies a more elusive condemnation, and one that is much more difficult to overcome because not unfounded. There is an earthy saying "It is easy to bear the other chap's pain"—as, indeed, it is easy to bear his poverty or his grief. There is a spurious fellow-feeling that does not speak of love or kindness to the needy but of formulas that advocate eleemosynary organizations to distribute surplus goods to the economically disadvantaged: "The easy speeches that comfort cruel men" (Chesterton 1906). Yet revulsion at this dainty, antiseptic philanthropy can itself lead to distorted protest, so that even to talk or write in wholly dispassionate terms about these distresses is condemned as a heartless display, as if no Philosopher or pharmacologist or mystic had any acquaintance with distress; or as if every surgeon operated for a perverse pleasure of cutting human flesh or breaking human bones. These accusations are rarely warranted. Certainly any bizarre exceptions are deplored.

Yet it is certainly true that a competent practice of Medicine, even an unreflective and unanalytical one, becomes possible only by cultivating a clinical detachment. The nature and function of this detachment are apt to be misunderstood by those who have never had to confront unending professional contact with illness, distress, grief, and often too their witless causes, ignorance and stupidity. But here we must recognize that in the ideal clinician and Medical scholar, at least, primitive sympathy is displaced by a far deeper concern over suffering. An effort to understand pain in its depth, coldly and dispassionately, has much more to offer than weeping and the wringing of hands. But it is much less indulgently perceived by shallow and impressionable minds.

Even so, there is the taunt that the dispassionate scholars come by their answers cheap. When pharmacologists, without more to do, undertake studies of a new drug that just might produce more relief than distress by properly controlled trials (which inevitably means withholding it from some of the patients), such procedures are too readily supposed heartless commerce in human suffering. (The protesters in their sentimentality too easily forget the horrendous side effects that may occur with another thalidomide.)[1] A Darwinist or a population geneticist may usefully explore the question of what the advantage of pain may be or how a population is the better for experiencing collective grief, and wonder how such questions might bear on the constructive management of these vicissitudes without doing more harm than good. But those asking such questions would be wise to do so behind closed doors if they would escape the anathema of those who see themselves as the champions of humanistic compassion.

THE ANALYTICAL INACCESSIBILITY OF PAIN

Existential knowledge of pain is at once vivid and visceral rather than articulate and analytical. The word *visceral* here is, of course, metaphorical; but not entirely. The pains that arise from viscera, in appendicitis or coronary thrombosis or an inflamed gall bladder, are distinguishable one from another. Yet though at times severe, they are notoriously vague. Moreover, they are incongruously localized. We all have plenty of experience of feeling the pain of a somatic injury and identifying it with a particular site; but we have no such experience in pinpointing visceral pain, which, in order that the conscious mind may grapple with it, has to be assigned to a spurious location. Pain of this kind is known as *referred*. The place to which such pain is referred in any particular instance is itself a kind of metaphor.

But even the pain in somatic (by which we mean nonvisceral) nerves lacks the precision both of quality and location that the most highly developed (epicritic) sensation of touch enjoys. Furthermore, its time relationships are vague and rather strange. Compared with the impact of touch, that of a harmful stimulus is relatively slow in onset, and it proceeds in two phases, one of sharp discomfort building up rapidly but not instantaneously, replaced some seconds later by a duller and more sustained discomfort.

It is not surprising, then, that precise information about this indefinite sensation is scarcely accessible. We proceed as best we may, by the usual methods of ontological inquiry discussed earlier, especially in Chapter 11.

ONTOLOGICAL SYNTAXIS, OR BOTTOM-UP INQUIRY

We have certain fundamental information that may help us to build up out of simple elemental components a coherent theory of how pain oper-

1. Just how easily it is forgotten is made evident in an outbreak of the disorder phocomelia in Brazil, where thalidomide is being widely used for a variety of purposes among patients, many of whom are apparently largely ignorant of this devastating side effect (McCluskey and Horizonte 1994).

ates. The scope of the topic is massive (Mountcastle 1980; D. D. Kelly 1981), and we must be content with a brief and naive statement of elementary facts.

Anatomy and Physiology

Contrary to what popular experience suggests, pain is not merely an exaggeration of normal sensation. There is not a single continuous scale of one sensation on which warm water is soothing, hot water invigorating, and boiling water painful. Pain is experienced in a special way, detected by special sensory organs, transmitted on special nerve fibers, and finding its ultimate sensorial representation in the thalamus (Bonica 1990). It is not experienced as painful in the higher centers of the cortex. In the latter respects it differs radically from sight, in which the retina is functionally to be viewed as actually part of the brain (the visual cortex). An even more extreme case is the sense of smell, which in evolution was originally the solitary role of the forebrain and still has no representation in the thalamus (Price 1990).

Pathophysiology

When the well-being of the interior milieu is perturbed in certain ways, for instance quantitatively, redress is attempted in the first place by homeostasis, a topic discussed in Chapter 8. With other kinds of perturbations, or more severe ones, the corrections take a different form. For instance, foreign bodies, including, but not limited to, the organisms that cause infections, are engulfed by scavenger cells and disposed of in various ways. Under more taxing injury there may be set in force more radical processes that constitute what is conventionally called *inflammation*. This phenomenon—the congeries of redness, local heat, swelling, discomfort, and impairment of function—consists of diverse mechanisms, cellular responses, antibodies, scavenging, reconstitution, and repair. Details need not concern us here. However, we fasten attention on the two last classic signs of inflammation: discomfort and impairment of function.

EXAMPLE 12.1. An acutely inflamed knee joint will typically be painful, and the pain is aggravated by movement. Accordingly, reflex contraction of muscles supporting the joint may oppose movement. The result is to interfere with the normal function of the joint (which is to move). In turn, walking becomes tedious and painful.

Now, these two features of inflammation are neither inseparable nor wholly independent. As to the first, the pain is most striking in acute infections, while many such chronic infections as tuberculosis of the interior of the lungs are typically painless. Conversely, one can find inflammatory disorders in which, other things being equal, the pain is severe out of all proportion to the inflammation (e.g., subarachnoid hemorrhage or dengue fever). On the other hand, a pain, even a severe one, unaccompanied by the confirmatory signs (e.g., the pain that occurs in tic douloureux or in migraine), would perforce be attributed to some mechanism other than inflammation.

The impairment of function in inflammation may be due in part simply to the immediate effects on the structure attacked. It may also be a protective disablement because the overcoming and the repair of the disorder may be optimized by prohibiting all unnecessary demands. Whatever the mechanisms, there is no doubt that the inflammation is disabling and may interfere with the ordinary means of survival, escape, ability to fight, and so forth. Clearly this protective inhibition of function reduces Darwinian fitness, at least transiently. To balance the evolutionary account, we are led—we might say we are forced—to believe that the capacity for local disablement and the pain must, on the average, make for phenotypes that are optimal; and this competition between short-term disability and long-term benefit calls for further and deeper analysis. Whatever the conclusion is to be, it must account for the concentration of pain in the acute phase of the process, with much less of the pain coming later. We shall have more to say about the issue in the section on top-down analysis.

For the time being, however, we may explore the consequences when this disabling mechanism following injury is absent because the sense of pain is itself impaired. We may cite three illustrations.

EXAMPLE 12.2. One classic form of the extremely chronic infection known as leprosy (Hansen's disease) is widespread loss of feeling, notably of pain. As a result, local injury goes unnoticed and must be dealt with by the inflammatory mechanism operating without the benefit of spontaneous immobilization. Widespread, severe anomalies may commonly result.

EXAMPLE 12.3. In certain systemic disorders of the nervous system, notably in one form of quaternary neurosyphilis (tabes dorsalis) and in diabetic neuromyopathy, pain sense is selectively lost; and injuries, even fractures involving the joint surfaces, may occur unnoticed, with gross physical distortion in the outcome (the so-called Charcot joint).

EXAMPLE 12.4. A more precisely analyzable disorder is syringomyelia (in some particular anatomical locations termed syringobulbia), a disorder disrupting the central fibers of the spinal cord as they decussate (i.e., cross over from one side to the other). Because of the particular details of anatomy, in a precisely defined region the sense of pain and temperature are selectively lost while the other senses are intact. Again, gross disfigurements of, say, the hands or other joints may occur.

We are led from these extreme consequences to suspect that the spontaneous immobilization and the "favoring" of the inflamed part that the pain demands have important selective value. Arguably the immobilization (e.g., in a stiff joint, or the abdominal rigidity of acute peritonitis) is a simple reflex, perhaps triggered by the input from the nerve fibers carrying pain. It is noteworthy, however, that drugs like morphine that relieve pain by mechanisms acting on the thalamus in the brain, and not on the peripheral nerves, may relax the immobility and (a notorious danger in acute abdominal emergencies) abolish or "mask" abdominal rigidity. So it would be oversimplifying the whole process of pain to treat it as a purely reflex, spinal, response.

ONTOLOGICAL PARSING, OR TOP-DOWN INQUIRY

To approach this problem from the most sophisticated levels of organization is Ethically and Psychologically more satisfying. There is the sense that by this route the challenge is not explained away by some glib mechanistic answer. No mere formula is being substituted for an authentic confrontation of pain in all its vivid details. That does not, of course, mean that the top-down approach is anti-intellectual or indifferent to understanding coherently the basic (and therefore, one hopes, remediable) causes of pain, including psychogenic pain. The difference in viewpoint lies rather in the allegiances of the inquirers.

EXAMPLE 12.5. Suppose that pharmacologists are addressing how pain may be rationally managed. Should a severe and inescapable choice arise for them between regarding *either* the neurochemical analysis *or* the patient's distress as the main topic, they would feel themselves much better equipped to deal with the former and, while respecting the latter, they would leave it for those more skilled in dealing with it. The motive for this narrowness of responsibility is not disregard but diffidence. The clinical therapist would be much more expert in addressing and making the clinical choice. That does not mean that the pharmacologist is heartless or the therapist sentimental. Arguably each is the better for being aware of the other's point of view, and, of course, both should aim for an ultimate reconciliation of any differences they may have.

In the familiar domestic analogy of "throwing out the baby with the bathwater," the issue is a matter of what is the baby and what the bathwater. In the matter of pain, what is the point of the point? Where does the greatest ontological density lie? We are far from being assured that even the Medical ethicist and the Medical metaphysician would agree on that point. Indeed, it is perhaps a meaningless dilemma. Perhaps all that is called for is a restraining wisdom lest a shallow success in one objective be mistaken for a deep and wholly satisfactory outcome for all.

We might best start this discussion of ontological parsing at the point where we left ontological syntaxis, although with very different ammunition to support the cause.

Pain as Distressing

First, the phenomenon of pain-insofar-as-it-is-a-distressing-entity (let us call it P_1) is distinct from pain-insofar-as-it-is-physiological-equipment (P_2). There is nothing absurd about the physiological statement that P_2 operates even in a completely unconscious patient. The surgeon making an incision in a patient too lightly anesthetized may expect a reflex motor withdrawal response. But that must not be mistaken for P_1, which is the unqualified ("default") meaning we attach to *pain* in most Ethical issues in human beings. We recognize at once that the theories of the eliminative materialists, such as Churchland (1984), face the same difficulties in accounting for the unpleasantness of P_1 as they do in accounting for consciousness. Perhaps these quandaries are all part of the same problem. It is vital to our analysis that any answer, to be acceptable, must explain coherently the issues, most especially the Darwinian ones, that are puzzling us, not simply explain them away. While we have yet to be convinced by any of these eliminative theories, we are just as dissatisfied with insubstantial black-box statements about property-emergence of complexity or, for that matter, smooth answers proposed by mystical humanism or natural theology. The answers all seem to offend against the principle of conterminality. They provide an ad hoc answer to the question but offer no enlightenment in any other field, suggest no useful corroborative inquiries, and above all are carefully spared the ordeals of verification, falsification, and authentication. They are rather like saying that the way to break into a safe with a combination lock is to know the right combination: undoubtedly true, but devoid of any deeper or generalizable insights. To ascribe pain to the "human condition" does not seem to be saying anything useful at all. Any appraisals we can now make are, of course, nothing like final. More refined theorizing may in time be more enlightening. But at present, theory is of little further value.

EXAMPLE 12.6. P_2 has certain similarities to mechanisms of avoidance, as blinking or other startle responses are, or flight from an aggressor. But blinking does not ordinarily cause distress, and the emotions of pursuit and flight (which are rather alike) are of a totally different kind from pain.

Spontaneous Rescue from Pain

This next element is in some ways so much more puzzling than the primitive matter of distress from pain that it seems to hint that there is more to pain than simple avoidance. There are undoubted mechanisms intrinsic to the body that protect against pain.

First, there exist well-established, extensively studied morphinelike substances termed *endorphins*, normally secreted in the body, that allay, sometimes almost wholly, the feeling of pain. They operate in emergencies—for instance, in the heat of battle. Injuries that would ordinarily be painful may pass almost unnoticed.

Second, there are two analogous mechanisms of dissociation that may render the individual insensitive to pain, namely, hysterical anesthesia and hypnotic suggestion.

Third, simple remedies exist. Counterirritation (even if it is only a soothing warmth) is effective. Acupuncture is more elaborate.

Fourth, and most elusive, much of what is perceived as pain may be changed by habituation and reorientation. Exactly how this is done is obscure, although there may be various motives that induce individuals to cultivate such changes.

EXAMPLE 12.7. There are certainly clinical disorders called congenital indifference to pain (CIP) in which individuals of not particularly heroic cast are quite undistressed by what in others would be painful stimuli. This anomaly appears to operate at a higher level of the brain and is not at all like the physiological loss of the sense of pain recorded in Examples 12.2–12.4. These conditions of CIP are rare but well known. Two forms, at least, appear to be genetically determined, the commoner form being recessive, the other dominant (McKusick 1994: entries 147430, *243000). No mechanism is known. It has been proposed that the cause is an overproduction of endorphins (Yanagida 1978), but there is little substantial evidence to support this surmise. Some degree of indifference to pain is a feature of the Riley-Day dysautonomia (McKusick 1994: entry *223900) and of various sensory neuropathies. But these are in many other respects quite distinct from CIP.

It is said that pit bull terriers have been especially bred to be indifferent to pain, so that, for instance, any ordinary means of prying loose their jaws are ineffectual. It would be interesting to know something about the genetic dynamics of such animals, notably their survivorship and fertility. It would seem that in the wild state they should have powerful Darwinian advantages.

Minor degrees of stoical indifference are commonplace and can be cultivated. It was a major part of the indoctrination of Spartan youth and of many North American Indian tribes. Milder instances are the habituation to the discomfort of walking barefoot, or the discomfort of stopping the strings against the fingerboard of a violin, mandolin, or other such musical instrument. It is commonly supposed that the fingers (or other tender parts) in time develop calluses; but habituation may occur much faster than that. There are many social pressures on the individual to *harden* the body (whatever exactly that term means) against cold or other discomfort. But again, whatever the motive, the actual mechanism involved remains obscure.

We cannot develop here this argument at the length it deserves. The important point to make is that there exist mechanisms for reducing both P_2 and P_1. These mechanisms might be so efficient as to override the Darwinian advantages of pain as a warning device. We may note, however, that one feature of CIP is the occurrence of Charcot joints of the type described in Example 12.3.

But much of pain that we may call pathological pain (P_3) to all appearances serves no useful purpose at all: tic douloureux, pain from intracranial metastases, proctalgia fugax, migraine. It is not easy to see why in such cases the systems of rescue are not promptly recruited.

The Imprecision of Pain

A further top-down challenge is to explain the imprecision of pain. The puzzling aspect of the imprecision is not so much in space as in time. When a person touches a hot object, there is a perceptible interval followed by a sharp pain, and then a period of several seconds of discomfort of quite a different kind, much more primitive in character and long outlasting the removal of the stimulus. No analogous pattern among other senses comes to mind,[2] including that of temperatures kept within harmless limits. Now, as a simple avoidance method—something to warn one against a harmful stimulus—pain seems extraordinarily clumsy and inefficient. It is not prompt; it lingers long after the message has been emphatically transmitted and reacted to, producing continued distress that often does not seem to have any evident further purpose. Where temperature is concerned, some of the gap might be ascribed to the time taken in the heating up and subsequent cooling of tissues; but the same continuation of the pain occurs after a blow, or a pinprick, or some such source of pain.

What possible advantage can this sluggish pattern have? Of course, we must be open to the possibility that the complexity of pain, however generated, simply requires an accumulation of stimulus to a threshold level by generating a chemical message; and that for some reason the message has

---

2. It may be noted, of course, that the perseveration of certain sensory effects may occur in the special senses—for example, "seeing stars" after a bright flash; having "ringing in the ears" after a sustained loud noise; the sense of vertigo after several days at sea; the sense of pressure on flesh after the pressure has been removed.

to have a long half-life. Yet pain from a single short-lived period of damage can last hours, days, even months.

Pain as Nonquantitative

We are all aware from experience that there are degrees of intensity in pain, from the barely perceptible to pain so intense as perhaps to lead to loss of consciousness. The physician becomes adept at distinguishing among the causes of pain by their characteristic changes over time and just how abruptly they appear and disappear: the characteristic smooth periodic waxing and waning in the severity of colic, the lancinating pain of dissection of the aorta, the throbbing pain of toothache, and so forth. Yet although pains can be ordered in severity, they are not amenable to any natural scale of measurement. No doubt one of the main causes is that pain is something that is felt but can be discerned by the observer only in the impact on the individual suffering it. The adept clinician learns, in fashions hard to codify, to distinguish among those who have somatic pain, those with pain as a conversion (and not merely manipulative or otherwise convenient) symptom of hysteria, and those who are consciously acting as if they had pain (malingering and the Munchausen syndrome).

The scientific analysis of pain from the top down is further complicated by the social and personal meaning of a painful sensation.

EXAMPLE 12.8. The pain of an accidental blow sustained by a boy in a physical sport may be accepted without murmur, although under other circumstances, such as deliberate and intentional punishment from an angry parent, it would cause deep resentment.

EXAMPLE 12.9. Without raising the red herring of the perversion called masochism, we can understand the totally other and healthy satisfaction embodied in Robert Louis Stevenson's paradoxical phrase (1881) describing the feeling experienced at the end of a long day of walking, "the body full of delicious pains." That sensation, should it arise without the antecedent of physical effort, would not be so gladly accepted, and might cause concern. Thereby hangs one of the great modifying factors. A pain may distress not so much in its intensity as because of accompanying anxiety that the pain may have some sinister significance; and even without any explicit relief, it is often assuaged by prognostic reassurance.

Pain, Homeostasis, and Humor

We have already mentioned the taboo about humor toward pain. But that comment calls for some modification. Homeostasis (as we saw in

Chapter 8) is a cybernetic process that conserves the interior milieu within acceptable operating limits. However, if it were so sensitive as to correct every slightest variation in, say, body temperature, it would consume an inordinate amount of effort. As temperature fluctuated, one would be continually shivering and flushing, dressing and undressing. Domestic thermostats that behave in this jittery fashion are wasteful and can become irritating. In practice, there is benefit from having, not a single acceptable level (the *homing value*), but rather a zone of levels that call for no adjustments (the *neutral zone*). This is the pattern described by Dilman (1981), a Russian gerontologist whose main thesis is that the degree of *laxity* (indicated by the width of the neutral zone) increases with age; and this seems to imply that unconstrained widening of the zone is harmful. We have designated this the Dilman model and have explored some of its genetic and mathematical properties (Murphy and Renie 1984). The optimal state is, then, neither too jittery nor too lax; and it is presumably selected in accordance with the overall cost of the system and the damage done. Just so, it is not uncommon to find that many body responses to drugs are not monotonic but involve phases that stimulate and others that depress a response. One effect of humor—perhaps the only one of Darwinian importance—is to buffer responses in the physiology, the emotions, and the responses to minor disturbances that in greater degree would cause the wasteful and often destructive effects of impatience and anger (McDougall 1924). Perhaps the threshold for pain operates in the same fashion. Carrying a small load is "no trouble at all"; then, as the weight is increased, "tiring," then "exhausting," then "painful"; and finally "excruciating," even "torture."

Merton (1948: 86), on what evidence we do not know—perhaps casual experience—has suggested that in the long run those who spend their lives trying to avoid pain always suffer most in the long run. That is not to deny that avoiding unnecessary injury is both advisable and effective. Perhaps the enhanced awareness lowers the threshold of what is called painful. Perhaps there are many counterparts, such as the appreciation of joy, or beauty, or good wine. It would be interesting to collect formal evidence on the point.

ONTOLOGICAL PARAPHRASIS, OR INQUIRY BY TRANSVERSAL

As we described the strategy previously, especially in Chapter 11, paraphrasis or transversal is an approach that does not attempt to change the level of complexity; it is neither a building up nor a breaking down. Rather, it is a restructuring of one complex experiential system as another, much as a translation from one language into another is. We shall start with a brief excursus on voice. This excursus is, if the reader pleases, broadly analogous with the grammatical treatment in Chapter 7 on the commensurability of fact and obligation as an exercise in grammatical mood.

The Voice of Pain

One of the methods of analysis by transversal is to inquire into the way in which we habitually confront the topic of pain, which is unwittingly slanted by the arbitrary grammatical constructions in which it is received. The argument here is a subtle one. In making it, we must presume a working knowledge of the grammar of verbs, notably their voice. We furnish a brief outline of these presumptions in Appendix 2.

EXAMPLE 12.10. One of the most interesting verbs in our context is the Latin *patior* (I suffer), which is passive in form but perceived as being active in meaning. It is noteworthy that the word *patient* is derived from it, denoting one who suffers, that is, one subjected to suffering or (in the other sense) long-suffering. What is even more remarkable, the very word *passive* itself comes from this verb. This last anomaly makes one wonder what grammarian decided that the verb *patior* is active (rather than passive) in meaning and therefore qualifies as a deponent verb. Why is it not simply a verb totally defective in the active voice?

In English we start out with the assumption, implicit and for the most part unrecognized, that all pain and suffering are inflicted on us, and that we are quite inert in the face of them. That may or may not be true. However, nothing is lost, and perhaps much gained, by opening the topic up for discussion. As we shall see later, it may throw some light on the puzzling evolutionary aspects of pain.

Pain, we are agreed, is a device warning of damage or threat to parts of a complex cybernetic system (P_2). Pain is also a distressing experience that we endure (P_1). Is there any more to it than that? What is the nature of distress? What do we mean by *endurance* of pain, and what are its dynamics? Is the experience of pain an active or a purely passive process? Is there really such a thing as pain without use or purpose? In this strategy of transversal we are not attempting to solve the same problems encountered in ontological parsing or syntaxis. We are looking for an answer that is no less complicated than the question but that opens the prospect of some new meaning, some new way, biological or Psychological, of looking at the problem that will allow us to approach the subject coherently. In doing so, it is necessary to clear up an ambiguity. We must distinguish between the voices of the encounter and of the use of pain.

The encounter of pain. All people have some degree, and choice, of control over their exposure to painful occasions. Some will *actively* seek pain for various reasons and motives: as a means of purging guilt or a sense of restitution for injustice; for ascetic mortification (like wearing a hair shirt); as a manifestation of psychiatric disorder, such as the self-mutilation in the Lesch-Nyhan syndrome (McKusick 1994: entry *308000.0018) or in masochism. Some may adopt a *middle* attitude, neither seeking pain nor taking any special trouble to avoid it: "taking troubles as they come." Others may be extremely *passive,* allowing pain to be imposed upon themselves. There is a mounting popular interest in the degree to which people of both sexes and all ages seem prepared to tolerate frank abuse, although the motives are no doubt mixed. This field of attitude toward encounter of pain is of growing public interest. As such, it suffers from the superficial judgments that make no attempt to comprehend what it underlies. It is a large topic that would be out of place here, and of doubtful relevance to Ethics proper.

The use of pain. Our interest in the voice of pain lies rather in the perception and the constructive exploitation of pain by the person undergoing it. Some see it in *active* terms. There is a long active tradition, which we commonly term Spartan or stoical, that sees pain as a means of "building character," of developing the seasoned soldier; as a means of acquiring the admiration of others; in less vain terms, as a means of cultivating freedom by emancipation of the spirit from the constraint of fear.[3] A large group, of more *middle* voice, may not see pain as a constructive means but may put up with it as the by-product of another activity that is desirable in its own right. It is sustained, as often as not, by the proverb that one cannot make the omelet without breaking the eggs. Much of long-distance running and walking are of this type, although again the exact motives are mixed. They include the sense of well-being that is associated with the "delicious pains" savored by Stevenson, to which we have already referred; it is also part of the cult of the sunburned skin. At the *passive* extreme in capitalizing on pain lies much that we may call pure misery, in which all pain is useless, meaningless, and to be avoided wherever possible but inexorably encountered nonetheless. This topic of use is much closer to our purposes here. Not that it is easy to understand, for it involves complex and much elaborated overlay of attitudes, policies, the strivings of religion, cult, social groups, the pharmaceutical industry, sports entertainment from football to bullfighting and, increasingly, professionalized athletics, and much more. None of these is at the heart of science or Medicine; rather, the concerns are how the forces of genetic selection have operated to produce the voice of pain and the appropriate social and other attitudes.

As a point of departure, consider (by way of analogy) Searle's approach

---

3. Compare "Endurcissez-vous à la peine et vous deviendrez fort" (Harden yourself to trouble and you will become strong).

(1992) to the nature and cause of behavior. He dismisses the extremes of eliminative reductionism: the claim that the behavior of an organism consists of its physical properties and nothing else. He likewise recoils from the idea of vitalism, essentially an unfettered dualism, epistemically a deus ex machina for which no corroborations are possible. Behavior, he says, is best understood as the result of neurobiological mechanisms. His view will not be uncritically accepted, especially by the extremists. But even if his proposal is of its nature not a final one, in the present state of inquiry it is *tactical* temporizing of the first importance.

EXAMPLE 12.11. Eliminative reductionism will demand that pathology is merely one stage of an unbroken chain of physical causality. A pathologist (however committed to materialism in principle) would refuse to see it in that light, and in our view correctly so. Epistemically, the belief in the unbroken chain of physical causality is at the present time an act of almost pure faith. What is worse, even if it were in some unimaginable way known to be true, it would still labor under overwhelming epistemic problems that quite possibly are permanently irresolvable.[4] What is even more disturbing, there are nontrivial reasons for supposing that, granted there is an unbroken chain of physical causality, the way in which a mind functions is incomprehensible to the mind itself, and then ultimate proof, or even ultimate statement of what is to be proved, may be forever inaccessible to us.[5] In the face of this conundrum, at least exceedingly difficult and perhaps insoluble, pathologists must deal with real-time problems. They do so, not in terms of particle physics, but in terms of well-attested empirical phenomena that yield coherent and useful statements such as "The jaundice was due to stenosis of the common bile duct resulting from a scirrhous carcinoma." Of course, that takes for granted such notions as *jaundice, stenosis, scirrhous,* and *carcinoma,* each of which might generate a list of unresolved details. Pathologists have a powerful sense that they are dealing with the corporate properties of complicated but ontologically dense systems, the behaviors of which are well known empirically even if not radically understood. And there are plenty of other respected academic disciplines, from music and astrophysics to philology and comparative embryology, of which the same claim (or complaint) can be made. There is even a certain mistrust, by no means destructive or anti-intellectual, of intruding the wrong kind of refinement in the mistaken supposition that it makes the statement more

4. The difficulty would take us into technically deep problems. In brief, it is summed up in a claim that we have heard ascribed to Poisson: "Give me four parameters and I will make an elephant. Give me five and I will make it wave its trunk." As the number of free specifications in the model increases, it rapidly becomes almost impossible to falsify.

5. J. Cohen and Stewart (1994) put the dilemma involved in a characteristically pungent form: "If our brains were simple enough for us to understand them, we'd be so simple that we couldn't."

"scientific." Witness the dictum "high-power microscopy, low-power pathology." Low-power microscopy discloses patterns of tissue organization that may be vital to diagnosis and interpretation yet may be wholly unrepresented in the electron microscope. Cosmologists trying to conduct their studies in a Wilson cloud chamber would be in much the same predicament. Had Beethoven taken to Fourier analysis, we all would have lost.

THE ETHICAL IMPACT OF PAIN

In applying the transversal strategy to the matter of pain, we may seem to be endlessly dancing around the subject without coming to any very explicit insights. The accusation is just. Because of the deplorable neglect of the subject, there is dismayingly little to communicate. We can see the force of that neglect by engaging in a purely illustrative skirmish with the Ethical aspects of pain. It reflects credit on neither the biology nor the Ethics. The industriousness of the physiologist is admirably scientific, and, as has been well said of the Venus de Milo, all there is of it is excellent. The same is true of the comparative physiology of pain among species. The ethicist too has concern with pain, but it involves so little appeal even to the fragments of information there may be from the other two disciplines, Medicine and science, that there can be said to be almost no useful ontology to invoke.

For instance, physicians, in making any decision about what they should do about pain, need to have some depth of understanding of how the whole needs of the patient are to be met. If the argument is to be that pain is bad, therefore they should combat it, therefore they should give morphine to the patient with the acute abdomen, then no doubt the pain will be taken care of; but because of masking of the critical signs, the wrong decisions may be made and the patient may die as a result. However, orthodox nontechnical opinion would argue that phronesis, common prudence, has been sacrificed to a mistaken compassion. The preferred course is in the active voice: the stance that the patient's distressing abdominal symptoms are to be resolutely turned into a vital gauge to sound management, even at the price of continued distress.

Well, but what of unnecessary pain? Is that too an overriding Ethical countervalue? A little reflection will suggest that that is absurd. Children who never played, never walked, never swam, would escape much pain that the usual child feels, but they would have a very narrow existence. Where, then, the limits are to be drawn is a matter of understanding the intimate role of pain in the process of development. Education is rarely—we would say never—without at least metaphorical pain; and the same is true of physical prowess, skill in the fine arts, and productive scholarship. There is merit in the claim that the deplorably low yield from our much prized institutional education is largely the price paid for trying to avoid the simple if unpleasant fact that education must go beyond "having fun." But the voice of this pain is no more than middle: it is a by-product of the learning, not the purpose. The belief of former times that learning could be enhanced by extraneous pain has left its semantic mark, so that *disciplina,* which originally meant teaching, now for the most part means punishment (*Webster's* 1988: sense 1). How far pain can be used creatively (and hence in the active voice) is arguable. Sadness seems to have active value. P. B. Shelley's line (1819) "I fall upon the thorns of life! I bleed!" seems to be a determined effort. But exclamation marks and all, it smacks of a rather effete sensuality that underlies his work, and that was common among some other Romantic poets and culminated in the frankly masochistic poetry of Swinburne (Ober 1975) and in Flecker's *Hassan* (Wilson 1990: 129). Newman (1865), a less suspect witness and one with much greater experience, sees matters very differently: "that sense of ruin that is worse than pain." It may seem that we have strayed a long way from our topic. But however much it strays from the scientific, it is the clinician's business to grapple with the reality of pain at all levels of the human personality. If nothing else, these extravagant instances should alert us to the perils of addressing all experiences of pain as something that may be resolved by right notions and a little common sense.

What does Ethics have to say about useless pain? That question answers itself trivially and by tautology. If it is useless, why, it has no merit; and common humanity decrees that if it is distressing, it should be combated. But who is to declare that pain is useless, and to whom and on what terms is the maker of that decision to be held accountable for it? The patient who of necessity is steeled to confront prolonged pain can too readily receive more harm than good from the injudicious sympathy of others. As to the bland, unreflecting, irresponsible view that pain is bad and we should, without any ifs or buts, eliminate it, that is what leads to much of the horror of the leper colony.

So perish all intellectual traitors.

SUFFERING

Common superficial judgments treat as interchangeable the terms *pain* and *suffering.* In themselves they are both more or less unpleasant states, uncompromisingly bad; and both call for relief. Yet as we shall see, they are in fact very different. Suffering is vastly more complicated and elusive, often more sustained. Pain is ambiguous and fraught with evaluative, and therefore Ethical, difficulties. Suffering is also, but it is much the more confusing.

We address the problem as coherently as we may. *The reader is emphatically warned to look for neither epistemic nor ontological satisfaction.* We shall have to raise many more problems than we may hope to solve.

Suffering as Distinguished from Pain

Over the last twenty years or so there has grown up in the literature a recognition that pain and suffering need to be radically distinguished (Cassell 1982, 1991; Fordyce 1988; M. L. Cohen 1991). These valuable writings merit special protection from the hatchetmen of criticism. They should be seen as pioneering efforts, as preliminary skirmishes with an important topic that is only dimly emerging from obscurity and is particularly vulnerable to the attacks of the narrow pedant. They may not fairly be assailed at this stage by shrill demands for precise definitions and inalienable epistemic principles. The shape that this line of inquiry eventually takes comprises matters to be discovered, not invented, nor imprisoned in premature and stultifying axiomatics. Those who imagine that such strictures are the normal, early, and presiding accompaniments of scientific discovery would benefit from reading Kepler's cosmology and how it adumbrated, but never quite articulated, Newton's principle of gravitation (Koestler 1960). Or, as a more recent example, they might read Chargaff's seminal discoveries (1951, 1952) of the stoichiometry of bases in nucleic acids that came so tantalizingly close to, but never quite articulated, the binary structure of DNA; or the remarkable speculative papers of Pauling and Corey (1951a–g) on the stable secondary structures in proteins before anything in the nature of necessary or sufficient proofs was available. Full precision and inalienable proofs are the late, and to our minds by no means the most important, aspects of insight and discovery in science.

From the early writings have emerged a number of tentative distinguishing features between pain and suffering, to which we have made a few ever more tentative additions. They are perhaps in large part self-explanatory:

Physiological pain is a sensation, at least under its metonymous[6] interpretation as a type of sensory modality (P_2). Unlike suffering, it may occur in the unconscious patient or the hypnotized subject without causing any

---

6. Metonymy is a rhetorical figure in which one entity is given a symbolic meaning from association with another, usually more significant, entity. Thus, to say that a criminal "was pardoned by the crown" is a metonymy, meaning pardoned by the authority of the head of state. Again, to desecrate any physical realization of the flag of the United States violates various state and federal laws. Interpreted literally, that provision is absurd, since a copy of the flag may in itself be the top of a birthday cake and submitted to the indignity of being eaten and the other even more degrading catabolic processes that ensue. But the flag connotes the sovereign majesty of the state, and hence is taken to merit respect and dignity. Metonymy has a pervasive and often grossly misleading effect on philosophical analysis. To say that pain and a particular electrical activity in nerve tissue are "exactly the same thing" (and even Philosophers have made that statement in so many words!) has something of this metonymous character: it treats this electrical activity as the point of the point, the gist, of pain, whereas all that the facts warrant is that in some conscious states the electrical activity accompanies the primitive phenomenon of experiential discomfort.

subjective distress. It can be more or less described (as a feeling of pressure, stabbing, burning, etc.). Suffering is a state that may be described (if at all) only in terms of metaphors.

Pain has geography, a physical distribution. It is localized typically to one particular part. That is true even of pain as a somatization of Psychological disturbance (e.g., chest pain as an expression of an anxiety). It occurs sometimes, as in the phantom limb, in a completely figmented part. It makes sense to ask a patient, "Where is your pain?" or "Where are you hurting" but not "Where is your suffering?" Suffering is a diffuse experience—diffuse not in the sense of being remote, vague, or indefinite but in the sense of being global. The same global quality characterizes consciousness itself, something that resides in an elusive domain of experience without in itself being in the least insipid or unfocused; and we are satisfied that neither state, consciousness or suffering, is intentional.[7]

EXAMPLE 12.12. An analogy—but only an analogy—that comes to mind is the word processor on which this manuscript is being composed. First, there is a screen. On it is displayed a fair amount of text. Second, there is a much longer document (of which the current content of the screen is part) that can be readily enough recalled but is too large to be displayed. Third, there is a large residual part of the computer that is represented by the hardware and is ordinarily accessible only to the systems analyst. The displayed part is something like the conscious mind; the undisplayed part is like the accessible unconscious; the hardware is like the inaccessible unconscious. However, there is always a preferred part of the screen, where the cursor is flashing, and this corresponds to the intentional part.

Suffering has history, pain does not. Pain is not present before the harmful stimulus is applied. When the stimulus and its ill effects are over, pain disappears, although perhaps slowly. Suffering is a different matter. The mere *prospect* of pain can cause suffering, but it cannot cause pain. The *memory* of pain can cause suffering; so can imagining a pain that one has not experienced. But pain recollected in tranquillity is not painful except in a metaphorical sense.

Pain is specific. The pain of burning differs from the pain of stabbing or of torsion. Suffering, however, engages the personality as a whole.

Pain is autochthonous, suffering is not. Except in loose metaphor, one may not experience another's pain from the outside. On the other hand, one can suffer with, and in a sense for, another by the mere fact of knowing that the person is suffering. This seems to be what McDougall (1924) called "primitive passive sympathy." If one person starts to scratch, others tend to scratch also; if one person yawns, others tend to yawn also; if one

7. The word *intention* has a technical meaning that is discussed in Chapter 13.

person laughs, others want to laugh as well. The relationship of love enhances this sympathy, this compassion, this fellow-feeling; and it is one of the powerful forces of nursing and the operation of hospice care for the dying. At the same time, we realize that intimate personal love, as between husband and wife, may interfere with the efficacy of clinical management and alleviation of suffering.

Pain has a metric. There is a useful sense in which the total pain experienced by several individuals is the sum of their personal pains. There are at least rough correspondences between the disability, the amount of medication, and the physiological activity registered in pain. This perception, crude as it is, involves the viewpoint that pain is generalizable—that there is a large component of homogeneity in the pains that are due to (say) metastatic cancerous deposits in the spine. But suffering does not seem to have that property. A grossly obese patient trying to walk may be helped by being given the physical support of other people at some discomfort to themselves. That seems to be an authentic sharing of pain. But no analogous method of sharing suffering comes to mind any more than there is a sharing of coma. It is so individuated that there is no common ground between M's suffering and N's suffering. It is, perhaps, in this area that solipsism has one of its roots: the lack of assurance that others grasp what the suffering is like because perhaps nobody else has ever experienced the same thing. The nearest to bridging this gap is perhaps the cultivation of fellowship such as occurs in Alcoholics Anonymous and kindred support groups. It is hard to say how far this is a genuine exchange of suffering, and how far a matter of moral support and exchange of encouragement. There seems to be no useful way of dealing with this problem epistemically; but ontologically it points up the shallowness of trying to deal with problems that are essentially individual and individuated by using categories that can exist only by being general. A distinguished surgeon, addressing the risks of gastrectomy, once said that a mortality rate of 1% does not mean that every patient contributes somewhat to the mortality but that the patient who dies contributes 100%. The exactions of doctrinaire positivism cannot accommodate this view; and so much the worse for positivism.

Suffering has context, pain does not. As we have noted with regard to R. L. Stevenson's description, what is suffering in one set of circumstances may be even a pleasant sense of well-being in others. We note in this context the puzzling aspects of the use of nonanalgesic drugs in the management of chronic pain (Onghera and Vanhoudenhove 1992). Such drugs seem to reduce suffering despite the fact that (by definition) they do not reduce pain.

Pain with Suffering

To distinguish carefully between pain and suffering does not mean that they are totally separate or that they can always be adequately dissected.

It is usual to apply the transitive verb *suffer* to experiences (typically, but not always, damaging) and the intransitive form to a separate component of associated distress.

EXAMPLE 12.13. "The patient suffered a blow on the head. Since then he has been suffering from recurrent headaches." There is nothing here that says that the patient experienced or experiences any distress from the blow as such at the site at which it was inflicted. He may already have been unconscious when it happened. His recurrent headaches may be so mild that he does not even consider taking an analgesic.

The phrase *to suffer from headaches* implies a distress that might be simply discomfort or perhaps apprehension about the possible sinister significance of the headaches. In this connection, for instance, it is interesting that in ordinary English—*pace Webster's* (1988)—the word *headache* does not mean the same thing as *a pain in the head*, though it is not at all easy to say exactly where the difference lies. Moreover, the one may be superimposed on the other. Migraine is a headache; and it may be provoked, prolonged, and aggravated by episodes of stress that may be represented by distinct tension pains. A headache may be organic, psychogenic or psychosomatic, or commonly a mixture of them.

THE ETHICAL IMPACT OF SUFFERING

If we are diffident about making any statement about the Ethics of pain, we are more reluctant than ever to address the Ethics of suffering, about which much less is understood.

EXAMPLE 12.14. Consider, for instance, one very special form of suffering, that of bereavement. It is commonplace that grief varies widely in form, intensity, and duration. No doubt there is often a ritual component, most florid in the histrionics of professional grievers. There is often a more respectful social ritual of decorous behavior that may nevertheless be out of all proportion to the real sense of emotional loss. When it finds its own true level, the grief may be brief and intense; the starting point of a profound depression; and occasionally a sane, but irremediable, sense of loss. Now, that surely is very strange. One must be a child or have had a very sheltered upbringing not to be well aware that all will die, and perhaps most often that death is heralded by signs of deterioration, evidence that it is imminent. Yet grief usually comes as if this inevitable event were a surprise and a shock. However, there is a growing sense among clinical counselors that grieving is in some ways a constructive process, akin to the orderly healing of a physical wound under professional supervision. In this view, those who, for whatever reason or motive, deny themselves due grief heal unsuccessfully and are in some degree disabled by that curtailment. At a deeper and more generalized level, very much the same demand for orderly and wise management is important in clinical depression.

EXAMPLE 12.15. Counselors in clinical genetics have the same, or at least closely analogous, advice for the parents of defective children. However much the parents love them, or try to love them, or try to believe that they love them, part of effective coping involves an explicit comparison between the child they actually have and the child they had hoped for and, as it were, have been denied. It is as if they must have a period of wholesome grief to heal the loss of the child who never was.

EXAMPLE 12.16. No doubt very much the same must be true of those who, though handicapped, are intelligent and resourceful enough to confront their own deficiencies. Sometimes the defects and their practical solutions, the cultivation of imaginativeness in devising new ways of improving a restoration of well-being, are all straightforward enough. Such is the case with blindness, deafness, defective and missing limbs, and much more. It is supported by the tradition of sharing these discoveries among affected persons. Subtler defects in psychic endowment may be much less accessible. The mentally backward may be happy and enjoy self-respect where the intelligent and the gifted may not. The greatest threat to the retarded may be those relatives, teachers, and clinicians who, for whatever reason, set unrealistic goals of achievement for them.

It is much more difficult to deal with defects of a deeper and less easily confronted type: addictions to alcohol, tobacco, and narcotics; displays of resentment or anger. Nevertheless, they may be tolerable on the common (although by no means assured) claim that such flaws are diseases and in some measure matters beyond the patient's control. They are thus to be handled as clinical problems. There are behavioral problems (lassitude, boredom, wandering attention, ready discouragement) yet more difficult to confront because they are not nearly so readily identified as diseases at all but fall into the treacherous domain of what many regard as moral defects. As such, they are quite beyond our scope here. Given all these constraints, there are no doubt ways of making the best of one's life. But wise planning calls more than ever for patient and reasonable assessment of the endowments and needs of the person concerned.

THE BEHAVIORAL IMPACT OF PAIN AND SUFFERING

All illness is liable to impinge on the behavior and the attitude of the patient. In some rare cases it may produce enjoyment, even exhilaration. There is a large popular cult of the adolescent with a leg fractured by skiing, hobbling around in a plaster cast adorned with the graffiti of friends in admiration of this ordeal of adulthood. We say nothing of the incongruous euphoria of the hypomanic.

Pain and suffering are particularly prominent causes of behavioral changes, which are curiously diverse. Most patients are more or less distressed by them and grateful to those who offer relief. However, there are impacts that have an important bearing on Ethics.

Most conspicuous of them is the fact that both pain and suffering are distracting. Indeed, a common term of bygone days was that a person was *distracted* by grief or suffering. This distraction may impede coherent judgment. The fact that freedom of choice and decision may be impaired is a matter to be borne in mind where informed consent is an issue. "I would give anything to get rid of this pain" is scarcely a frame of mind in which measured decisions may be made. Although most patients positively welcome care and attention to their pains, there are patients who are stoical in their attitudes, demanding little relief, occasionally antagonistic to analgesics. It is unwise counsel to interfere with this attitude without very good reason. For the clinician to be more sorry for patients than they are for themselves is more often than not damaging, even demoralizing to both. There are occasional patients who treat their pain as a matter of mystical importance; but this attitude is often shallow and may very occasionally generate an attitude of spurious mysticism of which the wise clinician will be wary.

However, such distress commonly causes resentment, depression, even frank nihilism. The targets of these attitudes may include those engaged in their clinical management, and resentful lawsuits for mismanagement are occasional and deplorable outcomes.

There are more devious consequences. In the drug addict, for instance, pain may be exaggerated or even frankly fabricated as a means of obtaining narcotics. Inasmuch as many such patients are fully aware of what they are doing, clinical discernment and firm management will function well. However, much of this manipulative use of pain is unconscious and manifested in hysteria, hypochondriasis, and kindred disorders that may be very difficult to treat.

This topic might be developed at length. It suffices for our purposes here to point out yet once again that the intricate issues involved are not adequately dealt with by shallow slogans about the relief of pain and the stamping out of suffering. Ethical issues are to be addressed in adequately formulated terms and a concern with the losses as well as the benefits of intervening.

A COMMENT ON THE PURPOSE OF PAIN AND SUFFERING

A proper concern about the principle of conterminality requires that we try to raise our assessment of pain and especially suffering above the level of unarticulated distaste, dislike, fear. In this situation we are hedged by two contradictory counsels that may be seen as Tory and Whig policies. The first is that we should be cautious and reluctant in tampering with a mechanism, clearly well conserved in the Darwinian sense, that even the most arrogant cannot convincingly claim to understand. The contrary opinion is that if we are fainthearted about changing anything that we do not understand, we might as well give up Medicine and take up some useful activity instead. These views differ in everything except that both urge decision and demand thought; and they take for granted that our big handicap is lack of understanding. In the event, even if there is nothing else we can do, we feel obliged to state the need for understanding and (lest this sentiment be totally void) give some indication of where we might look for better understanding. Each cobbler to his own last. We shall as usual try to confine our comments to what science and Medicine may have to say.

Existential arguments from comparative biology and Darwinism have weight and must be respected. But they are vulnerable, especially so when the basis of the inference is something that does *not* happen. It is of the greatest importance, then, to understand some of the limitations. Genetic and Darwinian selection are indeed selection: a preference among *choices that are available*. The superficial suppose that if there is great utility from such and such a property, then it will in time occur and be selected for. But in the first place, that property must be *possible and feasible*. It would be helpful to have a gland that turns base metals into gold, but we must seek it elsewhere than Darwinian evolution.

Then again, it is common for the superficial to talk as if in the selection of a trait there were necessarily only one simple matter, a single advantage to be considered; but there is no reason to suppose that that is in general true. To be sure, there are a few "typical" examples that are endlessly paraded in textbooks, such as the selection of the sickle-cell gene as a balanced polymorphism because in the heterozygous state it protects against falciparal malaria. But, as so often, the "typical" examples have a distressing habit of turning out to be most atypical. When the sickle-cell example was discovered (Allison 1954), there was a wide expectation that it would be the first of many. Forty years later we would be hard put to give many other confirmed instances of human diseases with inordinate frequency due to balanced polymorphism.

Again, notwithstanding much arm-waving about exotic inborn errors of metabolism, we know very little about the detailed dynamics of genes, and we know even less in the more complex species. We do not make that point in any combative spirit. Rather, it is a frank confession of our corporate ignorance, and indeed somewhat to the professional embarrassment of the authors. The genetic basis of disease is by no means a simple matter of identifying genes and showing that they do indeed cause particular diseases. Much more serious effort than that must be made to put the claims on a firm basis: in particular, how exactly the putative gene causes the disease *(pathogenetics);* how the dissemination and survival of the mutant form operates *(evolutionary genetics);* how the frequency of a deleterious trait in a population is rationally accounted for *(population genetics);* and much more.

EXAMPLE 12.17. The genes that regulate the development of the fetal heart present all manner of interesting challenges. For example, there are theoretical models of how they *might* work (Manasek et al. 1984; Clark 1984; Kurnit et al. 1985; Murphy, Berger, et al. 1988), but hard evidence is still lacking. So far there has been little success in determining the number of genetic loci involved. But there are two solid black-box data. The defective genotypes that cause congenital heart disease (CHD) are, by genetic standards, highly deleterious. Yet they are bewilderingly common. Serious CHD occurs in 1 in 130 human babies. The latter, particularly, goes very much against the grain of classical population genetics, which would predict a frequency of perhaps 1 in 10,000 or less. How surprised geneticists may be about these facts really depends on how much faith they have in naive theories of selection. The pediatric cardiologist's stance might be that, if possible, all CHD should be prevented; and that opinion is probably well founded. The careful geneticist, however, might want to know first what price might have to be paid in deleterious effects elsewhere in the genome in order to achieve that goal.

When we try to apply these precautionary statements to pain and suffering, we must confront the distasteful question, Is the object of the Ethics and the policy it prescribes to *do* good or to *feel* good? The question is frank to the point of brutality, but it cannot be sidestepped in anything intended to be a scholarly inquiry. (It may, of course, be a false dichotomy.) It is in no way sweetened by the fact that we make no claims whatsoever as to how the questions about suffering might be rationally answered. We can merely attempt to open up a few naive possibilities for discussion. Suffering is, of course, the more difficult to grapple with, but also the most pressing; the management of pain, although still pragmatic and empirical rather than deep and rational, at least operates from a vast experience.

With no pretensions to scholarly system, we offer three possibilities about the genetic dynamics of pain and suffering.

First, suffering, which gives every sign of being a subtle and abstract system, may be still in the process of fine-tuning and development and yet be in need of much perfecting. It is possible that suffering is a mechanism by which the noxious dimension of experience is usefully and constructively converted into beneficial knowledge and wisdom; but at the present stage it still has distressing effects.

Second, we are so committed to the idea that pain is a warning device, a restrictive impediment of behavior, that we may be overlooking the possibility that it may be a teaching device. Perhaps the physiology of pain, and especially its prolonged aftereffect, is a device to ensure that the lesson is properly learned. "Burned child dreads the fire." Indeed! But that tells us, among other matters, that the child will be much more careful next time.

Finally, it may be that suffering is one of the inescapable prices that have to be paid because there is no possible—or at least available—means of achieving the purposes of pain without distress. Endorphins, we know, will allay pain by a natural process. But in fact they seem to do so only for acute pain under special circumstances. It is possible that too extravagant a use of them will vitiate the manifest benefits of an intact sensory system of pain.

13 Respect and Intention

We continue to address more complicated topics in the intimate and intricate domain of the human being as an intrinsic participant. We find ourselves stepping from one compartment of a Chinese box into a larger one in an extensive—for all we know, infinite—set. We are no longer, so to speak, treating with fundamental ideas but are setting out to analyze human beings (including ourselves) thinking about fundamental ideas. Just as Medical science and practice are more than Medicine and the elements of physical science, so Medical Ethics and its underpinnings are obliged to become more than a compendium of methods and arguments or even a system containing both. Medical Ethics must also address human beings thinking about and applying these methods and arguments. (Needless to say, this development taxes our understanding, grasp, and insight, our dispassion and frankness, even our courtesy and diplomacy. What we are looking for is not a parading of colorless prescriptions about behavior by those who are, or fancy themselves to be, in a preferred position attained by deep reflection and experience. Rather, we seek a recognition that even if the ideal system were indeed established beyond cavil, the Ethical perspective, if it is not to degenerate into meaningless attitudinizing, remains a dynamic process: not an alien indoctrination, but an inquiry to be vigorously acquired as a process of convinced self-education.)

In dealing with the human being as subject, we are obliged to consider now two peculiar topics of human phenomenology: *respect* and *intention*. The terms share much the same problems in analysis. Both are ambiguous, with peculiar etymological histories. Both, though in wide and popular use, have been taken over by theorists and endowed with peculiar technical meanings. Both bear on Ethics, but in a distinctively personal way. Both lay the ground for vital, but yet more elusive, analysis to follow.

RESPECT

The word *respect* is originally from the Latin *respicere* (to look back). (It is interesting that according to Shipley [1984], the root *spec* is related by metathesis, i.e., by Spoonerism, to the Greek stem *skhep*, to which we owe the word *skeptic*.) It has undergone an elaborate development. We identify three steps in its fleshing out.

First, in its oldest sense, *respect* is a rather cold term taking due note that there is a setting or background, an orientation aided by a dispassionate assessment of merits or their absence (*Webster's* 1988: sense 1). When mathematicians speak about "differentiating Y with respect to X," they mean that the behavior of Y is being examined from the standpoint of X and of changes in it. To be sure, this treatment puts X in a preferred position, but that implies no partiality. The force of the expression is analogous to studying the behavior of Mars from the viewpoint of Earth. That choice by Ptolemy was quite natural; but it so happened that it led to gratuitous complexities that were to be simplified so beautifully by Copernicus. In spite of vapid moralizing (some ancient, some modern) about Ptolemaic cosmology, the Copernican revolution had nothing to do with deciding whether the Sun is in some way more worthy than Earth (setting aside the question of what on Earth it could be more worthy of). Indeed, Newton's theory of celestial mechanics shorn of its gratuitous absolutism and Einstein's extension of it to electromagnetism some two centuries later have long since declared that the question of which goes around the other is a pointless, and perhaps even meaningless, debate.

Second, *respect* as an attitude to somebody or something acknowledging importance or excellence is a later meaning.[1] Just as in the calculus Y is studied with respect to X, a lawsuit must be conducted with respect to (the point of view of) the bench; and in the ceremony of the court, the advocates will from time to time expressly acknowledge that fact. So this deference has come to acquire a secondary sense of honoring the wisdom and other excellences of the learned *office* of the judge, even though the judge be demented and irascible and everybody knows it. In ordinary social contact, the use of this word *respect* has a less ceremonial character but instead denotes sincere approval of good qualities (*Webster's* 1988: sense 2). A minor extension of this meaning lies in the appraisal that so-and-so is a *respectable* person, worthy of that kind of regard because of virtue, not primarily because of office.

Cantore (1977: 141 ff. and passim) identifies respect for truth as "typical of scientific research"—a sound, if rarely articulated, observation. He extends it to the point of reverence and kindred sentiments. His usage is perhaps to be identified as the worthiness that attaches to truth itself.

A third and more elusive meaning of *respect* is much closer to what we use it to mean here and shall address. It is the sense hinted at in the second

---

1. A curious but noteworthy feature of the attempts of dictionaries to define *respect* in this sense is that the synonyms used *(esteem, defer, regard, admire, appreciate, consider)* all seem to show exactly the same shift from what was originally a completely neutral and cold assessment to the later sense of looking up to someone or taking special care to please or to meet the needs of that person.

meaning by the phrase "the *office* of the judge": the recognition that respect attaches to a kind of Platonic ideal of the person-in-office rather than to the merits of that actual person. The common phrase "respecting the privacy" of a person, for instance, is not necessarily any statement about whether that person acts in a way that conduces to privacy—too often, the very opposite. The same is true of that set of respects that are called rights (see Appendix 3). They are often perceived as an inalienable attachment to personhood, the personality that the individual ideally achieves, even if it is severely compromised by, for instance, gross mental defect. Big Ethical questions attach to that cloak of protection and how it is to be effectively conserved.

It would be out of place here for us to trace or discuss the many possible theories of the origin of these social and legal guarantees embodied in respect of personhood: whether they are to be seen (at the one end) as spiritual attributions or (at the other) as a set of conventional Legal fictions invented as the building blocks for the regulation of the public good. As Holmes points out (1881), the original significance and purpose of a law may be so obscured by the passage of time that the theorist may be taxed to discern any germinal principle that may be invoked in delimiting its area of application.

We note arising *ex nihilo* a sense of respect, often cast in the form of rights, for living forms of lesser standing than human personhood—for animals and, to a milder but not a trivial degree, for trees and even plants, both individually and collectively (in the case of endangerment of a species); for the environment (seen as a common resource); on cultural grounds for human artifacts (extending from archaeological specimens to historic buildings, works of art, and even purely instrumental objects such as the tools of painters and writers or their preliminary sketches or drafts). In consequence there are being generated a graded set of attitudes (none of them indulgent) toward vandalism and wanton and heedless damage.

To understand something of respect and how we are to introduce it into the Ethical context, we shall try to understand where it takes its origin and wherein it resides. Three promising lines for analysis are complexity, richness, and organization; and we shall attempt to analyze each in turn.

COMPLEXITY

As a starting point, consider the following problem.

EXAMPLE 13.1. A telegram is to be sent to Paris by a parsimonious but exact Philosopher conveying the instructions on how to play American football. The French, we shall suppose, know nothing of the game or of any game from which illuminating analogies may be drawn. Telegrams cost money, and there is thus a demand for brevity. Except for conciseness, there is no interest in the vocabulary, whether official or slang. On the other hand, the rules and goals of the game must be communicated quite clearly.

A measure of the complexity *of the rules* will be given by the length of the telegram. Of course, the complexity *of the game* (comprising all the tactics that may be developed and used while staying within the rules) is much greater; but it is not to be communicated, for many reasons. Doing so is likely to stunt the (almost inexhaustible) inventiveness with which such a game will be played in France. The ideal reasoner will be able to deduce all the known tactics and many more besides (to be kept secret for the great occasions). Many other matters that do not win games are designed to entertain the crowd, as for instance the parades at halftime, which in their new setting might have their own Gallic quality. The television commercials might not be accommodated with the customary reverence.

There are thus two components to this complexity: the first, essential or *paradigmatic rules;* and the second, *germinative tactics.*

EXAMPLE 13.2. The human mind may operate in analogous fashion. The usual distinction is that *education* is paradigmatic, loading into the mind only the *hardware* (without which it cannot operate some *software*), containing a few useful common methods; and the rest of the mind is adequate free space devoted to much practice in solving problems for which no explicit methods have been provided. There will be plenty of practice, under which mysterious germinative methods will be cultivated. In contrast with education, *teaching* loads the hardware, masses of software, and provides little else. We shall have more to say about this example below.

EXAMPLE 13.3. In early years, operating systems in computers stored large tables of logarithms and other common mathematical functions. It soon became clear that it is far faster and vastly more economical of space to store not the tables but the paradigmatic devices (algorithms) and to compute afresh the specific value assumed by the function each time it is needed.

Now, as studies in artificial intelligence make clear, it is difficult to say in general how far computers can solve problems that are not stereotyped. Sometimes, of course, the solution may be simply a matter of searching (for instance) an exhaustive table of known integrals. Sometimes it may be no more than recovering several pieces of apposite information, and from their union and confrontation a solution is rapidly put together. But the germinative process in actual human minds may depend on a repertoire of devices—cultivation of the sense of analogy, the recognition of patterns in a complex assembly, and so forth. Sometimes there are routine drills that the reasoner may recognize and employ. Polya, a distinguished mathematician, has given coherent accounts of how one might go about solving certain classes of problems (1954). In contrast, other mathematicians (Poincaré 1913; Hadamard 1954) have found that details are often worked out in their unconscious minds by processes to which they do not have access. There seems little doubt that such skills come from understanding, knowledge, and practice. Naturally, they are not to be adequately gauged by naive tests for knowledge of fact and method. The best performances by computers fall short of this inventiveness of outstanding human minds. Nevertheless, we may reasonably look for continued development in computers in solving problems in sophisticated Logic. But the mathematicians' habit of generalizing, of constantly seeking more fundamental insights and constant practice, develops a Chinese box of progressive amplification that is effective. To the inexpert, unfortunately, this expansion commonly seems exasperatingly far from the practical world.

Phenomena at least as complex lie in the infinite subtleties of language, which continually expose the crassness of standard didactic grammars. Any word processor with a speller is adept at seeking out the puns that (often cryptically) enrich so much of poetry. Much of the interminable quest for Miltonic allusion could benefit from programs to search compilations of all the mythical figures from Adam to Snow White who got into trouble from eating apples of doubtful provenance, or who achieved distinction from golden keys. No doubt constructing lists of ear rhymes and eye rhymes is simply a matter of searching techniques. But the truly creative aspects of poetry and music are much more elusive events.

There is much more to complexity than mere numbers, which too easily divert attention from the essence of complexity. A giant computer may perform billions of computations, or a wind tunnel handle vast numbers of gas molecules. The formation of a crystal involves immense numbers of operations, yet since the same pattern is repeated over and over again in the course of the process, it is easy to describe succinctly their pattern of steps with great precision. Here there is grand multiplicity of operations; but that in itself has little to do with complexity. Indeed, every Statistician knows the paradox that for many systems, as the sample size increases their corporate behavior becomes progressively easier to describe with ever higher precision. There is no finite sample size at which the utility of information from an infinite population becomes saturated. However, that statement calls for some careful attention to what we mean by *information*. The possible confusion recalls the mistaken belief about trench warfare in the First World War that command of a space of military significance increases without limit as more and more arms are concentrated on it (Hart 1936). The military lesson was grudgingly learned, and trench warfare had no role in the Second World War. Instead, the comparable myth of saturation bombing became common.

No. Complexity is not the outcome of multiplicity but quite a different matter. It seems to depend on deployment of limited resources to encompass as much freedom as possible. It is difficult to grasp or express that more precisely in simple language; but it is akin to the notion of degrees of freedom in the paradigm. To find it, one maximizes what is known in a vector space as the rank or the dimensionality of the space spanned. Cast in rather different terms of causality, the formation of the crystal involves a great many parts, but they are highly *redundant in operation:* all are doing the same thing. But complexity offers low redundancy in operation with *high diversity in deployment.* A single end may then be attained by several different pathways, so that though the one fails, the whole will not.

EXAMPLE 13.4. The need for efficient homeostasis of blood glucose is vital because of the unique importance of glucose to the brain, the functioning of which requires that the glucose level not sink too low; and the delicate balance of electrolytes and osmosis may be imperiled if blood glucose stays high for too long. Many factors—starvation, strenuous exercise, overdosage with insulin—may lead to hypoglycemia. Multiple mechanisms exist to restore depleted blood glucose; they include several hormones, autonomic tone, an increased sense of hunger that prompts the person to seek food, and sometimes sophisticated medical care. These diverse patterns operate in so intricate a fashion as to challenge mathematical modeling and physiological analysis of the system as a whole. Yet probably not more than twenty factors (if so many) are involved.

RICHNESS

As Hardy said of mathematics (1967), it is much easier to illustrate richness than it is to define it. An idea or a system is rich if there is a striking contrast between the economy of the structure and the multiplicity and diversity of the consequences. Of course, these terms are relative and elusive.

We may cite three illustrative properties of such a system.

Diversity and Unity

What we recognize as diversity is often an artifact due to failure in our intuitions. The class of quadrupeds is easy to grapple with because, despite the differences in size, habitat, diet, and intelligence among mice, elephants, otters, and sheep, all have four legs and hence mechanical similarities in the way they walk. So is the class of mammals because of their way of feeding the young, although it is less intuitively obvious that the whale is more like the kangaroo than like the dogfish even though both the whale and the dogfish are marine animals and give birth to fully developed young whereas the kangaroo does not. In mathematics it is both interesting and, in a curious way, satisfying to find that such diverse figures as the point, straight line, circle, ellipse, hyperbola, and parabola, although apparently of quite disparate shapes, are all examples of the conic section; that is, if we bake a cake in the form of a simple cone and slice it once at random, the cut surface may take any of these forms. In the more subtle ideas like the fractal (Mandelbrot 1977) or Chaos (Gleick 1987; Devaney 1989) or angular homeostasis (Murphy n.d.-a), one is shocked and exhilarated to find the diversity in the repertoire that emerges with only relatively small variations in the values for the specifications.

Richness in Relation to Complexity

The discernment of complexity is related closely to the foregoing and readily flows into it. If the teasing out, the unpacking, as it were, of one of these rich processes leads to remarkable diversity and ornateness, it is perhaps to be expected that the richness of the outcome indicates that the process is complex. In the world of empirical inference, we are faced with not the process but the results of it; and perhaps the first step to understanding it may be to try to guess how complicated the instructions for the germinating process may be. Here again, intuition seems to be a poor guide. An elaborate result may prove to have a simple cause, a simple result a complex one. It is very slowly that we have grasped the importance of that strange dissociation. Knowing much about the workings of the brain but very little of how it is generated, we expect the genetic coding to involve a great many genes. But that is not necessarily true. We may be profoundly shocked when we discover that a simple process suffices to produce an outcome that is both intricate and reliable. (Indeed, other things being equal, the simpler the process, the more apt it is to be reliable.) To grasp this disparity, one plausible, even obvious, mental adjustment at the outset may help.

Unwittingly we tend to suppose the order of events as follows. Evolution faces a challenge to form some intricate pattern, such as the development of the heart or the brain, and having done so must cultivate, cost what it may, a mechanism for doing so with high reliability. Now, whatever kind of image that may be, it is certainly not Darwinian. Evolution does not "set out" to do anything. Change occurs randomly. If the change is an advantage, it is more likely to survive and be perpetuated. But it survives because it survives, not because it has accomplished some important strategic advance. Indeed, it is not part of the theory that there is any particular objective: survival on any terms is survival, and the change is not the purpose of evolution, but evolution the result of the change. If some other random change had survived simply as a result of enhanced survival, evolution would have taken a different course. Once one makes those statements, they will seem obvious to the point of triteness, and unworthy of taking up space. But they are commonly overlooked for all that.

The scientific challenge is to reconstruct what in fact did happen in evolution. If evolution started at A and ended at B, the question is not to discover how the problem of getting from A to B could have been "solved." It is rather to reconstruct what did happen, and what (if anything) can be learned about the process and mechanisms of that evolution. Just so, the role of the historian is not to decree how history was destined to turn out but to discern what did happen. Evolutionary science is just like history, except that the evidence is not the written documents of the historian but the prehistorical evidence of the fossil record and the conservation of the genetic code. In the event, the reconstruction is often extremely difficult and painfully conjectural. But in the case of the diamond, despite its elegance and reliability, these intricate questions and patterns do not occur.

Illumination

From these sets of properties—unity-diversity and complexity—emerges a third phenomenon: the possibility of a simple account for *ontogeny,* the diverse development of the individual member of a species. How exactly can change at one nucleotide lead to a person with six fully developed fingers rather than five? The answer is not at all obvious. Indeed, the challenge is so preposterous that none would believe it possible were it not for the fact that it does occur (McKusick et al. 1964), and any theory about it, however farfetched, however much an exercise in pure imagination, however lacking in empirical support or difficult to verify, must perforce be taken seriously. If it were possible to prove that there are three and only three theoretically possible and fully satisfactory mechanisms to account for the event, then it is not the slightest help to dismiss them all as extremely unlikely, for under pain of abandoning rational explanation we must accept at least one of them as the actual answer.

Of course, to describe how such illuminations are attained is to write an exhaustive history of scientific discovery. It must suffice here to point out how often the major scientific advances have an unmistakable character of beauty. Indeed, the distinguished physicist Dirac was quite unencumbered by any supernatural beliefs whatsoever, yet he demanded beauty as a hallmark of scientific truth (Hovis and Kragh 1993). From this elusive, but nevertheless profoundly authenticating, beauty flow conceptual economy, insight, the capacity to cultivate new intuitions. In all likelihood, it is this quality that informs the theories of esthetic unity.

ORGANIZATION

Organization, the third and last hallmark of respect, is the most elusive of all, and yet the most important to our topic. The issues may be put on the table by stating a problem.

Example 13.5. Compare the contents of a garbage heap with some acknowledged work of art, say the Taj Mahal. Randomly permute the components of the garbage heap, and nothing of significance is lost. Randomly permute the components of the Taj Mahal, and whatever pile of rubbish emerges will make no sense whatsoever. Now, clearly the issue here is not merely one of complexity. To make a *precise copy* of a garbage heap would probably be every bit as demanding, even as to expense, as to make a precise copy of the Taj Mahal. To give a *precise description* of the garbage heap would probably be much more difficult, because the components are probably smaller and much more heterogeneous; and the whole would be denied the economizing artistic constraints (such as symmetry, proportionality, grouping of masses, hidden harmonies and rational but nevertheless obscure germinating processes) that underlie all great art. Certain scientists might perhaps receive bribes (we would choke over calling it funding) to undertake a search for these artistic constraints in the garbage heap; but they would do so with dismay and little hope.

The ontology of what exactly free-floating organization may be is not at all easy to address, still less define. Utility and purpose are issues, but often demeaning ones, and difficult to apply to human beings. An old criterion of life, "growth plus differentiation" (now overshadowed as a criterion by discernment of chemical markers), lends something to the analysis. The word *differentiation* rather begs the question, however, since to define it in terms that would distinguish it from mere diversification is not easy, especially since it may often be misplaced and then become quite pointless (as in the dysplasias). Organization must certainly involve the uses and abuses of complexity: the fostering of freedoms that serve no useful purpose is at best pointless and at times harmful; there must be some rate of exchange between complexity and richness. Intuition suggests that a highly organized system is likely to exhibit a high level of emergent properties; but that notion is not easy to state more precisely, still less to prove or verify. For the same reason there must be enough *hard-wiring* and redundancy in the system to ensure that it develops and operates within acceptable tolerances. For higher organisms there must be enough capacity to learn from experience and, in human beings, to accommodate reflection, adaptation, prudent experimentation, and in general to rescue the whole from what the popular cant calls lockstep.

To continue with this argument, we consider further some conceptual terms, broached earlier, that will also color future discussions. We shall subsist unabashed on metaphors from elsewhere, unabashed because in many places they are nearer to literal reality than to vivid poetic imagery.

Hardware

Hardware, taken over as a technical term, denotes the permanent structures and features of a computer. Operations and functions contained in the hardware are commonly called *hard-wired* (e.g., even in most contemporary hand-held calculators the means of taking logarithms or trigonometric functions are hard-wired). These terms may be used metaphorically for the features of the human body that do not have to be learned but will automatically be built in and activated in normal ontogeny. In the domain of behavior, such structures are usually called *instinct.* There have been endless semantic attacks on this word because of the not very successful attempts either to define it from the analysis of its evident characteristics rather than its innate (i.e., nonlearned) character, or to locate where in the nervous system it is executed.

Software

In computers, *software* denotes optional material (text, programs, special mathematical functions) that may be added to a computer. Typically, it is designed to operate unchanged and, indeed, usually cannot be changed by the user. (It will, of course, change if damaged and may cease to work entirely.) In behavior, this term is used metaphorically to denote habits that may or may not be able to draw on an instinctive background but are typically learned by social conditioning (such as eating, sleeping, excretion, walking, manipulating toys, etc.) or systematic indoctrination (elementary teaching).

Unallocated Space

Unallocated space is that part of the computer that is occupied by neither the hardware nor the software but may be freely used to assemble text, programs, and automatic devices at the ingenuity of the user. It may lead to material that is appropriate software, but the main intent is to provide space in which the user may practice solving problems by assembling and concatenating the resources of the computer. In the metaphor, the human counterpart is the cultivation and the exploitation of resources to understand knowledge and address problems of an unfamiliar kind—what is connoted by that much-abused word *education.* An imaginative step further gives us a glimpse of understanding as to how a finite Chinese box might be generated by these means. An essential component of both the use of the computer and education is (in a profound ontological sense and not as mere metaphor) the freedom in imagination, cognition, and volition that is constrained by nothing but the demands of truth itself. Indeed, this freedom allows the Chinese box the space to develop and in turn to foster further freedom. But it takes both freedom and energy to get the process started in the first place and to keep it from collapsing. The analogy with a Random branching process is enticing. These ideas may be endlessly elaborated in the light of further information and understanding.

RESPECT AND HUMAN ETHICS

This difficult topic of respect lies at the heart of Medical Ethics. Its ontology requires special attention, for undoubtedly it is the area in which the (often intrusive) feelings run highest when Ethical issues are in question. These feelings touch closely the quality of humanity, the topic in which dispassionate analysis is hardest and from which human disengagement is all but unimaginable.

As we stated above, movements demanding recognition of rights for animals, plants, and nonliving things have been advanced *ex nihilo*. Conterminality, insofar as it adduces nothing that is not contained in the bald statement of the putative right, is as always condemned. On the whole, parsimony is desirable although not an inalienable consideration. Positing rights that are trivial by reason of particularity, redundancy, or multiplicity is to be deplored. This implied criticism is no insurmountable obstacle. Proliferation of rights contributes nothing to the dignity of Ethics. Putative rights in trivial causes without precedent, imitating and extending the concept of human rights, have little value. Even well-entrenched precedent alone is not enough. The price is now being paid for trying to construct a shallow-rooted theory of human rights out of compassion, or from transcendent values, or from political sentiment. Had there been some ontological purpose in the first place (see Appendix 3), it might be much simpler not only to develop and extend these proposals but also (what is at least as important) to rescue them from the grosser absurdities.

As to the finer things—the preservation and cultivation of the beautiful, the true, the rare, the common goods and pleasures—we can only fleetingly applaud them, and then declare them (by any reasonable criterion) outside the limits of the underpinnings of Medical Ethics.

INTENTION

The origin of the term *intention* is an even more involved matter than that of the term *respect*. The root (*Webster's* 1988) seems to be the Latin word *tenuis,* which is related to *thin.* From experience, thinning leads to the associated notion of stretching out, reaching beyond what is immediately accessible, and sometimes breaking. Hence the words *tend* (so easily, but falsely, related to *trend*); *tendency;* and, as a kind of physical association, *tension* and *tense,* which in the first place had the sense of fragility but later became colored with a sense of excitement, perhaps because many endeavors of excess stretching lead to disappointment and disaster. The prefix *in-* adds a flavor of eagerness, which is mild in the words *intend* and *intention* but becomes very strong in the words *intent* and *intense.*

INTENTIONALITY

Loewy (1989) attributes to Kant the notion that *intention* denotes very much what the layman would suppose it to mean: a deliberative identification of purpose. The term *purpose* needs to be considered carefully. The situation, however, has been somewhat confused by the word *intentionality,* which seems to have originated with Brentano (Edelman 1992) in the context of consciousness. It has been addressed by many modern writers on the mind-brain problem (Searle 1983, 1992; Churchland 1984; Edelman 1992; Shaffer 1993).

The Concept of Intentionality

The very term *intentionality* seems to indicate (Searle 1992) that the grammatical voice[2] of awareness is not passive or middle but active, and in consequence it demands an object. Thus, one of the ways in which a person is distinguished from a machine is that a feature essential to a person is intentionality, that is, the positing of an object of awareness. A machine may perform an operation repeatedly and in fulfillment of a sharply defined purpose, as a printing machine producing a newspaper does, provided that the purpose has been designed into it; however, that is not the operation of true intentionality but rather, in Searle's phrase (1992: 78–82), *as if* intentionality.

From our standpoint, this idea of intentionality is not, prima facie, objectionable, although Brentano's original formulation was prompted by metaphysical demands rather than scientific perceptions. It remains to be seen how useful the idea is. Moreover, the claim that awareness *must* have an object seems to be a strong one; and no accumulation of individual examples may be regarded as proving it true or even making much of a claim that it is a universal need. It is affirmable but not falsifiable, and as such it presents epistemic problems. Since it has some importance to what follows,

---

2. In the sense used in Chapter 12. For further treatment, refer to Appendix 2.

we shall try to lay bare some of the difficulties that arise. These developments raise some interesting questions that may turn out to have a much wider area of application. In particular, they may help to clarify the meaning of *intention* in an Ethical context. If human consciousness demands an object, then it appears that every human Act is linked to a particular object, and linked to a particular purpose of the person acting.

An Aside on the Character of Assertions

To set the stage, we note how the character of an assertion relates to the relevant evidence; for the moment we leave the specific topic of intentionality.

EXAMPLE 13.6. As applied to human beings the word *heterozygote* denotes somebody who, at a particular locus, has two different alleles. A typical step in genetic counseling is to note that the Probability that a gene will be transmitted to any particular offspring is ½; and if both parents are carriers, the Probability of both parents transmitting the gene so that the child is homozygous and therefore affected is ¼. The *segregation ratio* for affected children is thus 1 in 4. Now, the definition and nature of the heterozygous state are chemical matters, and statements about them are strictly ontological; and the fact that there may be methods for discerning them is neither here nor there. The methods have no impact on the meaning of the statement.

EXAMPLE 13.7. Consider now the statement "poet: one who writes poetry; a maker of verses" (*Webster's* 1988). We might argue about what is meant by *poetry* or *verses,* but let us gloss over that nicety. The affirmation may seem to be of much the same kind as that in the previous example, but it is in fact very different. When in the first flush of romantic ardor Gray (1750) wrote about the "mute, inglorious Milton" who died wholly unfulfilled, was he speaking of a poet? It seems to us that common usage would exclude the mutely inglorious from the ranks of poets. The working of the ordinary language is that a poet is not someone who has skill but one who has already written poetry. On this scale there are no potential poets, only accomplished ones. The radical difference between this example and the previous one is that the meaning being defined refers, not to a state that in principle exists permanently (like maleness or femaleness), but to one that in fact exists, that (like dutiable goods) has been declared. The ontological tenor of the statement is thus inseparable from empirical evidence, and hence the statement is at least in part an inescapably epistemic one.

EXAMPLE 13.8. Consider the phenomenon of *ascertainment,* as the term is used in genetic analysis. There are lethal autosomal recessive disorders in which the sole sources of genes available to children are heterozygous parents and (much more rarely) new mutations. Affected children must have inherited the gene from both parents, and hence *a couple at risk is a couple who have already had an affected child*. This example, like the one about the poet, is a statement that is in part at least based on empirical evidence. It may be difficult to pinpoint how exactly that judgment can be reconciled with Example 13.6, which is very similar. Both of them revolve around Mendel's Laws, and both involve the heterozygous state. The problem lies in the elusive nature of the phrase *at risk*. Risk in this example is a matter of the inference that the parents are both heterozygous, and it seems that that claim is not falsifiable. If the couple have shown that they can have one homozygous child, then (from the genetic standpoint, at least) they have shown that they can have others. But while the Probability of having an affected child is exactly the same in a heterozygous couple who have had several children, all of them healthy, the risks are indeed different.[3] Risk here is in part an epistemic statement, and so is not the same as the strictly ontological statement that the segregation ratio is 1 in 4. This divergence is the basis of the (easily enough resolved) paradox that the genotypes of the progeny are determined independently, and yet every time a healthy child is born the recurrence risk changes (Murphy 1979b). The epistemic component in this risk lies in the uncertainty about the parental genotype (i.e., the sample space is unclear).

Likewise, the mortality rate in myocardial infarction is not the same as the mortality rate in necropsy reports of myocardial infarction (Murphy 1997).

Intentionality (Continued)

What, then, are we to make of the statement that one cannot have awareness without intentionality—in effect, that "being aware" is meaningless in the middle voice? If it is supposed to be an ontological statement, then to have acceptable scientific standing it should be falsifiable—that is, if it is false, one should be able to prove it false empirically—for the first item of business is to address how the data are to be treated epistemically.

Appeal to the commonplace of even the best writers, "My mind went blank," may be brushed aside as mere cant. That rebuttal does not help much. It is rhetorical and invites rejoinders of the same ilk. Should a counterexample of nonintentional awareness arise, it might be automatically dismissed as "not true awareness," throwing the entire onus of proof (under severe scrutiny and cross-examination) on those who put the ex-

---

3. It is not difficult, for example, to imagine mating patterns in which the zygote (the newly fertilized ovum) cannot divide and no fetus results. The risk is then either zero or undefined.

ample forward. This tactic is a kind of semantic criticism in which no attempt may be made to define what "true awareness" is, other than insisting on the necessity of an object. If some state is dismissed as not awareness solely on the grounds that there is no object, why, an object will always be necessary. But that rejoinder is a tautology, and the kindest name we could give it is "a definition."

In any case, the demand for an object may be met by the claim that an object is always present in the unconscious mind. This escape hatch may be true. But the fastidious would insist (as in all such pentheric cases) that at the very least the original proposition as stated has nevertheless been disproved by the counterexamples; and it should be withdrawn in favor of a new and properly formulated proposition.

Levels of Intentionality

This matter of the object is an important one. Searle (1992: 130) says flatly, "Most, but not all, consciousness is intentional." If that is so (and we believe it is), we may usefully call nonintentional consciousness zero-order intentionality. Edelman (1992: 112) is less decisive: "Consciousness shows intentionality; it is of or about things or events."

But there is no dispute about the existence of higher levels of intentionality, including self-contemplation. There is, first, the awareness of ordinary things, intentionality of order 1. Sometimes the focus is a lavish process, a kind of mental exercise or warming-up device, such as one sees in the young child or the inebriated. Edelman (1992) sees it as a characteristic of "non-linguistic and non-semantic animals."

Edelman goes on to say that there is "higher-order consciousness" such as self-analysis of one's awareness and behavior. As we address still higher-order processes, it becomes abundantly clear that there is less and less to be gained by black-box methods and the cant of objectivity, while more and more is to be gained by analysis from within, what we recognize as *reflection*. In particular, there is much to be gained from expert guidance by those accustomed to exploring the elaborate and subtle mechanisms that evolve for the maintenance of psychic homeostasis (see Chapter 8). These mechanisms are in part spontaneous and in part deliberately cultivated. We can scarcely be surprised at these developments and the rapid decline of doctrinaire reductionism. That one can never hope to construct a simple model or even a simple set of coherent techniques for analyzing an essentially complex system verges on tautology. It seems to point directly at a Chinese box that will certainly be intricate and perhaps intractable. We shall meet it again in Chapter 15.

INTENTION AND ETHICS

Since Ethics is indeed concerned with human activity, it may well be asked whether Ethics should deal with intention, and, if so, where and how. We must be particularly on our guard against confusing an accessory and heavily Medical theory, the practical deontological prescription, and the demands of conscience in all its senses. How to use and abuse a piece of scientific apparatus is no doubt an important matter to the manufacturers if their good name is to be preserved. But that is not the task of the scientist. Intention is a basic aspect of Morality; and it is also treated in many texts of Philosophical and scholastic Ethics. But these matters are outside our purview, and we express no opinions about them here.

We recognize two ways of using the term *intention:* the intention that the individual person has in acting, and the intention that is, or would be, reasonably imputed by others to particular behavior. Indeed, this brief discussion of these two aspects is a foretaste of matters that we address in Chapters 14 and 15. A closely related topic is the consequences of an Act, whether viewed as a component of a consensual or a consistential Ethics, or simply a concern over the potency of Ethics. In general, the consequences of an Act may be foreseen from experience of similar Acts. The nearest to a gold standard for Ethical behavior that we may hope for is consensus among reasonable observers.

However, individual observers may have their own personal, idiosyncratic[4] interpretations, which reflect their psychology and differences in kind and range of experiences (see Chapter 15). Very occasionally, the best interpretation is found to have been highly idiosyncratic, the insight of genius. But while some few solutions may be manifestly absurd, there is no infallible way of discerning a priori the soundness of any particular interpretation.

At times particular persons may have objectives that differ from what is imputed to them or ascribed to courses of action they may consider. Their objectives may depart radically from the gold standard, even ignore it totally. This is a delicate topic, but one that merits brief discussion.

The Flat Surface

We are obliged to be careful about the reasoning before we brave the full fury of the blast.

The goal of the Ethical analysis is to define a uniquely good or at least optimal solution. Let us suppose that there are many possible answers to

---

4. The word *idiosyncratic* has various unpleasant connotations, from the obscure to the deranged. We need hardly point out that we use the term in a completely neutral sense as appropriate for anything from fingerprints to handwriting that is distinctive and personal.

the problem in hand. (That assumption, at least, can hardly need to be documented.) Not all answers will be equally good, but every one that has at least a few serious proponents will have some evident merit, and the courtesies of debate will demand that we treat it with respect. Let us further suppose that there is some reasonable way of comparing merits, and that it can be cast in metrical terms. That assumption is rather more demanding, but we are prepared to regard it as nonetheless a useful one. We then plot a map on a surface, the height representing merit, and the location on the plane[5] being the corresponding ontological structure. This display we may call the ontological-ethical graph (OEG). Now, we cannot arbitrarily impose constraints on the OEG (e.g., that it be continuous or smooth). In the ideal outcome, one single point is dazzlingly high above the rest, like a radio transmitter on the top of a mountain. Those familiar with the properties of contour maps may find such maps a helpful image here.

However, several solutions may be equally good, or almost so. We may hope that all the competing answers will be clustered together so that we have grounds for believing that there is an ontologically cohesive answer. But we have no assurance that that is true. Competing high points (i.e., plausible explanations) may be very widely separated.

EXAMPLE 13.9. For instance, there might be a first reasonable argument that the Ethical way in which to care for conjoint ("Siamese") twins joined at their heads is to do an immediate operation that separates them. But in certain instances, at least, it will involve major risk to one or both. Once the operation is successfully completed, however, the outlook is good. A second reasonable view might be to wait until the babies are somewhat stronger and then do an operation in multiple stages. One can imagine any number of intermediate proposals. All will be in much the same region of the OEG. Another proposal may be radically different: that the twins not be separated at all but be reared together. They will have serious handicaps, but they will avoid the perhaps high risk of disability due to brain damage. A third and prudent proposal might be to delay the operation until the twins are old enough to understand the risks and make their own decision. These three courses of action might have comparable merits; and they may be espoused by sane and competent clinicians who differ in their perceptions of a single set of agreed facts. It might be that almost all solutions other than hopeless vacillation are about equally good. Then it seems reasonable to conclude that there are no weighty Ethical imperatives other than that of avoiding frank incompetence. If that conclusion is acceptable, then it is fitting that proponents respect one another's decisions.

---

5. Or a hyperplane or a manifold, or some more complicated structure.

Reason and Purpose

The nice distinction between *reason* and *purpose* was made by McDougall (1924), a kind of prepared stronghold against the Freudian erosion of epistemology by the inchoate and nonfalsifiable claims for a purposeful unconscious. We outline it briefly. In behavior, reason comprises the analysis of the interrelations between Things, of insight into the consequences of Acts, of the appropriate behavior if certain ends are to be attained, and so forth. Motive comprises the moving forces that provide the instinctive promptings to act to some purpose. Without motive, the wisest and most convincing decisions are impotent. The most powerful urges serve no purpose if not canalized by reason. The commonsense comparison of this reciprocation is with car, driver, and fuel. Fuel is the motive. The components of the car—steering, pedals, and gears—are the effective mechanisms of behavior. The driver is the reason, and the itinerary the purpose. Just how far this model can be verified or authenticated is a pragmatic and open question. How far it is ontologically sound is a question at the intersection of Medicine and Philosophy.

Intent

In dealing with intention so specifically, we prefer the term *intent,* which has a more technical, less ambiguous connotation. We recognize two kinds of intent: constructive (i.e., imputed) and idiosyncratic intent.

DEFINITION.   *Constructive intent* is the construction or interpretation that a consensus of reasonable observers would put on the objective of the Act of a reasonable person.

This sense of the term *intent* implies that behavior can be analyzed within a general system that takes note of the characteristics of the person acting. Individuals may have quite different constructive intents, influenced by age, sex, and occupation.

DEFINITION.   *Idiosyncratic intent* is the objective that a particular person in a concrete situation wishes to attain.

Because the functioning of the unconscious is complex (see Appendix 1), idiosyncratic intent can be fully inferred only a posteriori, if then. A consensus may be grossly incorrect. Idiosyncratic intent cannot be the basis of an Ethical principle, still less of an Ethical code.

EXAMPLE 13.10. A man is crossing a street in the direction of a restaurant, the only building on that side. The constructive intent of the Act is to reach the restaurant. Let us say that his idiosyncratic intents are to eat and (because of personal favors from the proprietor) to patronize the restaurant. The motives may be a desire to eat and friendship with the proprietor. The reason may be that he needs food to sustain life and good health, and that he receives a discount on his meals there.

EXAMPLE 13.11. A surgeon is devising an operation to repair a heart valve. The constructive intent of the Act is to repair the valve. The surgeon's idiosyncratic intent may be to perfect the procedure. His motive may be his desire to gain professional recognition, or financial gain, or to please a benefactor who suffers from that condition. His reason may be that the patient will die if the operation is not done, and that operating provides the opportunity to develop new techniques.

We perceive Ethics to be a system of analysis to help in resolving conflicts in situations presenting options. The idiosyncratic intent of the person acting is not in itself germane to Ethical analysis any more than the soundness of a mathematical argument is affected by whether the mathematician is bored with it. That remains true even when it can be argued prudentially that cultivating good intentions makes it easier and surer to behave ethically (e.g., in an emergency or when distracted).

We have to admit that clinical practice is a living, existential engagement, so that the idiosyncratic intent of the individual practitioners will have some, perhaps small, impact on the communal mainstream of clinical practice. But this impact is buffered by the momentum of professional standards of practice. Moreover, individual physicians may be aware that they are unusually sensitive to certain demands or biased in handling them. They may see fit to disqualify themselves from dealing with relatives or close friends. In this fashion extraordinary emotional involvement is kept from becoming part of prudential clinical judgment.

Moreover, the consensus on which Ethics is based is attained externally. According to this view, the Ethical standing of an Act does not depend on the idiosyncratic intent of the individual acting. A morally praiseworthy idiosyncratic intent is neither sufficient nor necessary to make the Act acceptable, and conversely. Two equally competent persons acting in the same way in the same circumstances have exactly the same Ethical standing.

In their deliberations many ethicists have included idiosyncratic, as well as constructive, intent. However, once idiosyncratic intent is explicitly introduced, there arise serious conceptual and practical differences.

Physicians are only too painfully aware of the harm done by well-meaning colleagues who have never learned to question motives or even to suspect the integrity of their own intentions. A patient is safer in the hands of a competent cynic who "sees through" everything (including even personal defects) than in those of an incompetent philanthrope who has attained little self-knowledge. This realization, we think, will prompt practitioners to keep their own feelings from affecting such decisions regarding their clients. But separating the material and the personal aspects of an issue can be exceedingly intricate, since confusion between them can occur readily not only at conscious but also at unconscious levels of mental functioning. In particular, the wisdom of experience is that clinicians do not attempt to make any professional decisions regarding near relatives that may inhibit the usual recourse to external standards established by consensus.

14 External Phenomenology of Responsibility

It is perhaps only responsibility that imparts anything more than an academic interest to the theory and practice of Ethics. Those with no sense, concern, or capacity for responsibility would be unconcerned with Ethics. The topics in this and the following chapter have for us proved to be the most difficult to deal with ontologically. For that reason we shall be content to move slowly, gradually elaborating the very simplest of ideas into what we trust will be somewhat more realistic terms—if not elemental, at least elementary.

The word *responsible,* though akin to the words *responsive* and *response,* is more than a biological term. Its religious origin is evident in cognates that include *sponsor, spondee* (the metrical form of the ritual chant), and John Bunyan's *despond.* It is a term of Legal importance as well. In the narrower Ethical sense, it connotes informed and searching choice of behavior. Nevertheless, it is to be seen as a summary statement of the deliberative conclusion reached, rather than an axiom or other fundamental structure of choice. Observable response (including elective inaction itself) may be considered the main gauge that Ethics or its equivalent is at work; and it is a topic of great richness.

THE FUNDAMENTAL PROBLEM

In a textbook on, say, mathematics, it is not ordinarily thought fitting to address, or even to mention, any deontological or prescriptive issues that might conceivably arise. In the writing of the book it is taken entirely for granted that the reader wants to know and understand about sound method and reliable results. The writer does not urge that readers should pay their bills, save their money, or compute their income taxes honestly, carefully, and accurately. Indeed, most such books are no doubt written with readers in mind; but they are about mathematics, and in their content there is no indication that it makes any difference whether there are readers involved at all and, if so, whether they are excited, challenged, interested, perplexed, bored, or endlessly wondering when something important is going to emerge. Readers overwhelmed by discouraging tracts will presumably take a rest, seek help, or give up reading the book. It is all one to the writer, who is focused on mathematics, not on how to stay out of jail or run for the Senate with an unblemished record of financial probity. There is nothing other than the desire to learn mathematics that impels diligent study.

Perhaps there are those who perceive Moral Philosophy and Ethics in much the same light. The exponents are not perhaps fanatically concerned with carrying out (as distinct from discovering) an appropriate course of action. It is the familiar problem from Chapter 7. Without other considerations, the nicest Ethical judgments do not lead inexorably to any particular action.

While all this detachment has merit,[1] we must look askance at any suggestion that Ethics is nothing more than an entertaining hobby, and that whether its students appropriate any of its content is an issue of no importance. The concern over lack of any existential commitment is, at this level, largely a matter of outrage that any serious-minded scholar should remain a whited sepulcher, decked out in much hard-won scholarship that is to have no impact whatsoever on the internal formation of the mind: all lofty formulas and no metanoia.

Nevertheless, to see the complaint of detachment exclusively in terms of these honorable sentiments is to miss what to us is ontologically much more important. Let us set aside sincerity and integrity and the nobler moral virtues. Ethics without existential engagements is dislocated. In our definition (Chapter 1), Ethics is the study, not of appropriate rules of human conduct, but of the making of decisions in concrete cases—necessarily, the study of human beings discerning appropriate decisions. Ethics without engagement is as anomalous as studying Medicine without any attention to, experience of, or concern for patients. It may be excellent biochemistry, or molecular biology, or mathematical theory, but there is simply no point in pretending that it has anything to do with Medicine.

A local minimum for misclassification—of species, for instance—on a metrical trait is achieved by finding a point at which the conditional Probabilities under the competing hypotheses are equal (see Chapter 10). But that is a mathematical fact, not an Ethical principle. Applying it to screening for metrical diseases would have to incorporate values and penalties of right and wrong decisions and accommodate phronesis, pentheric issues, and the like (see Chapter 3). The basic difficulty lies in making a satisfactory statement about whether human beings are, or are not, inside the system being studied.

At once we perceive that both the main terms are ambiguous. *Human beings* may denote those doing the studying but may also denote those within the subject matter of the study. The distinction is preserved in many other studies: in clinical practice of all kinds, the patients differ from the

---

1. We mistrust any scholars-in-a-hurry, ethicists and physicians included.

clinicians. In politics, the representatives differ from those represented. In social anthropology, the scientists differ from the subjects studied. The ambiguity spills over to the term *inside,* which seems to denote the content of the field of study. Now, of course, it is a common and *asymmetrical* device implied in the scholarly point of view to allow one group to study another by constituting two strictly distinct groups. Judges study criminals. Physicians study patients. Historians study earlier human beings. Sometimes, distance is lent to this disturbing asymmetry by introducing an abstract theory, or by using evidence that is about neither human beings nor their attributes but is nonetheless the result of human behavior. Instances include the study of trade figures in economics and artifacts in archaeology. Popular cant would call these intrusions "objective evidence."

But the boundaries are always precarious. At times, judges too may commit crimes. Physicians may become patients. Historians may study the histories of historians. There is always the latent possibility that at some stage professionals in any of these fields begin by looking at something apparently quite outside themselves and (metaphorically speaking) end up by having to examine the backs of their own heads. Looking at the field as external observers, they find that they themselves are inside it. At a certain stage that ambiguity may cause radical confusion.

EXAMPLE 14.1. The analogy that comes to mind is geometrical. Intuition prompts the "obvious" belief that a leaf of paper from a book represents two quite distinct, consecutive pages (i.e., has two sides). One cannot trace a continuous line from one page to the other without lifting the pen or crossing an edge. By that test, however, the famous Möbius strip (Figure 14.1) has only one side and shows that the intuition that a leaf has two pages, if applied to pieces of paper in general, is not sound. Likewise, there is the intuitive belief that in every closed three-dimensional figure one can distinguish unambiguously between what is interior and what exterior. The Klein bottle shows that that belief is also not in complete generality true. Yet in both instances the properties are global only, not local. In any isolated *part* of a Möbius strip, there are two pages; so that in a sufficiently large strip, in finite time, one may never recognize the intrinsic ambiguity at all. It will be clear that the ambiguity between global and local properties is not changed by distance but tends to be concealed by it. The original intuition may be vindicated in any particular Möbius strip by cutting it transversely at any place and allowing it to untwist. But, of course, that maneuver radically changes the topology.

In much the same way, the real ambiguity about what the object of Ethics is and what the Ethical method is, and how they differ, can much of the time be glossed over by expanding the ontological loop—for instance, by introducing a great mass of technical detail between what the students

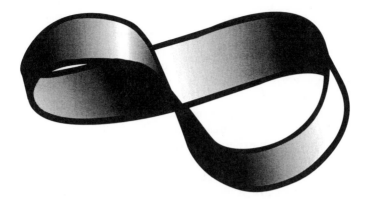

Figure 14.1   The Möbius strip. If a pencil is put anywhere on the surface of the strip, it is possible to draw a line connecting it to any other point without lifting the pencil or crossing the edge of the strip. By this criterion, the strip has only one surface.

of Ethics are addressing and the point at which it extends to include themselves and their very discussions about the distinctions. Eventually these students will be studying themselves studying themselves studying what was originally supposed to be outside themselves. The whole is like the difference between successive coils of an infinite spiral staircase. Indeed, such is the depth of the ambiguity that the expressions "the content of Ethics" and "the scope of Ethics" are indifferently used to mean either of these two quite distinct things. It is like confusing the measurement of the size of a molecule with the essentially molecular structure of the scale on which we measure it.

There is some risk, in a sufficiently complicated pattern of this kind, of losing track of what is reality and what not. Interesting use of this ambiguity has been made in serious literature by such writers as George Macdonald (1895) and Christopher Priest (1983). It may be this expansion that has forced upon us some of the false preconceptions of Ethics in rational discourse. The polarized, and perhaps wholly artificial, schema of Ethics presented in Chapter 2 may have arisen in that way by (as it were) cutting a Möbius strip. In it there appears to be an antagonism between (for instance) axioms and consequences that we ordinarily have to try to resolve in an atmosphere of cut-and-thrust, mutual recrimination and criticism. Consistential Ethics, though both reasonable and accommodating, smacks a little too much of treaty, of compromise as a means of resolving a frank tug-of-war. But if the Ethical Möbius strip had been preserved and not artificially sundered, neither polarization nor compromise would have been necessary, perhaps not even possible. After all, the Möbius strip is topologically homogeneous. It has no preferred interior parts: the twist does not occur in any particular place but is a property of the whole strip, and any part of the strip would be equally accessible to any other part of it. The ethicist might start equally well at any point. All serious work, however exclusive, on any true component of it would cosmically be an impartial, nonpartisan, contribution.[2]

Tantalizing though this prospect is, we think it wiser, for the present at least, to adhere to the more classical uncoiled schema: axioms-theory-verification-speculation-experiment. This less adventurous device, undertaken in the interests of tractability, is the equivalent of cutting the Möbius strip. Thus, two arbitrarily distinct relationships occur. The one is the rational system available to the disinterested theoretical observer from Mars (of whom more later). The other is the human being inside the system and actually addressing real problems.

It is on the basis of this rather reductionistic parsing that we shall apportion the contents of the current chapter and the following one. In Chapter 15 we shall try to make amends by addressing briefly some tentative conceptual approaches that might eventually enable us to repair the damage done by implicitly cutting the strip.

THE MEANING OF *RESPONSIBILITY*

In our analysis there are three main pertinent but radically different ways in which the terms *responsibility* and *responsible* are used: as a device for the identification of accountability or liability; as the problem of determining the capacity or skill to act; and (in a more narrowly Ethical sense) to characterize the behavior of a particular person in a particular encounter. They are not closely related, the first being a matter of undertaking, the second of endowment, and the third of performance. That disparity does not prevent them from being confused.

Responsibility as Accountability or Liability

Preliminary disclaimer. The discussion in this section has a superficial similarity to, and may be mistaken for, a Legal one. We explicitly disclaim any such meaning. Even the word *contractual* is to be understood in a non-Legal sense (to designate explicit, informed, and adequately deliberated undertakings by a freely operating person in right mind). Legal analysis of responsibility is a technical field in its own right, of which we claim no expert knowledge. No doubt for good reason, Legal problems

---

2. This analogy might have a wider role in rescuing us from the more fatuous partisan disputes about the relative utilities of knowledge, experiment, interpretation, and imagination in science generally. Those actually involved in science will every so often complete a circuit of the loop.

of responsibility are often based on what are clearly fictive constructions that we shall not in general accept. (We may remark incidentally that much harm has been done to Medicine and Ethics both by accepting uncritically and without protest Legal decisions; and by radical failure of the Medical theorist and the clinician to inform the law.) Likewise, we are not in any way attempting to furnish analogous review for any other field of technical competence. Last, it should not be necessary to state yet once again that we are not attempting to prescribe Moral, deontological, or Ethical principles. The broad topic we are discussing is meaning contained and implied in common, nontechnical vocabulary; the principal tools are lexicological.

Types of accountability. A person who is somehow to be held to account for a particular activity may be said to be responsible.

EXAMPLE 14.2. On every ship under way there is ordinarily an officer responsible for the command of the ship. Note that in this sense the adjective is best placed after the noun it modifies: "the officer responsible," not "the responsible officer." (As we shall see in due course, the latter expression may be ambiguous.) The nature of the liabilities is diverse: failure to discharge a responsibility may leave the person open to civil charges of negligence or criminal charges of recklessness; to political impeachment; to moral condemnation; to social ostracism.

The natures and origins of various forms of accountability may be distinguished:

1. *Voluntary accountability:* Voluntary accountability is that which is gratuitous and undertaken without any obligation. It may be *explicit,* stated in a formal contractual agreement, as in a married couple legally adopting children. Or it may be *implicit,* as in the responsibility that parents automatically incur for their children by voluntarily begetting them.

EXAMPLE 14.3. A particularly vexed problem about which the voice of Medicine has been deplorably silent is the Medical good Samaritan. The passerby seeing someone in need of Medical attention has no legal obligation to offer help, but many will see fit to do so. The clinician, having more to offer than most, will perhaps feel under more sense of obligation. The law in its wisdom offers no support, even moral support, to those undertaking this voluntary accountability.

2. *Involuntary accountability:* The accountability is involuntary when the natural choice has been preempted for reasons that are beyond the control of the person concerned.

EXAMPLE 14.4. The responsibility of parenthood, even if only implicitly assumed, is ordinarily freely undertaken. The mother of a child conceived as a result of rape may explicitly forgo, but may not evade, the responsibility. However involuntary her motherhood, she may not simply abandon the child (once born) to fate. The one possible exception is that she undergo voluntary abortion.

EXAMPLE 14.5. The same applies to military conscription to fight a war, which, it need hardly be pointed out, has perplexed many consciences.

3. *Ineluctable accountability:* The problem here is subtly different from involuntary accountability. The accountability is not merely accidentally and extraordinarily acquired (as in the foregoing cases) but lies in the very essence of the personhood concerned. It is such that from the very fact of the explicit existence, there is no escape from accountability. Here there is no natural redress. It is ordinarily socially impossible for a person to revoke all statehood.

EXAMPLE 14.6. Thus, any particular person might not have existed. Hence arises an Ethical counterpart of the classic ascertainment problem in genetics (Weinberg 1912; Li 1970; Murphy, Meyers, and Rohde 1987), to wit: the only cases that can be said to have Ethical substance are those in which the person concerned is de facto alive. Had an individual not existed, the question of accountability from, or on behalf of, that nonexistent individual would be ontologically void. Conversely, the fact that the individual issue has arisen can only mean that that person exists and, as a consequence of existing (having had no anterior choice about being born), has responsibility for the care of his or her own life. This responsibility cannot be abdicated, since there is no ontological redress against the consequences of that person's existence; and suicide, far from being a remedy, is a crime against which cogent forces are Legally warranted, and it is a crime that may incur penalties (although not, presumably, capital punishment).

EXAMPLE 14.7. A person has no control over aging. Nevertheless, at the age of Legal majority the person has no option but to assume certain civil responsibilities (for debts incurred, voting, liability to military service, etc.) except by proof of Legal incompetence.

The measure of accountability. Explicit, contractual accountability is a binary process. The contract is either fulfilled or not. For instance, in Example 14.2 the captain is understood to be at all times completely in command of the ship, even when asleep. However, not all accountability is contractual. If on the high seas the captain as a result of illness becomes incompetent, or otherwise is not effectively in command, there may be no other contractual accountability; yet some person or persons on board may in some measure be held accountable to act in the captain's place. This would normally be the next highest ranking competent officer, who in signing a contract will at least implicitly have undertaken the obligation to fulfill this role if needed.

EXAMPLE 14.8. Now suppose that, as a result of an epidemic on board, the only available person may be a passenger, whose only contractual obligation is the usual one for passengers to accept the authority of the captain in certain matters. There can be no question of an implicit contract at all to supervise or save the ship and passengers, other than what might, in the tradition of Rousseau, be called a social contract of the kind implied under *ineluctable accountability*.

EXAMPLE 14.9. An analogue arises in the surgical operation. The principal surgeon has a clear contractual responsibility for the patient; an assistant has at least an implied contract. Should that principal surgeon become incapacitated or die suddenly during the operation, the assistant would clearly have to assume a responsibility at least implied by the original agreement to participate in the operation. The degree of responsibility would then depend on the assistant's competence and Legal empowerment. An assistant who is a medical student, for instance, would only under the most extraordinary circumstances have either the obligation or the title to complete the operation but would certainly be required to seek or send for somebody competent to take over. But even a student nurse, if left as the only person capable of action, has the responsibility to make every reasonable effort to ensure that the patient does not die there and then. It is difficult to believe that this duty is even an implicit contractual responsibility. The responsibility of other surgeons in the surgical unit (e.g., department) would be implicitly a weak contract, while that of a surgeon who happens to be at hand would be more like a social than a Legal contract.

Hypallagous responsibility. While, formally, responsibility is strictly predicated of persons, in the sense of accountability it is sometimes used in loose, even trivial, fashion to ascribe it hypallagously to impersonal objects.[3] We must note, however, that the reductive materialist and the proponents of "strong artificial intelligence," while acknowledging the idea of hypallage, would balk at the idea of its being demonstrated on the epistemic grounds implied here.

3. We remind the reader that in the rhetorical figure hypallage, or transferred epithet, an adjective is transferred from the term that it properly qualifies to some other noun. "A man should be prepared to die for his native land, even if he has never been there" is hypallagous. *Native* means "born in that place (country)." In the example, it must properly apply to somebody other than the subject of the sentence (perhaps an ancestor).

EXAMPLE 14.10. The expression used in the sentence "A front wheel blowout was responsible for the accident" has a verbal, but no evident ontological, relationship to what we have been discussing. It is merely another way of saying, "The cause of the accident was a front wheel blowout." But, of course, the very existence of the tire, its being fitted to the car, the periodic inspection of it, and so forth all involve intervention from human beings, to whom some responsibility (in the sense of accountability) will be imputed.

Responsibility as Capability or Skill

The term *responsible* denotes a person with the current capacity to exercise an appropriate skill in a competent manner.

EXAMPLE 14.11. The sentence "Small wonder the shipwreck occurred; there was no responsible adult on board" would ordinarily be taken to mean either that there was no adult on board or that none aboard was competent to form judgments and act on them.[4]

We are hard put to formulate in nontautologous terms what constitutes the ontology of capability. We shall be content to cite multiple criteria that provide predominantly an evidential characterization. This in some measure reflects the multiplicity of the term. The evidence of capability is of two types:

1. *Inherent qualities:* Inherent qualities arise by virtue of native endowment, such as manual dexterity, facility in communication, experience, and intelligence, and a clear insight as to what the implications of a course of action would be. Other things being equal, a mother of several children may reasonably be supposed to have greater (albeit informal) skill than a childless woman in taking care of a baby. This presumption could be readily overtrumped by relatively slight evidence to the contrary.
2. *Formal qualifications:* Since unselected persons concerned cannot generally be deemed to be impartial judges of their own competence, in serious matters it is usual to impose a requirement of formal qualifications, documentation of professional training, or training in a skill or an art. Legal recognition is conferred by licensure after proper training, often ending in a formal exami-

---

4. This example illustrates the point we made earlier about the placing of the adjective. The meaning of the order "adult responsible" would leave no doubt that the word *responsible* is not a term of praise but a designator of office.

nation. There are, of course, innumerable specialist qualifications that need not be considered in detail here.

Our concern is with ontological issues, not with Ethics, still less with forensic Medicine, so it is undesirable to confuse criteria. Legal entitlement is neither a necessary nor a sufficient condition for actual competence.

EXAMPLE 14.12. In the course of time, the formal qualifications and the practical skill of the physician may be grossly out of proportion. The issue may be a physical impediment: the cardiologist can no longer hear soft aortic diastolic murmurs, the orthopedist is no longer strong enough to perform certain maneuvers. However, more subtly the loss of competence may involve a more serious defect such as forgetfulness or erosion of professional judgment.

One must also recognize that competence involves, and must be adjudicated on, the relationship between what the person professes to be competent to do and actually can do reliably.

EXAMPLE 14.13. An abdominal surgeon does not profess to be, and is not expected to be, skilled in the assessment of the functioning of the parietal lobe of the brain; but a neurologist is.

Responsibility as Quality of Behavior

The term *responsibility* is also used as a descriptor of the quality of behavior.

EXAMPLE 14.14. One may say, "Considering that the boy was only ten years old, his performance was surprisingly responsible."

This sense of the term clearly has both a degree and a contrary. One may, for instance, talk about a child as being "very responsible"; or of an adult as being "extremely irresponsible." It may be applied either to particular Acts or to habitual conduct. Clearly such use of the word is an expression of approval or disapproval. It is mentioned here largely because it is occasionally a distraction and a source of confusion.

EXAMPLE 14.15. By common usage, the contrary of *qualified* is *unqualified*; the term *disqualified* implies explicit forfeit of professional standing. But the opposite of a *pertinent* comment is not an *impertinent* comment, for because of semantic drift *impertinent* is no longer the opposite of *pertinent* but rather has the meaning of *impudent*. The words *internal* and *external* are opposites, but not *instant* and *extant*. Likewise, the opposite of *responsible* should be *irresponsible*. But while the former word is fairly neutral, the latter is condemnatory. An onlooking surgeon does not say, "I am irresponsible for that patient." Even to say, "I am not responsible for that patient" is not wholly free of the taint of insouciance. The moral accretions to the term are such that one is driven to such circumlocutions as "That patient is not under my care, and I have no grounds or authority to intervene in his management."

Commentary

These three perspectives on responsibility—namely, accountability, skill, and commendability—quite naturally delimit what is imposed on the person. Responsibility as accountability explicitly defines a limited set of negotiated obligations and nothing more. Responsibility as capability denotes what the individual is demonstrably qualified for. Its moral force is more social and often highly personal. As quality of behavior, responsibility is prompted much more by social approval than by formal requirements or sanctions; and it is scaled to the expectations appropriate to age and the attitude of the reasonable citizen.

EXTERNAL AND INTERNAL COMPONENTS OF RESPONSIBILITY

It is now appropriate to identify the basic components of what is called responsible behavior. They appear to be of two kinds, external and internal.

The *external* phenomena are those aspects of behavior that can be identified by detached, and otherwise uninterpreted or uninformed, observation. The classic epistemological image is the intelligent observer from Mars: the scholar with no personal experience of participating in the type of response, and having no indoctrination as to what is fitting. External phenomenology, insofar as it has a body of method, might almost be seen as behavioristic, but without any hint of the self-sufficiency implied by analytical and Philosophical (as distinct from empirical) behaviorism (Copleston 1967: passim; Flew 1989; Searle 1992). The objective is not to make any unwarranted claims for the method but to find out how far this deliberately restricted approach can usefully be pushed.[5]

5. This disclaimer is important to what follows. We have no wish to suffer the painful misinterpretation meted out to Descartes's exercise in the *Method* (1637) as if he had been pushing some exclusive and comprehensive Philosophy rather than making a formal exploration inside a deliberately parsimonious axiomatic structure. Even his explicit disclaimer did not suffice to ward off this misinterpretation.

The *internal* phenomena are identifiable chiefly by the actions and reflections of the person or persons being observed, and the reflective and deeper analysis of the actions and the reflections of the observed, surmounted by the observer's reflection on both. The phenomena may sometimes be so recondite that while they necessarily influence the particular outcome, they can be recognized by nobody except, perhaps, a posteriori. However, the domain of analysis given here is necessarily (although not exclusively) experiential. That is, the internal phenomenology must meet the ordinary canons of systematic but empirical scientific inquiry. No doubt the distinction between the external and the internal is somewhat arbitrary.

From the standpoint of the observer we may consider phenomenology at various levels of decreasing transparency and increasing complexity.

EXAMPLE 14.16. To focus matters somewhat, let us consider a typical street scene:

1. The primordial data are largely material: buildings, stores, traffic, pedestrians, parked cars, and so forth.
2. The observer can infer more or less orderly behavior from the physical positions and motions of the people, and thus make surmises. For instance, most people do not park a car within twelve feet of a fire hydrant. Those who do are apt to find written messages left on their cars by uniformed policemen. By their effects, these messages must have undesirable, even ominous contents.
3. The observer may then speculate as to why some people conform to the patterns recognized and others do not. Perhaps there are factors other than ignorance or inability; and individuals are *moved* by certain considerations that can conveniently be named (in technical Latin) *motives*. But there are limits as to how far motive can be analyzed by observing behavior alone. If the subjects may be individually questioned, it will be much easier to discover and analyze their motives. For instance, those who refrain from parking at a fire hydrant may say that they do so out of respect for the law; or to avoid sanction; or because the needs for ready access to the hydrant in the event of fire are evident; or even because in case of fire their cars so parked might be damaged.
4. But although authentic motives exist, subjects may be unaware of them—which suggests to the observer a still more intricate line of behavior such as conditioned, instinctive, or unconscious behavior.
5. Even so, the observer may finally encounter situations where sentiment rather than discernible motives prevail, as in dedication, or unquestioned obedience, or love.

What we have called external phenomenology concerns levels 1 and 2, whereas what we have called internal phenomenology concerns levels 3, 4, and 5. Discussion of the use of this fictional device of the detached but intelligent observer who can explore levels 1 and 2 will complete the current chapter.

EXTERNAL PHENOMENOLOGY

We may capitalize on a convenient analogy with the drama. We begin with the characters.

The Agent

The Agent, the entity confronted with making a decision, is ordinarily a human being of major interest to the study. It seems irrelevant to the main discussion of human Ethics whether in fact nonhuman beings, such as animals or prehuman species or other reflecting intelligences, are capable of making responsible decisions; in the present context, at least, we confine the discussion to human beings.

The Agent may be an individual, or a coherent group of people acting jointly, such as a married couple or a family. A corporate group may function as an Agent only in a much looser sense, despite the manifold decisions of great impact emerging from or within such groups. There are also more and more situations in which decisions are operationally made by computers, although a computer is not ordinarily thought of as an Agent. But this last extension may be illusory. The computer will perform as programmed (even if the program involves mathematical Chaos in which machine noise in the computer may figure prominently); and while it may decree a decision in a particular case without intervention, the human Agent has at least implicitly decided to intervene at the level only of broad policy, not of individual decision. It seems a specious argument that accountability resides with the programmer only if the decision is deterministic; and hence that the stochastic or other indeterminate component in the execution of the program relieves the programmer of any burden of responsibility whatsoever.

In the real world it may be difficult to identify a personal, responsible Agent, especially in the actions of such groups as business corporations, military establishments, governments and agencies, perhaps even society as a whole. The computer may have to serve as the only identifiable Agent. It may even happen that no responsible Agent whatever can be identified externally, either in the sense of capability or in the sense of imputability.

The computer, seen strictly from the standpoint of external phenomenology, could be as much an Agent as a particular human. If the only component used in the decision, whether from the computer or from a human expert, is an unambiguous calculation, then the computer, if properly programmed in the first place, is less likely to make a mistake than a human adviser. The human being, it may be argued, furnishes the illative and phronetic safeguards, although it is an open question whether their use on the whole gives fewer or more palpably absurd answers. Computers have become so sophisticated that the question may be asked whether the computer as Agent and the individual human as Agent can be distinguished. The cognitive aspects of this issue is the famous problem embodied in the Turing machine (Penrose 1989, 1994; Turing 1937) and embodied in Searle's model of the Chinese room (1992). Arguments on the point deal with the Psychology of programming. Some doubt may be cast on whether the human being has more "freedom" or "insight" than the computer; but these are ontological matters yet to emerge from studies on internal phenomenology. Still within the purview of external phenomenology may be one important presumptive difference between the computer and the human as Agent: predictability. It will be argued that the responses a computer is capable of making when presented with specific data are all quite predictable from the known program,[6] whereas a particular human response may occur that is not predictable from what has up to then been understood about human response patterns.

A Note on Ethical Freedom

The notion of Ethical freedom is important but elusive. Some degree of unpredictability is a necessary feature of freedom, but it is not a sufficient one. Human freedom is being trivialized if it is to be identified with nothing more than the exercise of wanton caprice. It is almost as much in peril if it consists of incontinent appeal to phronesis, illation, and pentheric protest. Apart from the impact of the Chinese box that we address at length in Chapter 15, in free behavior there is the more subtle question of judgment as to what is to be deemed relevant, in effect, a personal choice of dimensionality. A clinician who has by chance some special interest in the fine arts, or the conservation of species, or history, or the academic discipline of law, may perceive as relevant to a particular Ethical problem some issue or insight denied to other colleagues. We say nothing of the yet more elusive, but perhaps to the individual very important, matters of sentiment, loyalties, and spiritual and mystical commitments that are, in a narrow technical sense, outside the domain of Ethics but nevertheless make major impacts on behavior without in any useful sense being capricious. But this argument may be irrelevant from the standpoint of strict external phenome-

---

6. We set aside machine noise, troublesome at bifurcation ("threshold") points, especially the more intricate effects of Chaos.

nology, especially if the question is to make judgments on the basis of the external phenomena. These subtle choices and judgments are clearly outside the purview of the computer acting only on hard-wired prescriptions.

It is not inconceivable that the decisions of a committee exhibit authentic emergence (q.v.). This phenomenon is familiar to the student of political history.

The Recipient

The recipient is the person (or object) on whom (or which) the Agent may exercise responsibility. (In Medicine the recipient is typically the patient or a relative such as a parent or a consultand.) The recipient need not be human or even intelligent; a person may be responsible for his children, for his dog, or even for his car. In the light of the analysis in Chapter 12, the recipient is likely to be operating in the Ethical middle or passive voice.

The Third Party

The third party is the person or object on behalf of whom or which the Agent is responsible for the recipient, and to whom or which the Agent is accountable.

EXAMPLE 14.17. A man is responsible for making sure that his dog does not bite a neighbor. Here the man is the Agent, the dog is the recipient, and the neighbor is the third party.

EXAMPLE 14.18. The third party need not be a person; the curator of an art gallery is responsible for the practices designed to ensure that mildew does not destroy the paintings.

The Agent, the recipient, and the third party may all comprise multiple elements, some of them human beings, some not. The three roles need not be distinct. The distinctions are made here for the sake of clarity, but they are often blurred, even totally artificial.

EXAMPLE 14.19. A man, for instance, is responsible for the use of his fists. Here Agent and recipient are the same person.

EXAMPLE 14.20. A diabetic may be responsible for taking insulin regularly because it maintains healthy carbohydrate metabolism. Here the Agent and third party reside in the same person, and the recipient is the regimen of insulin.

EXAMPLE 14.21. In the taking of daily exercises, all three roles are vested in the one person.

Additional parties to the action of the Agent may be considered. Society at large, a party to any action taken by one of its members, arguably constitutes a *fourth party*. However, all other parties at interest may be grouped as third parties.

The Amicus

We take this term from the practice of courts of law. *Amicus curiae*, the "friend of the court," is a person, not a party to a lawsuit (neither plaintiff nor defendant, judge nor jury, advocate nor prosecutor), who nevertheless offers to submit ex gratia an argument or testimony in the interests of promoting justice, and also perhaps to establish by precedent a legal position for an argument, principle, or notion. The characteristic posture of the amicus is impartial, detached, noncommittal. One would hope that all Philosophers might be looked on to adopt this attitude. But clearly that is not to be expected of those (including many Philosophers) who have a cause to plead.

In Classical drama the counterpart of the amicus is called the *punctum indifferens*, that character who sees everybody's point of view and is a dispassionate dissector or at least reference point for the issues. For completeness we have to admit the possibility that in the midst of an Ethical matter, there may exist parties who are not weighed down by prejudice, anxiety, or the demands of advocacy. Clearly this role can scarcely be fulfilled by the observer from Mars whose existential perspective on the internal phenomenology may be grossly underdeveloped.

The notion of the amicus is probably clear enough; but it may not be at all clear in what way the role of the amicus is sufficiently distinctive to merit particular identification. Is the amicus nothing more than another Agent engaged in merely a different set of Ethical confrontations and (as it were) intruding into other people's business purely for the fun of it? The answer is yes and no. The amicus is not perceived as a distinctive human being prohibited from addressing personal Ethical issues. To the contrary, if the amicus is to spare the time to aid and inform any or all interested parties, there presumably must be some nontrivial ulterior motive for so doing. What is more, the kind of deposition the amicus can make is likely to be based on personal experience of a similar problem. But the amicus, by definition, is not a party to a particular dispute and therefore is in a position to cut, at least temporarily, the Möbius strip.[7] Further, the ami-

7. In so doing the amicus can escape from trying at the same time to make a personal decision and make a self-analysis of the personal process of making a decision. This peculiar process is taken up at some length in Chapter 15.

cus, from personal experience, is perhaps able to engage a sense of the existential values involved while avoiding the abuses or other deplorable features of much of the current practice of parties at interest. The Ethical brief would aim to amend without incurring the charge of self-seeking.

The Setting

We turn now to the Ethical setting. But first we have a technical problem to deal with.

A note on imminence and immanence. Since *imminence* and *immanence* are both relevant to our discussion, similar in form, and widely different in meaning, we pause for a brief statement.

Imminence has the meaning "threatening" and as such connotes danger and immediacy. The common meaning of *immediacy* is one of time: that some dangerous event is likely to take place at any moment. However, that is rather too narrow an interpretation. The threat may denote closeness in time (the eruption of a volcano exhibiting preliminary signs); place (domicile on the San Andreas fault); economic instability (in the South Sea Bubble or the Wall Street crash); the flood of undigested data (in biological science); psychological peril (viciousness of the associates of a child); debasement of the language (with critical breakdown in communicating information in an emergency). It is not only that a disaster will soon occur, but that if or when it does, the parties under consideration will be heavily involved and damaged.

Immanence comes from the Latin verb *manere* (to remain) and has the sense of indwelling, latent, inherent, permanently pervading.

The concept of the ethical setting. Responsibility exists not in the void but in some actual experience, encounter, or confrontation. A clinician may have a general sentiment or policy of responsibility toward retarded children; but this commitment, and the observer's appreciation of it, extends only to those children in whose professional care the clinician participates. In this sense the setting is incurably personal and particular. It comprises all those particulars available to the external observer.

We must make a distinction, clear but readily overlooked, about the Ethical status of this setting. It is too easily, and mistakenly, supposed that the introduction of a setting converts an issue in Major Ethics into one in Minor Ethics, or even into casuistry. That is a radical confusion. Ethics has no domain of expression other than an existential world. But that does not mean it lacks fundamental abstract form. By analogy, an abstract formulation of art is an analysis, not of particular paintings, but of the notion of a painting and not (for instance) of mathematics or perceptual Psychology. Or again, the idea of a Random variable X (conventionally written in Statistical theory as an upper-case letter) is a representation of a quantity that may vary, whereas the outcome (i.e., the result of executing the Random process) will assume some value x (a lower-case letter) that once realized is what it is and does not vary. The discipline of Statistics, however theoretical, cannot deal with formulations that do not, at the very least, involve the idea of the realization of a (perhaps purely hypothetical) experiment. In its theoretical form it may not at any stage confront lower-case quantities. So let it be with Ethics.

The immanence of the setting. The setting is, in effect, both the information immediately to hand and its entire set of implications for the ensuing action as perceivable to the external observer. But a situation may contain much that has not yet been observed or inferred. Deeper analysis of the consequences may be obscured by corporate ignorance of knowable fact or theory; inherent indeterminacy; or the hiatus that may lie between what can be formally deduced from known axioms and what may be inferable from unlimited experience of observation.

In the ensuing action, matters of immediacy and urgency in time and space may dominate. Physicians are concerned, first of all, to meet the requirements that appear to be immediate in time or space, or of greatest magnitude—although these may be associated with only part of the authentic immanence of the setting.

EXAMPLE 14.22. Neonatal asphyxia is an imminent disaster, and no effort is spared to induce breathing. Even if normal breathing is eventually started, however, and the imminent threat to life averted, the prolonged anoxia may have caused serious brain damage and the immanent risk of mental deficiency that may only later become apparent. At the other extreme, the excessive use of oxygen in the premature may deal with the imminent problems of anoxia, but with a latent risk of blindness from retinopathy of prematurity (retrolental fibroplasia).

EXAMPLE 14.23. A combination of factors—geography, overpopulation, and political villainy—leave devastating famine as an immanent problem in central Africa. Experiences in recent years have shown that when the problem becomes an imminent threat, it is not to be overcome by the existence of an adequate supply of food, or the means available to distribute it to those in dire need. Those who would solve the problem are harassed at every turn. The scale and intensity of the famine are such as to make our domestic concerns over malnutrition seem trivial. There are those who dispute whether malnutrition is an immanent problem, an ineluctable recurrent defect that could be prevented if the desire to do so were taken seriously. But the practicing pediatrician or obstetrician in Baltimore certainly sees malnutrition not as a vast disaster on the other side of the world (where clearly it is inaccessible) but as a physically imminent local problem that must be grappled with one way or another. However unbalanced the comparison may seem, the minor demand on one's own doorstep has a higher priority than the vastly larger problem about which one personally can do almost nothing.

Tomorrow's minor snowstorm poses a more prominent problem than the threatened consequences of global warming fifty years hence. Partly, but only partly, that priority is fueled by mistrust of the soundness of predictions about the latter threat, over which the physical theorists are by no means agreed. But again, there is the sense that imminence adds a particular pointedness to Ethical problems.

The most immediate concern of the physician is with those matters that are required to preserve the freedom of choice necessary for more lasting matters. Most obviously, if the recipient is not kept alive *now*, then long-term Ethical questions about that respect are futile. In such critical occasions, the imminent will override all else. Nevertheless, it is necessary to have a practical sense of the total implications of the Medical setting. Such breadth of vision is not likely to come exclusively from instantaneous response to the particular crisis. It comes, rather, from sober reflection on the broad policy of management. Present facts, severally and jointly, bear on the consequences of current policy, which are more or less predictable. The long-term and overall outcomes are immanent in this information.

Outputs and Results

Unless the Ethical dimension is to collapse forthwith, the Agent reaches decisions and carries out Acts that have results.

Decisions and acts. In the external sense, the Agent's decision is observable only in terms of the Act or Acts performed, whether there is an explicit decision or an implicit pursuit of a policy. Rather than being executed in one indecomposable, irrevocable jump, in general the policy is continually readjusted, with more or less immediate feedback. Just so, in sailing a boat a course is maintained by "trimming" from moment to moment rather than once-and-for-all decision and by dead reckoning. If the Agent made an irrevocable decision, the result would be an Act in the narrowest sense and would itself be outside this cycle of feedback. Such a discrete Act is rarely encountered in Medicine. The nearest example we can think of is virtually irrevocable procedures such as an amputation. We have discussed this pattern in some detail in Chapter 6.

The very notion of responsibility implies that the Agent is able to change the outcome of the situation by intervention: *there must be some Act that makes a difference.* Just in what situation the Agent is able to influence the outcome is hard to say in many cases, as we shall see in Chapter 15. But there are certainly situations in which any effective Act is prima facie denied the Agent, for reasons that fall within external phenomenology. We mention two cases.

EXAMPLE 14.24. The Agent may be devoid of means of affecting the fate of the recipient or a third party. The familiar example is the fatal disease "for which nothing can be done."

EXAMPLE 14.25. The Agent may be able to do something that makes a difference, but for reasons of the state of knowledge, epistemology or ontology, there may be no means for deciding whether it would be harmful or beneficial in the particular case.

An important qualification is called for:

• The efficacy of an Act and its relationship to outcome have nothing whatsoever to do with consequentialist Ethics (with which, however, they have been confused).

Consequences. The observer from Mars will quickly discern that the approval or disapproval of an adjudicator for the activity of the Agent will in large part be determined by what the consequences of that activity may be. However, this formulation of the problem may be vague because to assess the consequences may be difficult; indeed, because consequences may occur in the distant future, a full estimate now defies analysis altogether. It seems that the Agent may be accountable for the consequences of an Act insofar as they could have been foreseen (although, of course, there is an internal element of awareness that limits how far the observer can understand and the Agent be held to account).

In any case, it is a characteristic of human knowledge, both rational and empirical, that for the most part the more immediate consequences are easier to grasp than the more remote. The barber careless in the handling of a razor increases the risk of cuts to his customers, and will be promptly sanctioned by society; this response is occasioned by the immediacy of the consequences. But an industrialist may allow his factory to pollute the atmosphere, and thus in twenty or thirty or forty years' time may be responsible for many deaths in the population at large, yet be less likely to come under sanction. The observer will note that many medical practitioners are deeply concerned with "getting the patient off the operating table alive" or "getting the patient's pneumonia cleared up before sending him home from the hospital." Nothing like the same concern is manifested for assessing what the long-term benefits of a particular operation for peptic ulcer may be, or whether it is to the benefit of society to have all children vaccinated against smallpox. And, indeed, the observer will be able to discern in full the impact, if any, only by tireless observation over a long time.

The Agents and the social critics, in their evaluation of the setting, may emphasize imminence over immanence. This emphasis can be costly in the long run (as some today are painfully aware), so that the consequences may eventually require reevaluation.

Sanctions. Certain behavior of an Agent is sanctioned—that is, treated by the recipient or the third party or by society as a whole in a fashion that can in no sense be said to be neutral, natural consequences of particular actions. A drunkard who dies of cirrhosis of the liver is suffering the natural consequences of this intoxication. But someone jailed for public drunkenness suffers what is not a natural consequence of alcohol but an arbitrary retribution by society. Sanctions may be distinguished as social, civil, or punitive. *Social sanction* involves a collective Act of society, under principles that have not been formally codified. Loss of friendship, contempt, ridicule, or social ostracism may result from behavior that is considered unacceptable even though technically it is not criminal. *Civil sanction* means that while behavior is not deemed criminal, nevertheless the miscreant will be liable in the civil courts. *Punitive sanction* means that in one way or another certain behavior will be regarded as criminal and be punished.

In general, individuals are observed to respond to sanctions in much the same way as to natural consequences. And although some people appear to ignore sanctions short of complete physical constraint, more behave as if sanctions were more important than natural consequences.

Feedback

We have noted that most decision making, at least externally, seems to proceed with continuous feedback from the results of the Agent's activity. We have also implicated a process of feedback in establishing a policy. Indeed, the observer can infer the existence of various channels of feedback among the results of the Agent's activity, decision, and Act. The observer can infer immediate, direct feedback from consequences and sanctions through ordinary decision making and formation of policy. With considerably greater technical difficulty, the observer can also infer less immediate impact by means of effects on the Agent, on the recipient, and on the third party.

15 Internal Phenomenology of Responsibility

In this chapter we grapple with what we may call the intact Möbius strip: the individual attempting to address Ethics not as a professor does—that is, not as an academic discourse about a topic "out there" from which the individual is safely detached—but, willingly or not, as a de facto participant, as someone caught in the toils. Our phenomenology of decision making has so far treated the individual as idealized and armed at all points. To attempt a more faithful representation with which any Ethically perplexed individual may have some hope of identifying, we must include those phenomena internal to the Agent that take an active part. The issues are twofold.

First, there are qualities—frankness, honesty, dispassion, fair-mindedness, thoroughness, practical sympathy, and the like—ascribed to perfect competence and ideal behavior that continually enrich Ethics with deeper and more constructive insights. The burden of making Ethical decisions must perforce start long before even modest accomplishment in these qualities has been attained. We must suppose perfection in them is an ideal to be pursued but not attained. Yet all informed opinion is agreed that individuals must ultimately take on the responsibility of developing, policing, and practicing their own personal, existential systems of Ethics. The arguments and ideas of others may be sources of knowledge, skill, and insight. They may be taken over holus-bolus by those who cannot, or will not, develop their own intellectual equipment. The latter group may, perhaps, labor under the delusion that such a strategy can be wholly sufficient and self-contained. However, the ontological notions of responsibility discussed in Chapter 14 will not allow that latter claim. While the person who devises an Ethical system is responsible for so doing, the *appropriation* of that system as a personal one is the ineluctable responsibility of the person who appropriates.

Second, there is what we shall call (taking it as a metaphor) the Möbius problem: the fact that the individual is neither wholly inside nor wholly outside the Ethical system; and, conversely, that the system itself is neither wholly inside nor wholly outside the individual. Rather, the supposition is that there is a seamless connection between the two, but not a wholly simple one because of a twist on the larger scale (Figure 14.1). This

Möbius problem imposes another constraint that is rather disturbing. We have been at great pains hitherto to avoid involvement in any topic that does not lie squarely in the domains of science or Medicine, or preferably both. But here we cannot wholly avoid two difficulties. First, Medicine is not confined wholly to scientific matters. Indeed, one needs little experience of authentic Medicine to realize the futility of supposing that it could be so confined, not because Medicine is shallower than science but because it is much deeper. Second, the discipline and the practitioner cannot be divorced even for purposes of discussion. We must recognize that all manner of concerns of those discussing the issues—tastes, education, hobbies, political affiliations, religion, national allegiance—must be respected and given a hearing. The discussants are to address whole-thickness decisions about real problems, not carry out pasteboard classroom exercises.

EXAMPLE 15.1. A nice parallel is given from genetics: the ambiguity between the organism and the environment. The immune system is concerned with (among other matters) distinguishing between *self* and *nonself*, which is a highly conservative genetic and evolutionary device. Ordinarily, then, the distinction is clear enough, and it may for most practical purposes be treated as if it were unconditionally true (despite the comment at the end of Chapter 8). But a well-known phenomenon is that DNA from a virus may become permanently incorporated into the DNA of the host; and at some later date it may be transferred to other individuals of the same or different species, certainly by artificial means (genetic engineering) and at least now and again spontaneously (e.g., in chimerism). Thus, in principle, at least, there is a shuttling backward and forward between individuals; and what the immunological vigilance operates on, and how, is conservative, but not to the point of absolute discrimination.

The resulting discussion of internal phenomenology, then, has a singular character because of its intensely personal nature. The analysis is not confined merely to cold abstractions, particularly since (as in Example 15.1) it deals with abstractions that are vulnerable. It is about (for instance) the professional endeavors of physicians and concerns the intimate particularities of the individual practitioner, who cannot reasonably aspire either to total dispassion or to exhaustive scholarship. It takes little experience or knowledge to realize that having the best intentions to carry out studies that are unbiased, dispassionate, sincere, and all the rest by no means guarantee that in practice one will do them that way, or even (especially in the light of psychoanalytic theory) that it is possible to do so. The task here is made no easier for us by the fact that, as always, our discourse is intended to be neither prescriptive nor adaptive.

We must hope that the inescapable involvement of the personal practitioner will not wholly undermine the Ethical endeavor, especially as any attempt on our part to "put it right" would merely replace the personal short-comings of the practitioner by the personal shortcomings of the authors. As a safeguard, we appeal to two guiding principles, already familiar from earlier chapters, although here the nature of the subject has induced us to narrow the limits we impose on our presentation.

First, we have been at pains to purge the text ruthlessly of whatever we can identify as our personal views and convictions. We appeal only to ideas, principles, and facts that would scarcely be disputed by thinking persons, concerning which unassailable empirical evidence has been or can readily be obtained.[1]

Second, so far as possible we keep the analysis in the indicative, not the imperative, mood. Ultimately the Agents are accountable for their Acts to their own individual selves. The only implied optative is epistemic: that (other things being equal) defensible action is the better for being delib-erative. If even that principle is to be in dispute, then the whole Ethical endeavor, even the most existentialistic Ethics, must be abandoned as with-out content or meaning.

This elaborate protection of freedom in structure does not mean that we shall reach no conclusions. But the conclusions are to be discovered in the course of the analysis; they are not put forward in advance as a theorem masquerading as open inquiry.

Furthermore, our concern here is not with Ethical content, methods, or prescriptions. Our goal is the more limited one of identifying the essen-tial features such as we have to respect in all (including ourselves) who can engage in rational discourse. Nor do we attempt to intrude anything of our own individual standards. Readers can make no sound inferences from our silence on details.

With these preliminary ideas in mind, let us address the internal phe-nomenology of responsibility.

STRUCTURAL ENDOWMENT

Whatever its ultimate ontology, the human mind is an incalculably rich nexus of structures, knowledge, logic, esthetics, ideals; political, social, and religious beliefs; culture; aspirations; nostalgia; folklore. It would be neither practicable nor to our point to attempt an analysis of all these essen-tially human components.

A minimal set of operating requirements for internal responsibility of any kind seems on reflection to be threefold.

---

1. Needless to say (in the spirit of our own assertion), we authors have no basis for claiming that our assessment in what follows is in any way to be given privileged treatment or immunity against precisely the same criticisms.

The first requirement is *an intelligence sufficiently cultivated to permit thought and the development and handling of abstraction*. This endowment may in human beings be disrupted, and the natural intelligence vitiated, at various levels of organization of the person concerned: anatomical (e.g., anencephaly), cellular (aneuploidy), biochemical (inborn errors of metabolism), defective physiology, gross pathology.

The second requirement is *an at least rudimentary sense of deontology*. By this we mean a grasp of the nature of obligation in particular types of confrontation that goes beyond the physical facts and Logical inference. Even in its most primitive form, the deontological apparatus is complicated. Progressive cultivation identifies some organized set of obligations that are to be taken seriously, a more or less sophisticated Moral sense, varying widely in its content. This attachment is, of course, in the optative mood as represented in Chapter 7. Moreover, while it is indispensable to Ethics, it is scarcely to be accommodated within science. The Möbius problem means that the unfolding of the human dimension may exceed all reasonable bounds.

The third requirement is *an acceptance of the possibility and authority of rational analysis*. This viewpoint is embedded in reasoning and to a greater or lesser degree in Logic. It is a feat of abstraction that we may hope for, but can scarcely expect to be fully developed, before at least the age of adolescence. The force of reasonableness is at first simple, but gradually, and with guidance, it incorporates deeper, more intricate and far-seeing aspects. Details laid down in the light of experience, reflection, reading, and argument vary from one person to another. The most elaborate level, which aims to iron out idiosyncrasies, is the development of a full Ethical theory; but in practice the most formal and scholarly Ethics, far from being unitive, has been extremely divisive, even radically nihilistic (G. E. Moore 1903). Professionals on the firing line will keep their own counsel, especially when it is necessary to make a concrete decision in real time. Our stance is to respect their diverse personal positions, and to promote reflection in general, without urging any particular partisan content or interpretation of an objective code.

PRELIMINARY PSYCHOLOGY

This book is in no sense a textbook of Psychology. So we must try to preserve an important but elusive distinction between what we may call scholarship in its broadest sense as a topic of discourse and Psychology in its present conventional sense. We might agree that an excellent scholar may be Psychologically deeply flawed, and conversely that Psychological excellence may exist with no guarantee of scholarship. The distinction is between the content of thought and the mechanisms of thought. Historical examples of the reality of this clash are legion and need not be addressed here. We can hardly be surprised, then, that the criteria and how they are organized are different, often almost totally different. The question of how wise it is to make and preserve the distinction between Philosophical Psychology and scientific Psychology is another matter that, at least by implication, must be examined in what follows. This section may be thought of as like a racial memory that began before the modern era of Psychology,[2] a time when Psychology was taxonomically a branch of Philosophy to be developed from introspection in the light of experience by ontological parsing (top-down analysis). In contrast, most modern Psychology is as much a branch of science as of Philosophy, frankly empirical in domain and developed by mixed epistemic and ontological syntaxis, parsing, and transversal.

We conveniently group components into three Philosophical classes of psychic activities: *affect, cognition,* and *conation.* Of them the now rather unfamiliar word *conation* requires a brief comment. It was first introduced by Spinoza (1632–77), although in a very different context, to denote that drive that is associated with continuing to exist, to survive (*Encyclopedia of Philosophy* 1967: vol. 7, p. 538). The pattern of analyzing the mind by the triad cognition-affect-conation, though implicit in Kant, seems to have been crystallized by James Ward (1843–1925) (ibid., vol. 8, pp. 277–78), and elaborated and developed by G. F. Stout (1860–1944) (vol. 8, pp. 23–24) and by William McDougall (1871–1938), who made it the basis of his hormic Psychology (vol. 7, p. 25). Despite the Philosophical cast of these writers (notably Ward and Stout), they nevertheless represent the transition between Psychology as Philosophical and Psychology as scientific. We do not imagine that, as such, they will be of major interest to modern psychiatry and Psychology. But in an atmosphere of tenuous connections, we much treasure what points of contact we may find.

These three aspects of the Philosophical model of the mind develop more or less sequentially, but not always evenly or equitably. We emphasize at the outset that the developments iterate endlessly and grow in complexity. There is no state in which the responsible mind can ever claim, on the grounds of age or experience, to have satisfied all three, or to have attained a permanent triumphal state of excellence.

Precisely for this reason, the discussion is centered not on a circumscribed *program* of development but rather on an unending *process* of development. In a very real sense, responsible Ethics depends not on application

---

2. This scheme is, of course, wholly out of phase with modern dynamic Psychology and psychiatry, and we shall duly qualify it later. But it provides a convenient checklist of ontologically analyzable components that have not entirely been trampled underfoot by the urge to uncouple rational discourse about the mind from the existential operation of the individual as a black box. The current topic is simply a device for discussion. It would be deplorable to suppose that in any way it could compete with, or displace, the largely empirical modern theory of mental health and disease.

of ready-made conclusions but on perpetual renewal by solving fresh problems and developing more refined principles and measures.

Affect

An endless sequence of stimuli evoking responses during fetal life, infancy, and early childhood gradually attain a level of organization perceived by the individual person as pleasurable or painful. These events become a cluster of feelings and thoughts that crystallize into cooperative attitudes to authority. Let us explore this from the standpoint of broad culture rather than empirical Psychology.

The first and usual attitude to authority may be a childlike trust: "Mother says" and, later, "Teacher says." Such trust may develop into an uncritical reliance on experts, textbooks, scientific opinion. One distortion that may result is that, by untempered indoctrination and imitation, the scholarly mind acquires an assurance that may degenerate into an unwarranted complacency. Over time, however, testing, external challenge, and internal conflict may forge a healthy self-criticism.

The contrasting distortion, born perhaps of disillusion, is an unpolarized set of convictions, procrastination, and withholding of even conditional assent—sometimes even militant doubt entertained not as a path to refinement of understanding or improvement of the standards of scholarship but purely for its own sake (skepticism). It leads to misgiving and provokes uncertainty, which may result in confusion and eventually hopeless indecisiveness. Such skepticism is typically directed not toward stringent evaluation of method, evidence, and inference (which are means) but toward knowledge and belief themselves (which are ends). A skeptical outlook of the latter sort is often deliberately cultivated by certain kinds of educators under the mistaken impression that that is how science develops. Nevertheless, systematic doubt, and, where appropriate, reservation, when directed toward proof and evidence (i.e., epistemological questioning, or skepsis), is an indispensable component of scholarship (Murphy 1981c).

These conflicting processes of affect run their course, and experience of applying them informs the mind. The preferred pattern is that there will emerge a fair balance between the need for self-assurance and the need for constructive guidance. If either is underrepresented, confident and warranted assurance is jeopardized and sometimes never attained.

Cognition

The attribute of cognition relates to intelligence, knowing, and human judgment. A cooler, more intellectual appraisal of authority (skepsis) is a safeguard against uncritical acceptance of judgment of oneself or others. It prepares the mind to grasp the Philosophical challenges. However, we would point out that an appeal to Philosophy, not as a discipline to help in developing critical judgment but as a quick path to the solution of the problems, too readily degenerates into the childish adulation of authority. The latter stance is replacing "Teacher says" or "The textbooks say" by "Philosophy tells us" or, worse still, "Such and such a philosopher has proved. . . ."

The desirable outcome is some sense of critical analysis and communication of insights. Properly used, Philosophy helps in the handling of knowledge and deepening of insights. But as Owen Barfield so trenchantly remarked, Philosophy is a *way*, not a *subject* in the didactic sense (C. S. Lewis 1955). Philosophy becomes a useless excrescence if it proposes to replace the analysis and cultivation of wisdom by promulgating the smooth answers furnished by soothsayers. To say the least, it seems unfair to treat great Philosophers as if they were sophists.

The results of these affective and cognitive components combine to furnish the mind as an instrument of thought with two valuable properties. The more abstract and disciplinary property is the acceptance of one's own fallibility, limitations in actual or possible command of knowledge, and the unwished, yet inescapable, intrusion of personal and often irrational attitudes. The more practical gain is the capacity to grapple constructively with pressing situations in the face of uncertainty. We might designate this vulnerable equilibrium between assurance and open-mindedness by the term *pliant confidence*.

Conation

In McDougall (1924), and in the sense we use the term here, *conation* is the striving for some end relevant to some Psychological encounter, even in the face of conflicting impulses as one judges necessary; it is a distinctly, but by no means exclusively, human characteristic. The rough-and-tumble of existential conation involves a concatenation of phenomena: knowledge and skill; competence; self-criticism and evaluation; and the continual urge to realize a goal. Together they may foster a distinctive deontological quality. There emerges a self-critical striving for deeper and richer solutions and the seeking of deeper understanding of the implications of attempted solutions. The human Moral conflict, for instance, is moved by the purely instinctual aspect of conation, but also by conation as a means of mobilizing the more elaborate psychic structures of purposive behavior and the yet more elusive Moral qualities of deontology. Nor do we imply that the levels of elaboration stop at that point. The ninth or tenth circuit of the Möbius strip might lead to some quite unanalyzable matters.[3]

3. Nonmathematicians are unlikely to encounter iteration except where it leads to convergence to some particular quantity. However, there is no reason why it should behave so. Unlike the common patterns in genetic population dynamics, evolution is apt to lead to open

The Resultant

Taken together, these three activities, affect, cognition, and conation, put the professional stamp on the thinking, feeling, striving, and self-critical human being: the sensible, well-balanced person in contact with reality, and not with mere theories of reality. Note again that these are qualities that the educator and the broad scholar will recognize and cherish without having (or even being concerned with) any technical knowledge of psychiatry at all. For the clinician in particular to preserve this stamp, a number of balances have to be carefully maintained, namely:

1. between punditry and guruism, at one extreme, and, at the other, a rootless vacillation with excessive appeal for the support of other practitioners;
2. between unwarranted hardening of ideas ("ideosclerosis") and frivolous pursuit of medical fashion; and
3. between idiosyncrasy to the point of eccentricity and sheeplike imitation.

The practical goal of the seasoned professional is embedded in Truman's motto, "The buck stops here" (McCullough 1992: 481). When faced with a decision, ideally the Agent is prepared most of the time to make unshared choices.

ONTOLOGY

In earlier chapters we have been dealing with an analysis of ideas, Things, and terms as objects of discourse that are external to the person. Here we must with some trepidation undertake a more challenging task.

The Central Problem of Self-Observation

In internal responsibility we encounter a singular phenomenon hinted at in Chapter 14 and now calling for further development: namely, self-awareness or (more formally) self-observation. The external phenomenology of responsibility required us to distinguish between the Agent and the recipient. There are two types of analysis that must not be confused:

1. In Chapter 14, we treated the Agent as the object of scrutiny, who experiences such and such, undergoes development, and so forth.

---

diversification. The same is likely to be true of the Möbius strip model of the mind or elaborations of it.

These topics are more complex than others we have addressed, but in principle not different in kind from them.

2. The principal difference in internal phenomenology is that the Agent has, in some measure, at least, to engage in a *self*-analysis (of motives, judgments of motives, intention, sacrifice, etc.), take it into account in making some decision, and accept the foreseen consequences. These are tasks that cannot be evaded and may not be delegated to another without abdicating responsibility and in this respect becoming less human. One perforce makes such a delegation in undergoing a general anesthetic or in preparing a power of attorney in anticipation of mental incapacity. It seems unfitting to abdicate responsibility, even briefly, for trivial reasons.

EXAMPLE 15.2. An analogy (though limited and physical) of a mental process invoking self-analysis was given by Bronowski in the matter of relativity physics: the physical conditions of the observer (in Bronowski's case, velocity and acceleration) have to be incorporated into the assumed equation to conserve invariance (Bronowski 1951: 83 ff.). That case has the virtue of definiteness; but it is unusually straightforward.

In Medicine, the observing clinicians intrude into the privacy of the patient (as physicists do in cosmology), but unlike the physicists they do so in an idiosyncratic fashion. Although physicians record findings in commensurable terms, each also introduces new dimensions of being that the particular interpersonal relationship involves. This novelty is particularly striking in psychiatric practice, where the Agent does not remain a detached and external observer of the patient but becomes part of the patient's mental milieu. Indeed, in transference the relationship becomes an extraordinarily intimate one, and even more so should countertransference also ensue.

The observation and analysis of the Agent by the Agent is at least analogous to an interpersonal relationship, unavoidably idiosyncratic, and in no way to be accomplished from the outside. Bronowski's proposition is pertinent but much too simple to be adequate for our purposes here. The level of consciousness of the Agent will no doubt be raised by considering it. It leads to the realization that the phenomena of self-observation and self-analysis involve a deep paradox that we must now try to address.

The Paradox of Indefinitely Many Levels of Judgment

Ordinarily, an epistemic or ontological analysis of some topic, X, consists of applying to X some framework, Y, comprising arguments, principles, and the like that are, so to speak, external to X, not part of it or dependent on it. That is, Y is treated as of a different order, and indeed higher than X; and Y calls on standards and methods that are also external to X, if only to power the analysis.[4] A judge at law, an umpire in a sport, or an examiner in a university is not on an equal footing with the litigants, the players, or the candidates. Rather, they are arbitrators. To them qualities are ascribed and powers delegated that are of a higher order, by which the judged must abide. In turn, their arbitrations are in general subject to challenge and may be overruled, but only by a still higher (appellate) authority, the arbitrations of which are thereafter binding, unless and until they are appealed to a yet higher authority. But these primary and appellate decisions are of their essence separable and separate. The judgment on appeal will treat the opinions of the first judge on their merits but not as having equal standing with the decision of the appellate court. Moreover, judges as a class may not pass judgment on matters in which they are personally involved: "No man may be judge in his own cause."

The constitution of this fundamental hierarchy of authorities is not at all obvious or straightforward, and we cannot undertake here an analysis of the many warrants (from the divine right of kings to the findings of empirical science) that have been put forward to justify it.

· The only thoroughly rational starting point is that, a priori, there is no preferred part of the system.

From sheer empirical fact alone no principle involving asymmetry or inequality in the treatment may be gratuitously intruded. There has to be created by consensus some higher, we might say appellate, system that may furnish the benchmarks of all orders.

We have, then, the general epistemological principle that no part of a system is *ab initio* superior to any other part; and that in points of dispute on an equal footing the "tie-breaker" is to come from a higher (superior, appellate) source outside that system. In an Ethical analysis, we may (for example) decide that survival and health are values to be promoted; but nothing in simple unadorned population dynamics of the kind discussed in Chapter 11 justifies that view. Indeed, naive Darwinian eugenics would expressly deny it: let the dead bury their dead. We can sustain the claims of professional hygiene only by appealing to a higher level of values.

Now, in the internal phenomenology of responsibility, this problem of multiple levels of arbitration is to be elaborated. A child starting with no judgments at all may have rudimentary principles instilled by a parent, and they may be quite adequate for many years of development. But, as we have said, the developing mind will come to experience its own misgivings, doubts, and questionings about the indoctrination, whatever its source—

---

4. These statements are analogous to and more or less in harmony with Russell's concept of levels of language (Russell 1940).

parents, teachers, textbooks, or other authorities. And once awakened, these questionings neither can nor may be ignored. At civil law, ignorance is no defense. At military law, orders from a commander are no warrant for criminal acts. Moral authority is no justification for blatantly immoral behavior. Appeal to the stature of an authoritative text can offer no warrant for swallowing palpable mistakes in it. We do not, of course, regard these traditional judgments as a formal proof of the inescapability of personal responsibility. The object of citing them is simply to show that, right or wrong, they are pervasive and, though not to be heedlessly accepted, are not to be heedlessly rejected either. There is certainly nothing very daring or innovative in our weighing their claims.

However, it is not at all an easy matter to understand how any such challenges can possibly emerge in the development referred to above. Nor do we have any prior reason for believing that the process by which they do arise is coherent, tidy, or efficient. The remarkable matter is that they emerge at all; and if we could analyze the process efficiently and accurately, this whole chapter could be handled in a more prescriptive fashion. Even so, the prescription would have to be persuasive in character rather than compelling. It cannot at the same time be excruciatingly explicit *(dogmatic)* and relentlessly directive *(assertive)*. The only moral force can come from the free acceptance by a discerning and understanding mind.

EXAMPLE 15.3. Suppose a physician, P, frequently encounters patients presenting with pain and wonders how to act, if at all. (The underpinning for the discussion that follows is laid out in some detail in Chapter 10, which should be freely consulted as necessary.) Let us suppose that P has been brought up with a stoical but rather unreflecting attitude: pain ordinarily serves a useful purpose and should not be tampered with; comfort is at most a minor value in life; pain strengthens the character; and so forth. As P understands it, the goal of Medicine is health, not simply, or mainly, the glow of well-being. So symptoms are important only as they throw light on the diagnosis of conditions that may impair health. A patient with recurrent severe headache consults P, who first regards the pain as merely another symptom that is to be viewed in the same way as obesity or lethargy or buzzing in the ears.

Now, from whatever sources—the protests of patients, the indignation of the patients' relatives, the criticisms of colleagues—P is led to call into question these more or less implicit, rather stoical, attitudes to pain. Although raising that question may lead P to seek other information, it does not in itself change the facts. Nevertheless, we shall suppose that P feels that the question, once raised, demands a serious analysis and answer.

The additional information perhaps merely confirms P's experience that pain is real and that most people experience it at one time or another. This conclusion seems clearly to demand an answer to the question of whether preventing or suppressing pain is itself a principle of Medical care. After all, P has already accepted, perhaps quite unreflectingly, the principle that the role of a physician is to promote *health*. Is *comfort* an objective to be considered as well as health? Is comfort perhaps part of health? But these questions are not about P's conduct or professional skill; rather, they are about the structure of the policy on which P has been professionally formed and which has hitherto seemed adequate. To accommodate an answer it is necessary for P to appeal to a new class of considerations, *values,* and to find a new system of analysis for grappling with them. It soon becomes apparent that values belong to an appellate domain of discourse (i.e., outside the mere facts of the symptoms). Perhaps P will be led to invent a personal set of values.

Moreover, the hitherto unique directive of health has an overriding relationship to the facts of symptoms and the facts of therapy. Hence, the physician not only has to set up a new explicit category of values but also must henceforth see that they are represented in the assessment of symptoms. As all these perceptions progress, P has to set up a rudimentary hierarchy of thought. But hot on the heels of that step comes the question, Are there yet other clinical values that should be added to health and comfort? P may be content to follow personal feelings about the claims in Medical practice of happiness or productivity or prevention or beauty or perpetual youth.

However, perhaps beauty is a trivial value, perpetual youth a mere vanity. Many discussions with colleagues have led to some misgivings that these attitudes are personal prejudices. (After all, in the domain of values, P has learned something from the need for revision of the personal viewpoint.) Perhaps a more analytical approach to values is called for. To answer that, a second and yet higher level of judgment must be devised that will rate proposals for what should be admitted to the class of values. Yet once again, the set of appellate principles for that decision must be something that is not on a par with the values themselves. But it is not at all obvious how the credentials for such candidates are to be developed and assessed.

P might appeal to what the patients feel they need; or might turn to the writings of the compassionate, the poets, the mystics. But each of these will from time to time assert claims that are disputable. Patients may have views of happiness that clash with readily ascertainable clinical facts—too large a diet or harmful use of alcohol. The poets may be rather too fond of hallucinogenic drugs. The mystics may be trying to defraud or manipulate their disciples meretriciously. What started as a private distress in a patient may at this stage have become a public or political issue. The difficulty is not so much that each such claim requires more or less serious consideration; it is rather that the evaluation of each claim is apt to call for a forum of scrutiny at a new height, a new kind of system of appellate principles.

Perhaps religious teaching has something important to offer. But religious teaching may be false, or obscure, or ambiguous. The same may be said of politics, or psychoanalytic theory, or the theory of empirical science.

Notice that this entire pattern of thought bears only a remote relationship to the ordinary hierarchies of practical knowledge *(phronesis)* and wisdom *(sophia)*. One may learn English spelling and grammar as self-contained skills in their own right without any knowledge of Shakespeare or Milton, or tackle income tax forms without learning abstract mathematics. But the picture we have painted seems to require the fully responsible physician to be constructing several, perhaps innumerable, levels of judgment, each impinging on the one immediately below, *and to be prepared to do so at all of these levels contemporaneously.* It is in this contemporaneity that the unique complexity of the system lies.

Countercurrent

In the foregoing we have supposed that the introduction of higher levels of judgment affects the decision only, not the data. So it is in the Legal appeal. The appellate court examines the Legal arguments and the judgments of a trial in a lower court but does not ordinarily collect its own evidence. But the change due to introducing broader issues in Medical Ethics is more pervasive. The idea that the facts (symptoms and signs) can be treated as quite separated from either the diagnosis or the management is unworkable. The following illustrative set of shifts of balance is by no means exhaustive.

Decision points. We noted in Chapter 10 that diagnostic resolving power is often so feeble that we must be content with making the working (epistemic) diagnosis that imposes the smallest expected cost or offers the largest expected gain. In practical terms, the clinician must be content to use the critical points so defined as if they actually constituted the true (ontological) diagnosis. But to change at a higher level the scope and concern of Medicine is to change both the sample space and the cost functions, which in turn shifts the critical points and thus the epistemic diagnosis. For instance, in genetic counseling, the diagnosis in a doubtful case of tuberose sclerosis is likely to be different if the issue is the patient's care than if the issue is the risk of transmitting this trait to the offspring, for this autosomal dominant disorder has a widely variable phenotype; causing perhaps no perceptible impairment to the person concerned, it may yet render a sib or son grossly disabled.

Scope. The higher-level process may decree that ugliness is a disorder. It is clear, however, that (in Medicine, at least) ugliness is not well defined. It is also highly debatable what kinds of ugliness fall within the domain of clinical intervention. No doubt there are disfigurements in which there would be no dispute. But while (in defiance of much campaigning) we might suppose that baldness in men is not disfiguring and calls for no treatment (especially any treatment with serious risk), it would not be nearly so easy to defend the claim that baldness is not disfiguring in women, this although there are some women who deem it attractive to shave their heads completely. What can one make in Medical Ethics of judgments that are so personalized?

Jurisdiction. A great many clinicians, perhaps the majority, see their field of activity as limited to the concerns—selected and on the whole rather well defined concerns—of their patients, and perhaps the concerns of a few of their patients' close relatives, from whom they may occasionally need cooperation and help. However, clinicians may choose to embrace professional responsibilities that go beyond that. For instance, we have known clinicians who undertook to monitor safety in toys and special areas of hazard like the strength of glass doors. Moreover, clinicians have had increasing numbers of Legal duties imposed on them. One such is the reporting of infectious disease. Another obligation is to notify the police of any evidence of physical abuse of spouses and children. An onerous task is to testify on the bearing of karyotypes in criminal trials even where the forensic use in itself not only is premature but also interferes with the collecting of sound evidence on its relevance (see Example 1.1). It need hardly be pointed out that the latter impositions inevitably change diagnostic evaluation, because the written diagnosis is apt to be Legally endowed with an absolute and literal quality that is often quite out of tune with its existential clinical significance or value. Yet again there are problems such as drug addiction, smoking, pregnancy in the unmarried adolescent, and gang warfare that have several quite distinct aspects, clinical, social, Legal, educational. They are being promiscuously permuted and inserted into inappropriate pigeonholes, making all manner of differences to Diagnosis and the uses and abuses that may be made of it.

Allegiance. Traditionally, and in the spirit of the Hippocratic oath, the clinician's allegiance is toward the individual patient and must be directed to fostering and championing what is best for that patient. The issue in deciding whether or not a treatment is appropriate is, then, a matter of balancing the good that will result to that patient against the bad that will result to that patient. However, the arrogation (political, commercial, and philanthropic) by outside agencies of the supply and regulation of methods of treatment (such as renal dialysis, the "artificial kidney") now requires that the diagnosis must include an assessment of priority, which, in an alien environment, is not merely a matter of whether the patient is in great need, or even likely to benefit, but concerns other matters (such as the importance of the patient) that may play havoc with diagnostic categories.

Eugenics. The technical possibilities furnished by modern developments, most notably in the various branches of genetics, have had gratuitous impact on the assessment of the patient. At the present time, for instance, it has come to be supposed that dementia is never caused by simple aging, by wear and tear, but is necessarily the result of an essentially abnormal state, most fashionably labeled Alzheimer's disease. Whether that claim is warranted, only more and better evidence will decide. However, that claim, true or false, introduces a eugenic dimension into how health is to be perceived. After many years of unbridled advocacy of the survival of the fittest (a naturally operating phenomenon, so it was supposed, that is to be advanced and sustained artificially by scientific intervention), the view among experts in genetic dynamics is slowly shifting to the idea that the best interests of the human species reside at least as much in variety of good phenotypes as in excellence—for, of course, what is termed excellent[5] is presumably optimal adaptation to the environment, and the latter slowly but inexorably changes. Insofar as clinical geneticists, pediatricians, or obstetricians allow eugenics to shape their assessments, recommendations, and advice, they must be beholden to the decrees of eugenic fashion. That source of guidance has been too often and too severely mistaken in the past to invite much confidence. And the slowly emerging field of pathogenetics, which is concerned with the imminent phenotypes, the crass or "bottom-line" phenotypes, and not with artificial gauges (Edelman 1992), suggests that the real criteria are something much more intricate than naive measurements of variation such as variance. But however wisdom might hope to argue the case, the impact of shallow journalism has had an unsettling effect on sensible clinical practice.

EXAMPLE 15.4. Parents often seek clinical consultations and even importune for treatment with growth hormone for their son on the grounds that he is "the smallest boy in his class at school." They blithely ignore the simple fact that in every class of boys, even one limited to promising basketball players, there must always be a smallest one. (That abuse is one of the rare arguments in favor of big classes at school. At least big classes reduce the number of "smallest boys," and hence the number of parents seeking absurd interventions.)

Ideation. Persons differ in thought processes as well as in body. Without doubt there are patients whose ideation is disrupted. But to be dis-

5. The relationship of excellence to normality is addressed in Chapter 9.

rupted is not the same as to be disruptive. It has been a recurrent abuse in certain political regimes to treat dissident opinion as psychotic and hence to warrant compulsory Medical intervention. Again we must be concerned at how far that political policy invades the domain of proper Medicine. We may congratulate ourselves that "things are not like that in this country." But the same abuses may be perpetrated less obtrusively and in many ways more effectively. For some years in the United States there has been dispute about prayer in schools. We do not wish to become engaged in this matter; but it is noteworthy that both sides accuse the other side of insidiously brainwashing the vulnerably immature. There seems to be no discernible attempt among those in power to undertake an analysis at an appellate level.

Pragmatic Counterparts

In practice, there are reasonable simplifications to this theoretically endless problem of the indefinite number of levels of judgment and the iterative give-and-take between the principles and the data. The inexperienced laity are forgiven for perhaps taking an oversimplified view of the whole problem of pain, or disablement, or mutilation. Those clinicians bewildered by the mushrooming complexity of the analysis will grow impatient and abandon the infinitude of courts of appeal in favor of common sense and common decency. The austerity of a personal system of judgments may be tempered by free debate with colleagues about these difficulties. Those learned in particular disciplines—in academic law, in Philosophy, in pastoral care—may have helpful contributions.[6]

Nevertheless, the need for the infinite set of courts of appeal will not disappear by being ignored. Nothing is gained by simply avoiding it. However, the problem of appeal is not entirely without precedent.

EXAMPLE 15.5. The value of the logarithm of a number can be expressed as an infinite series; and strictly speaking, to evaluate it would require summing an infinite number of terms. As is well known, however, the task is carried out in practice by evaluating perhaps five or six terms, which are commonly identified by combinations of the simple terms.

In the same way, the infinite recession of courts of appeal may in practice be dealt with by a small number of groups of levels. For one thing, it is not at all clear that there is a strictly ordered set of levels. There is likely to be a wide range of sophistication in the inquirers, and it is doubtful that

6. But a word of caution about experts. They may be identified in two ways, either by what they know or by what they do not know. The latter kind too often attain their serene judgments not by deep and sound endeavor but by taking their own arbitrary shortcuts that may turn out to be disastrously misleading.

any one person can cover a great range of levels. It is scarcely practicable to expect those grubbing around in the foothills of Ethics to be able to grapple with the higher subtleties of how the doctor-patient relationship may be abused or intricate issues of confidentiality be betrayed. Reforming the reprehensible Sarah Gamp[7] and her ilk would have to attend to many elementary habits, practices, and ethical principles before undertaking the professional niceties of the pupils of Florence Nightingale.

COMMENT. Ontology does not itself furnish answers to the questions of internal responsibility, not even cursory ones. It seems to us much more profitable to treat the ontological analysis as rather opening a partial *insight* into the complex nature of the ideas involved. It points up the perils to rationality of accepting shallow solutions on no grounds other than that they may provide a source of recommendations that appear practical and explicit. It is a traditional function of Philosophy, of *philo-sophia,* to protect wisdom, not to manufacture smooth and superficial solutions to intricate and inadequately analyzed problems.

MOTIVATION AND THE UNCONSCIOUS

In Chapter 13 we decided that in making Ethical decisions, personal (as distinct from metaphysical) intention has no proper place. In the Psychology of making and acting on a decision, however, it is vital. We argued at length that the Agent's intention has no ontological relationship to the Ethical standing of the Act as such. A mechanical act is conceivable even if the Agent (or, even more so, some surrogate device) has no intention whatsoever and is indeed incapable of forming one. For instance, a baby or a semicomatose patient or a patient suffering from chorea may indeed make a movement, even though it is not what we would call an Act. But here we are considering concrete decisions being made by real Agents. As a matter of empirical Psychology, motivation is then of the essence, driving and shaping the process. The essence of the decision does not come into existence if there is not at least some conative activity, however ineffectual.

What obscures the reality and coherence of this issue is that the Agent may be quite unaware, at the time, of many motives that are driving the decision. They are part of the unconscious mind (see Appendix 1). Commonly the lack of awareness is deeper than mere ignorance of the motive. Many even sophisticated people remain ignorant of the complexities of their motivation. Barriers may subsequently be lowered, enabling the Agent to understand something of the mechanism. The Philosophical Psychology

7. Sarah Gamp was a dirty, bibulous, and incompetent practical nurse in whom Dickens satirized her profession in *Martin Chuzzlewit* (Dickens 1844).

of Ward, Stout, early McDougall, and before the researches of Janet and Charcot, supposed that the epistemic and ontological issues in serious discussions are out in the open, or at least should be to scholars who have thought about them seriously. Psychoanalysis reacted to the opposite extreme, to the point at which epistemology in particular was being dismissed altogether. Scholarly balance would require a more measured judgment between these two extremes, which (at least as candidate universals) are equally unsubstantiated. This topic is a deep enigma; once some glimmer of understanding emerges, a whole hierarchy of cognitive problems arises. A first self-scrutiny for motives may be misleading because deeper motives still interfere with the devices by which one attempts to understand oneself. These interfering or predisposing motives may in themselves come under self-scrutiny, but by mechanisms that are distorted by yet deeper motives. And so on, in indefinite regress. For instance, being afraid of the ignominious criticism that a flawed decision might bring about, or being unwilling to trust one's judgment, may be a protective device to avoid confronting and resolving unpleasant decisions. On the other hand, repressed concerns (see Appendix 1), while they would not be perceived at the point of decision, may emerge later and provide insight and possibly lead to new and valuable considerations.

DECISION MAKING UNDER CONSTRAINTS

The Möbius property of the internal phenomenology of responsibility in the Ethical conclusions reached after many circuits of the loop tautologously implies that in the early stages, Ethics will be more naive and unfocused.

EXAMPLE 15.6. One image that by its sheer implausibility has informed much of our own deliberations is the hypothetical analysis of a child deliberatively admiring an apple in a neighbor's tree, considering that it would be pleasant to eat, weighing whether it would be wrong to take it, devising means to do so, considering when to eat it, and much more of the same. Now, undoubtedly this dissection has a certain conceptual utility. However, it wholly leaves out what we mean by "a child." The formulation is not so much an account of a greedy child stealing an apple as one of a meditation by a covetous Philosopher.

Our criticism here is not gratuitously anti-intellectual. In time the Philosopher no doubt furnishes the better prescription for deciding how to act (although at that stage the theft, by its very measured character, may be all the more deplorable). But those Philosophers who write for eternity are not often pressed by issues of immediacy. Experience of clinical practice would make short work of decisions dominated by this timeless, leisured, untroubled disputation. And good riddance. It is not enough that Ethics should deal with the theory of behavior that is in some sense exhaustively circumspect. It must also embrace the contemporary theory for making arbitrary decisions; and all decisions are made in context. In a work that is not directed at Ethics as such, this example is the first encounter we have had with the subject of how a decision is made in the context of time. Arguably the ontology of time merits a chapter in its own right. But at least we must give it more than a cursory comment.

Decision Making in Real Time

It is not easy to think of decisions and Acts being other than inextricably embedded in continuous, dynamic time, with duration (as distinct from the mere ordering of discrete events, which is the way in which they are usually portrayed). The conduct of a chess game is discrete, and the intervals between moves may be treated as having irrelevant length. But in the real world and away from the games, concrete examples are not easy to find. Perhaps indeed they cannot occur. If that is so, we suggest a working principle for our disputation at least:

* Time is of the essence in Ethical formulations.

Just so, the wisdom of the ages notwithstanding, time is of the essence in spatial statements and cannot be unequivocally separated from them. Note that this principle is not merely saying that Ethical decisions take time (which they certainly do). It is saying that time is one of the component dimensions of the Ethical formulation. Yet it is a remarkable fact that, traditionally, in large part time has been excluded from the essential components, the authentic apparatus, of Ethics. When the ethicist is faced with an irremediable lack of information, the most demanding Ethical analysis must do the best it can with what knowledge there is.

EXAMPLE 15.7. Suppose that the diagnosis in a patient is in doubt and there is no prospect of resolving that doubt. The decision must be made in the face of the gaps, even if the decision is merely "to wait and see."

Now, before we go further, we note that there is a radical confusion to be avoided:

* The quality of the Ethics involved is not compromised by these limitations, although the quality of the decision may be.

No Ethical decision may aspire to be better than the optimal, even if the optimal falls far short of the ideal. In general—there are occasional exceptions—one can imagine more favorable contexts for making judgments;

but when applied to decisions, the more favorable may be a luxury one can ill afford. Arguably the inferences are metaphysically more correct. By waiting long enough, one may attain dead certainty, the price being that the patient will certainly be dead. It would not be the first time that inappropriate *rigor mentis* has led to inappropriate *rigor mortis*.

Now, certainly there has been at least a casual awareness that time presses and that it may be necessary to take action before all the data become available. However, there is little formal recognition of the fact that *thinking also takes time*.[8] Granted this fact, it is easy to see the absurdities that result in the Ethics. Any computation that can be done on a computer can also be done by an unaided mind, but usually very much more slowly.

EXAMPLE 15.8. Suppose that the appropriate solution to a problem calls for sophisticated analysis such as a multidimensional time-series analysis.[9] In an emergency the inexorable mechanical delays involved in computer analysis are perceived as an acceptable excuse for forgoing it. In some cases, at least, that seems a perfectly reasonable *indulgence-in-principle,* not to be seen as a concession or a mitigation.

However, unaided clinicians who, faced by analogous constraints, cut short full examination are granted no such indulgence-in-principle. They are regarded as at best maintaining an inferior standard of Ethics and may even be at risk of suits for malpractice. That an Act had to be carried out "in the heat of the moment" is perhaps seen as a mitigation for an imperfect Ethics rather than as an acknowledgment of an optimal decision under pertinent constraints of time. We suspect that all of these details are as obvious to others as they are to us, so much so that they border on the trite. But they are rarely explicitly stated, the supposed shortcomings being ascribed to human incompetence in the clinician rather than identified as ineluctable components of the Ethical problem itself.

We suggest an Ethical principle:

• The absolutely best Ethical decision made within ten seconds may be different from the absolutely best decision made in a day.

This principle means what it says. Let us develop it a little. The tradition in Statistics is to distinguish conditional regression from multiple regression.

8. Those who have applied for research funds that would provide time with some leisure to think, read, and collate, as distinct from scurrying around accumulating data, are well aware how forlorn their chances are. But whatever the meretricious exigencies of politics, scholarship should be made of sterner stuff.

9. The CT scan is one such radically different discovery in which the computer is so central that it is built into the scanner itself. But elaborate diagnostic devices are rarely so well organized.

EXAMPLE 15.9. The blood pressure expected for a person of given age, weight, and sex may be represented as a function of these three variables, known popularly as predictor variables, or more precisely as regressor variables, or simply *regressors*. After appropriate adjustment for scale, the importance of each will be roughly given by the size of the constant by which it is multiplied in the formula. Sometimes, however, one of them—say, weight—may be regarded as a nuisance variable or *covariable*: the investigator has no interest in the effect of weight, which is merely confusing the study of those factors that are deemed of interest, which we shall call regressors-in-chief (age and sex), and is said to be *confounded* with them. The usual strategy of analysis is to make a statement of the effect on blood pressure of age and sex, *corrected for weight*. In other situations the regressors-in-chief may be age and weight, and sex is the nuisance variable. Or perhaps weight is the only regressor-in-chief. It all depends on what the object of the study is.

In optimizing a diagnosis, the time variable is habitually treated as at most a covariable. But there are plenty of cases in which, even if all the diagnostic features were treated as covariables, time would be seen as a regressor-in-chief.

EXAMPLE 15.10. For instance, time might be diagnostically of the essence. The diagnosis may depend on how the cardiac rhythm changes over time. In formulating the problem, there is, then, in principle no method of dispensing with duration. This is not to quibble about the difference between "no duration" and a few seconds. The cardiologist may require a Holter monitor study over twenty-four hours or more to be taken and subsequently analyzed on a computer in order to make a diagnosis.

EXAMPLE 15.11. Time might be therapeutically of the essence. Delay in operating for a ruptured ectopic pregnancy, perforation in a diverticulosis, or an extradural hemorrhage might have devastating effects. In this view, time has twin effects. In increasing the certainty of the diagnosis, it is a benefit. In postponing urgent action to cut short the disease, it increases the risk of death, a detriment.

Again, the particular characteristics of the Agent are themselves, as confounded variables, very much to the point. Some can reason more rapidly than others, or they have better intuition, or a specialist's store of relevant experiences denied to others, or perhaps more knowledge of a compiled and assembled sort. Others may reason more rapidly because they have more set convictions, or less inclination to take account of subtleties, or even less skill. Yet the implicit demands on the clinician (who faces unyielding constraints) are self-defeating.

Decisions under Stress

The press of time leads to existential stress. This stress is not a matter of a heavy load of decisions and interventions that the clinician in any field is called to make. Rather, it is the sense of inadequacy (perhaps wholly unwarranted) that one may feel while still being expected to act. This incongruous feeling makes it harder than ever to maintain the poise that is already under siege from the load of work. The experience of trying to deal singlehandedly with three patients simultaneously demanding lifesaving action is at the time distressing, but it is nonetheless an enriching experience.

There is another sort of stress, however, in which time constraint affects the quality of judgment itself. There is a mounting sense among physicians in certain settings that they are overworked, with the result that the fine edge goes off their critical judgment (Samkoff and Jacques 1991).

Stress and Psychologic Regression

Whenever the Agent is under stress, there exists the possibility of Psychologic regression of the personality [10] (i.e., the tendency to return to an earlier, more familiar, but not quite appropriate level of judgment in reaching a decision).

EXAMPLE 15.12. Suppose that there is a massive civic disaster such as an earthquake. Because the emergency services are inadequate, the Medical and surgical care of the victims has to be handled by far too few clinicians. Much boldness, even ruthlessness, is called for. The regression of hopelessness may pass unrecognized; or it may be condoned by those present. The clinicians are clearly at risk of making incompetent decisions. In orderly, quiet practice, clinicians confronting some dilemma may consult with a colleague (if readily available). Nevertheless, the need for a consultation may be a difficult judgment to make with certainty. By default, to act in good faith is reasonable when no another opinion or judgment is available under the constraints of time.

Discussion of this disrupting component of the phenomenology of internal responsibility opens the way for what is a much more complex and much more delicate final topic, which we broach with some trepidation.

TEMPERAMENT AND JUDGMENT

Differences in temperament among clinicians, and more broadly speaking differences in personality, are considerable and commonplace, and very

---

10. Psychologic regression is not to be confused with Statistical regression (q.v.).

much to our point. What is likely to be neglected is how far such differences are acceptable behavior and when they are to be seen as disordered. Shallow theorizing supposes that all well-balanced persons share much the same features that indeed constitute what is meant by being well-balanced; and that disparate behavior is to be taken as a sign of inexperience, although in fact it may be due to personality differences. However, diversity in itself should not be a matter of surprise. Indeed, there are many arguments and sentiments—from orthodox Darwinian theory to apocalyptic theology and even popular proverbs—in favor of variety.

It is hard to deny that very different but nevertheless stable behavior patterns are represented in well-functioning societies.

EXAMPLE 15.13. Over the years there has been much dispute among clinicians as to the most appropriate methods (combinations of surgical operations, radiation, chemotherapy, hormones) of dealing with cancer of the breast or the cervix uteri. We noted in Chapter 6 the disputes over the analogous problems of managing carcinoma of the prostate (Whitmore 1956; Sheldon, Williams, and Fraley 1980; Chodak et al. 1994; Lu-Yao et al. 1994; Whitmore 1994). There is no need to go into details; but it is quite clear that several different groups of experts obtain excellent results by radically different methods, and that usually they end up with strong preferences. If we may suppose that the main evidence comes from studies that are large, representative, competently carried out, and honest, one reasonable inference is that most groups are more competent at the method they prefer than at another; indeed, that statement seems to be a tautology. In the event, it seems that not only skills but the ordering of skills may vary. But then it seems absurd to make any exclusive claims as to which system is best unless proper attention is paid to what the characteristics of the clinician are. But given that, mere diversity among the successful methods is not of itself evidence of unreasonable idiosyncrasy.

An individual pattern is often referred to as a *temperament* (from the Latin *temperamentum,* a balance). More broadly stated, it is a personality style that informal judgment suggests is familial; and it is presumed, but not shown by standard and orthodox methods, to be genetic. Certainly it is molded by culture, environment, and experience.

Satisfactory groupings or measures of personality suitable for self-analysis are hard to attain and harder to defend. Nevertheless, many such categories and measures are in wide use. Ayurvedic practice in India has for centuries recognized several mind-body paradigms useful in assessing a person's physical and mental functioning (Bugra 1992). Jung's classic division (1921) into "introverted" and "extroverted" has long been entrenched even in the lay literature. Diverse modes of learning or communicating—verbal, optical, kinesthetic—are distinguished in clinical Psychology. Some ascribe differences in behavior to experiences and impact in everyday living. The Myers-Briggs psychometric system (1980) is a favorite example of contemporary methods for self-evaluation in group settings. It uses four pairs of variables to gauge temperament quantitatively—introverted-extroverted, sensing-intuitive, feeling-thinking, and perceptive-judging—comparable to those that Jung addressed qualitatively early in the century. We note also the more intricate, if less popular, system of Costa and McCrae (1992).

No doubt but diversity in personality collectively provides clinicians a welcome depth that can accommodate a wide range of demands and meet diverse, often conflicting, even mutually intolerant expectations from patients. We have no ambitions to assess temperament or to propose a grand strategy for its cultivation. It will be obvious from what we have already said that the devices for self-analysis develop according to the needs and maturation of the individual. That does not mean that these devices are all idiosyncratic; but it makes for some reluctance on our part to press particular categories or psychometrics upon the individual person. Moreover, we suppose that, whatever rules of behavior irreproachable Ethical theory may lead to, the Psychological setting of the individual will not be explicitly considered by them.

Temperament nonetheless remains a facet of internal phenomenology that impinges pervasively on the actual decisions the physician (Agent) makes in the course of professional work. It is involved as well in the stance that the patient (recipient) assumes in the course of being treated. Insofar, but only insofar, as the genetic perception of the observer can be formalized, the collective wisdom of genetic inferences offers prospects for examining the impact of temperament in the clinician on the nature of clinical management. At the time of writing, however, genetic models of the brain and intelligences are far too rudimentary to provide even the broadest information.

16 The Main Perspectives

SOME REMAINING PROBLEMS

The overwhelming contemporary tasks of scholarship now are to discern and communicate illuminations as they are made. A massive increase in new Medical and scientific knowledge, inquiry, and writing has caught scholars almost wholly unprepared. Yet long before the prodigious technology of computers, the insistent, immanent demands of that increase were there to be seen, though with little inkling of its urgency; certainly little effort was made to grapple with it. Occasional efforts have been made to organize an encyclopedic knowledge in a field, none more so than McKusick's remarkable catalogue of Mendelian traits in human beings that we have copiously quoted in this book (McKusick 1994).

There is no hint that the exactions of information are subsiding, or any real prospect that, for all their scope, computers, faster retrieval, global networks, and the information superhighway will furnish any adequate solution. Nor should we expect that they could or will. The methods by which anywhere in the world we shall be able to retrieve within a matter of minutes a copy of any publication whatsoever will no doubt come in due time. But though they will avert much waste of time and effort, these technologies will hardly make a dent in the problem, for the rate-limiting steps are essentially human — how many hours the same kind of mind takes to read, criticize, and evaluate the same kind of paper — and that labor will remain unchanged. If a computer can do the reading and the analyzing, then the load will indeed be lightened; but the limitation will always be the speed, efficiency, and accuracy with which the mind can assimilate what it needs to know. Moreover, the computer search will find and obtain copies only of what we instruct it to find. But the genius of scholarly discovery involves, among other matters, indefinable skill in discerning which papers in which subjects may be germane to a particular inquiry. We mentioned in Chapter 8 the astonishing and deplorable isolation of pockets of inquiry on normality and disease, and their apparent ignorance of each other. We shall return to the topic later. These human communications will be no faster; but we shall do very well if they get no slower, for there has been virtually no effort to anticipate the problems from this great outpouring of intellectual substrate. Everything seems to have conspired to the contrary.

Consider. More and more, the specialist has been lionized, and the generalist is more and more a figure of fun, a dilettante who may grasp a good deal but has no precise technical knowledge. With typical postprandial rodomontade, all deplore the decay of the so-called Renaissance man. But in sober moments all treat such a polymath as a pariah. It is so much easier to be a successful specialist. Conspicuous progress is so much more readily displayed on one little cabbage patch than in a broad landscape: "Down to Gehenna or up to the throne / He travels fastest who travels alone" (Kipling 1892). The specialist indeed travels alone, unencumbered with the task of making sense of knowledge in a full-thickness view of life. This truancy is not merely indulged but encouraged by the attitudes of those on high. The gurus teach that any intractable obstacles can be avoided by calling them meaningless problems that may be safely ignored (as the more extreme positivists have done). Yet there are those who would plead that trustworthy and careful crossties are more than irksome constraints: they not only offer the greatest hope of general enrichment and utility but also force us to confront the most intellectually challenging consistential tasks. We agree. Poincaré said that mathematics is the art of giving the same name to different things (Bell 1937). Indeed, it is. But so is Philosophy, and science, and the greater humanism, and Medicine, and the academic discipline of law, and anything that can be called serious scholarship.

The indications are that the world we know contains simple processes with complicated properties—all those phenomena that we call pleiotropy and property emergence and the workings of cellular automata and Chaos and fractals. It also contains complicated processes with simple properties, like kinetic theory of gases, Galton-Fisher theory, evolution, and cosmology. The possible patterns are known to us in various ways: from mathematical, Probabilistic, and genetic modeling. But our secure empirical knowledge must be discerned through a thicket of epistemic difficulties. We have not only the technical difficulties of estimation to deal with but also the much more elusive task of the proper use of the illative sense (q.v.), and the robust scientific culture to recognize when a promising conjecture is making exorbitant demands on mitigating devices and special pleading. In the absence of bedrock evidence at the genotypic level or some such high-resolution etiology, discerning natural groupings of (say) bodily types is in perpetual peril; and when there is much epistemic or observational noise, the difficulties are aggravated. One merely has to think of both the inconsistencies and the lack of progress in some of the most venerable claims (including the very names of the diseases) to realize how much of a challenge there is, especially as the standards of proof become more exigent than ever.

It is scarcely surprising, then, that we know nothing as yet of complicated processes with complicated effects. Because the human mind falls short of the computer in its power to store, retrieve, and process facts but nevertheless can imagine and see hidden connections and interfaces, the angels must be on the side of coherence, of rising above gritty details to the vision and enterprise to confront data in the large. But that is an undertaking that will not run itself. Eventually genius will out: whenever scholarship comes to an impasse, there has always been somebody large enough to do what must be done in the face of every discouragement and neglect and preposterous and arrogant strategic planning. Even so, there are better and worse ways of preparing for these labors of Hercules.

Yet in the ruthless pursuit of success—not achievement, success—the ideal of this broad and liberal education has been an early victim. Some broadening of vision, even if it does not go beyond the strictly scientific landscape, may still provide a coherence of thought and outlook that may rescue us from the slick cleverness of technical training. It is the cliché of all clichés that to give a man a fish is to feed him for a day, but to teach him to fish is to feed him for a lifetime. To be a self-subsisting scientist, it is not enough to have closed knowledge and stereotyped skill. There must also be the agility in the arts of keeping both alive and green.

We make no apologies for the sententiousness of these criticisms, for they cut directly to the heart of the Ethical undertaking. We have no reason to believe that the active challenges in Medical Ethics have escaped these erosions of vision and universality. We ourselves are, by training and interest, equipped best to grasp the Medical and scientific issues. Some years ago a group of us became interested in Medical Ethics, in reading the established authorities, inviting discussion, and trying to enlist the collaboration of ethicists. We had little insight into the enormity or even the true nature of the problem.

Some of the basic problems had already been partially uncovered by some forty years of theoretical studies, raised and prompted in a desultory fashion by certain changes in the main perceived goals. The shift of emphasis in epidemiology from nutrition and infections to cardiovascular disease, respiratory disorders, and cancer; the mounting clinical preoccupations with chronic, rather than acute, disease; the untold impact of the genetic revolution; the belated encroachment of applied Statistics and experimental design; preventive Medicine—these are some of the major disturbing factors. They brought to light some glimmering of the generally unsatisfactory and imprecise understanding and definition of disease, fitness, the acceptable range of normal health, and other topics that Medical ontology comprises. The need for precision in these issues is not nearly so pressing in clinical practice; but the mounting pressure, good or bad, to perceive Medicine as a branch of science directed to the study of disease, rather than as a compassionate profession concerned with the personal problems of individual people, demanded a whole set of new standards and orientations.

It soon became clear that the slow and exceedingly patchy progress in Medical science is not a mere blemish but a radical flaw in the understanding of Medicine. The gold rush for infectious causes of diseases had largely played itself out. So (despite much contributing refinement) had the vitamin deficiencies and the overt endocrine diseases. Seen as a fundamental defect in the theoretical formulation of Medicine, this sluggish advance was quite disturbing enough. The amassing of data on heritable traits in humans has long since made it clear that there are more genetic causes of abnormality than there are known diseases; and yet paradoxically, in most of the major common diseases no coherent genetic pattern has been discernible, even where there are strong black-box indications of a familial component. What we have found out so far has done little to rescue genetics from its unhappy image as the frivolous study of the exotic. Yet it is all within grasp, though at a price. The terms of the new growth are dismayingly unfamiliar. There is a widespread but unfounded hope that it will all go away, or that it will settle down into some neat ideas that do not raise a bump on the orthodox ontological landscape. In clinical practice we shall then settle back into that false, fleeting, perjur'd dream of "business as usual." Meanwhile, the dialectic is so foreign as to have made little impact on the traditional pillars of Medical theory.

•   Who would change Medicine must first change anatomy, physiology, pathology, and clinical practice.

The plight of Medical Ethics has been no better.

EXAMPLE 16.1. It is in hindsight astonishing that when cardiac transplantation eventually proved to be feasible there were in place no coherent criteria for defining death of any Legal or even clinical standing (this though for a hundred years or more, physicians had been signing death certificates that in the particulars they affirm are Legally binding). Cardiac transplantation produced overnight a hasty criterion of electroencephalographic inactivity, a deus ex machina that had almost never been used and is still not used except (tautologously) as a medico-legal safeguard in invading donors of hearts. It would be interesting to know exactly what Medical ontology was invoked in the argument to defend this criterion.

EXAMPLE 16.2. It is even now astonishing that the greatest impetus to amending the terms of informed consent came not from the clinical professions but from the public through their politicians. Even now there is much unfinished business as to what constitutes informed consent.

Such embarrassing instances could be multiplied. However, in this divisive age it is not at all clear that other professions are doing any better. The Legal defense of insanity (see Example 6.2), even viewed narrowly on its forensic merits, was woefully underexplored and is still far from satisfactory. Defects in the safety of both structure and materials in public buildings (brought repeatedly to light in several spectacular earthquakes) still haunt us. Although the perils of (for instance) lead paint have been known for a long time, removing the cause proceeds sluggishly.

In this book we have no ambitions to list all the pertinent shortcomings, still less to propose how we might correct them. Our modest and narrow goal is to begin a process of constructively and faithfully shaping and promoting the encounter between Medicine and Medical science on the one hand and Ethical theory on the other. Because of our own areas of knowledge, we have put almost all our effort into advancing inquiry into identifying, exploring, and ensuring an authentic contribution to the common discussion from the Medical and scientific side. The argument is that if an ethicist is to explore Medical Ethics, it is vital that the Medical setting necessary to support it be safeguarded against misrepresentation and omission of essential details. The temptation has been to cast the typical Medical issues as a handful of essentially small one-line statements. This preposterous distortion has been imposed in order to sustain the delusion that they can be annealed appropriately with some almost detached Ethical principle that has, perhaps, a long and honorable history of unexamined use in a totally different context. Even an almost irrelevant, untested set of rules might lend *some* little help if there had been any exchange of views. But the discussion (when it has existed) has rarely reached the level of authentic dialogue.[1] Too often even the shallow pretense of a dialogue has not even been put forward. More and more the content of Medical Ethics is a mere pastiche of Legal decisions in the formation of which no spontaneous informed Medical or scientific input is tolerated. Notorious instances are numerous.

EXAMPLE 16.3. As we noted in Example 1.1, the intrusion of the XYY syndrome as a psychiatric defense for violent behavior at a stage (Borgaon-

1. We are particular as to the meaning and use of this word. A *dialogue* is a symmetrical exchange between two or more parties under rules of inquiry freely accepted and endorsed by all participating and directed to mutual benefit and support in the pursuit of truth. Symmetry implies the right to unlimited mutual cross-questioning. In contrast to the scholarly dialogue, a deposition by an expert taken in a court of law is objectionable on the following grounds. (1) The rules of procedure may do violence to the opinions and standards of the deponent. (2) The deponent is the only party to take an oath, or liable to prosecution for violation on that count. (3) The advocates are, by their very title, not concerned with discovering the truth, not even strategically, but are frankly arguing a case, sometimes with open hostility to the deponent. Indeed, the hostility is hypallagously transferred from the advocate to the expert ("a hostile witness"). (4) There is no redress against the conduct (as distinct from the rulings and judicial decisions) of the judge. (5) Neither an impasse nor an indefinite suspension of the decision is an admissible outcome. In our view such a procedure is not a dialogue, nor even an acceptable part of a dialogue. That view puts under the very strongest suspicion Ethics based on the decisions of the courts. We may add that this rejection implies no criticism of the Legal trial qua due judicial process on its own warrants. It was never intended as dialogue in the first place and should never have been treated as if it were.

kar and Shah 1974; Hook 1975; Hamerton 1976) when there was virtually no sound empirical clinical or scientific evidence on the matter was outrageous. The fact that it was even admitted as Legal evidence, with the attendant perils from liability, interfered almost fatally with subsequent epidemiologically sound studies that might have furnished reliable scientific information.

EXAMPLE 16.4. Cases sub judice until recently have called to light radical confusion in the scientific bases of many forensic experts on paternity testing and proof of personal identity.

EXAMPLE 16.5. Jurisprudence has been led to very bizarre judgments in issues arising out of criminal and civil trials concerning prenatal testing and fetal damage. The anomalies arise out of the lack of any coherent theory as to whether at any specified stage the fetus is, or is not, Legally a person. Until this gap is remedied, Medical Ethics (as distinct from forensic Medicine) should pay scant heed to Legal opinions.

EXAMPLE 16.6. In theory, there has been value in exploring the Legal standing of the "brain-dead" person being maintained (in some sense) alive wholly by artificial (extracorporeal) means. In practice, it seems to have unnecessarily complicated the conduct of cases about which physicians of all ranges of conservatism and radicalism implicitly agreed.

SOME SOLUTIONS PROPOSED

There have been some attempts to deal with this hiatus between Medicine and Ethics. They merit a brief discussion.

The Drinking Party

One kind of answer proposed to these needs for dialogue has been the three-day symposium of experts whose noninterlocking papers will be published in due course. A three-day symposium is three days better than no contact at all. But there is little evidence that any serious creative interchange takes place at such meetings or even that they inspire any serious dialogue. They may, probably do, promote research severally by participants. They set the tone for granting agencies in pointing out areas worth developing. But there has been a misplaced trust in their capacity to get work done where it is needed at the interface between Ethics, Medicine, and the biological sciences. It is like the touching belief that reading the menu is a useful way of dealing with hunger. It is well to recall that *sumposion* (symposium) was the Greek word for a drinking party.

Interdisciplinary Studies

The way to do research in an interdisciplinary field is to do research in the interdisciplinary field. Now, this problem is not at all a new one, nor is its domain without record. Much might be learned first from disciplines that have compound names.

EXAMPLE 16.7. Sir George Pickering, as a solemn warning to his students about the dangers of taking commercial names of drugs at face value without critical inquiry, used to teach facetiously the proposition that no drug with the syllable *card* in its name has any action on the heart (G. W. Pickering, obiter dictum).

We might take the example as a watchword. There is a mounting tendency to establish interdisciplinary studies by inventing new disciplines with compound names. They have the professed goal of integrating two disparate disciplines.

EXAMPLE 16.8. We are tempted to extend Pickering's warning to the dictum that no compound discipline beginning its name with *bio-* has any authentic concern with life. When biochemistry or biomathematics or biostatistics or biophysics was founded, the intent was to undertake a study at the point of contact between life and some severe academic discipline, with fidelity and accountability to both fields. Now, *life* is a very simple term for an extremely complicated notion with sweat on its brow and mud on its boots. As such, it can be only a very coarse-grained sketch. Shipley (1984) gives as the origin for the word *life* something protected in grease (a cognate of the word *lipid*); and its Greek counterparts *bios, bia,* and *bie* connote force, energy, and way of life, but emphatically not animal life, which is *zoe* (Autenrieth 1876; Liddell 1889). We must, then, not expect too much worthy scholarship from such a lowly start without extensive and serious scholarship to prepare the way. But working at interfaces, like riding two horses at once, is notoriously unstable. Like any hybrid strain, the progeny born of the compound discipline only too rapidly revert to being pure scientists or unabashed naturalists. We must be wary of the prospects for the fashionable replacement for *Medical Ethics,* namely, that ominous term *bioethics.* That is not at all to deny that bioethics has made useful contributions. It calls attention to the need for the clinician to understand and cooperate with the law of the land (a useful perception that used to be part of forensic Medicine); to the need for professional courtesy, sympathy, compassion; to the need for a constructive curiosity about the background, the handicaps, and the constraints under which patients must face their disabilities. These are all excellent qualities, needed (and too often missing) in every profession. So is some kind of awareness about how the corporate wisdom of a profession proposes to deal with problems that all its members share. So is some concern to revive common sentiments that are important yet always in danger of being blunted by sheer habituation in the practitioner of any profession. These are all important components of professional conduct.

However, we quarrel with the idea that these important issues have much to do with Ethics as such or with Medical Ethics in particular. Insofar as their content arises in clinical Medicine, they are matters that should be cultivated within the profession. Agreed, there is a political comportment that bears on appropriate professional conduct; but it should be picked up casually and informally, by example and by indoctrination in the course of the practical apprenticeship in that profession. No doubt a practical politician must cultivate certain qualities. But the claim that political theorists should take the elementary course on *sarcopiesma*[2] and a laboratory course on kissing babies, coping with hecklers, and the need for cosmetic dentistry and expensive haircuts, rather than learning these matters by trailing around with a successful politician, would (we like to think) be perceived as ridiculous. Insofar as a code is imposed on Medicine from the outside and without any avenue of appeal, it will always be suspected and resented; and the clinician will wonder with some suspicion about why the responsibility of conserving and energizing them should devolve on a branch of Philosophy like Ethics. Setting that matter aside, there seem to some sinister implications in deciding conduct by decree. The technical and sometimes extremely exotic aspects of the total Medical problem should surely have some place in formulating the decrees. Expert testimony should be responsibly taken from those who have acquired the professional skill and have reflected seriously and in depth on the full implications.

Medical Ethics should be more robust. There is a common prejudice that it is a rare politician who can think beyond the next election; and the concerns of the laity are driven by emotions that are patchy and often ephemeral guides to the good. There are enough instances of long-term Ethical drives in matters that are not personal but prescribed for the faceless population—such as the impact of smoking or the change in the age composition of the population—to show that such drives can be sustained and be effective. However, they are perceived by the outsiders as of minor importance, even though they have a vastly greater impact on life and fitness than do discussions about whether liver transplants should be available for all. Nor can the Medical profession itself be congratulated for its foresight. All these customs bring to light a great gap in the scope and concerns of Ethics. How much serious Ethical concern is there with preventive Medicine? We do not imply that the extension of concern in this direction is an easy matter to deal with; it depends heavily on Probabilistic

2. "Pressing the flesh."

statements of what are purely hypothetical cases rather than confronting the quiddity of actual personal disaster in real people. Too many people of all ages enjoy a Certitude that they themselves are immune to the risks of smoking and alcohol and other drugs, hazardous driving, and all the other preventable causes of disease and disability. Yet those who have worked in accident rooms, city morgues, and departments of physical rehabilitation know a different story. Unfortunately that different story cannot compete with the sad stories on television or in the newspapers about a crying child or an abused woman.

There is no intention here of belittling real emotion or delicate sentiment. They should be seen, however, as prompting inquiry that will increase knowledge and understanding, not the action that ready-made ethics-by-decree demands. What can be done is a matter to be discovered, not enacted. No doubt it is a fine prospect for most people to live a healthy life of average length 120 years; but as an Ethical principle it useless, even if the means of achieving it were known. However, if conclusions about conduct are to come from inquiry rather than decree, there are powerful ontological and epistemic pressures to be seriously addressed. Something that might be clearly desirable and, at a naive level of inquiry, readily attainable may on serious examination turn out to be utterly meaningless.

EXAMPLE 16.9. In Chapter 11, for instance, we addressed the question of not only allowing people to be free but compelling them to be free. Impassioned advocates of freedom are apt to overlook the fact that what they wish and what persons of a type very different from themselves wish (or, at a more disheartening level, what they *think* they wish) may have almost nothing in common. There are many people who do not at all want to be free, at least in the sense that the advocates mean by the term *free*. At the present time there seems to be in Russia a countercurrent, a nostalgia, for the good old days of the communist regime when the disaffected did not have to spend their time making their own arrangements about food and housing.

It is quite obvious that the opinions throughout the world about oppression are formed from the writings and the speeches of the articulate and motivated. But the latter are a far cry from being a representative group in any society. In particular, they include more than their fair share of those who prize freedom. Can they be justified in demanding (and imposing!) this freedom on all?

PATHOGENETICS

Lest this discussion become too diffuse, we take a topic that has been of interest to us and that throws some of these points into high relief. *Pathogenetics* is a portmanteau word—in Lewis Carroll's terminology (1872)—

coined to avoid the clumsy phrase "the pathogenesis of genetic disorders" (Pyeritz and Murphy 1991; Murphy and Pyeritz 1996). Unlike *etiology* of disease, pathogenetics deals with the detailed pathways and the ensemble of causation rather than with the particularity of causes. How is some genetic anomaly in the DNA or the cellular structure or the chromosomes explicitly converted into a phenotype that is recognizable as a (clinical) disorder? Stated like that, it seems to be simple in principle, however much pettifogging detail might have to be cleared up before the whole process is understood. There is more to it than ingredients (the traditional fare of etiology), more even than a recipe (how the parts are compounded, the added component that defines *pathogenesis,* or "disease production"). The full account of pathogenesis also includes the inner workings of the system in health and disease, what in Chapter 4 we identified as turning an almost totally black box into a totally white one. It is only by this means that one can provide a rational cure or (a quite different issue) presume to improve on the health of a stock by something better than hit-or-miss.

We cannot do more than sketch the topic here. But at least we can identify something of what bearing pathogenetics may have on Medical Ethics.

The Genes

The genes and their impact are ubiquitous and popular and need no champion. They exhibit a number of contrasting characters that are of the essence. A little leafing through McKusick's catalogue (1994) will suffice to demonstrate both their richness and how the compendium grows apace with each edition. They are a hive of variation: the more closely we look, the more evidence we find of diversity *(allelism)* at each component *locus,* so that among the offspring of the same two parents there is a virtually unlimited number of combinations possible. This allelism in the *genotype* (or particular assembly of genes) is the very embodiment of individuality. What it does to the external or black-box appearance of the person is identifiable with the *phenotype.* We can clarify these relationships by an analogy from Aristotle's ontology.

EXAMPLE 16.10. The genome (namely, the assembly of genetic codes that is the paradigm or blueprint for the ontogeny of a species) is pretty much the counterpart of Aristotle's *essence.* The genotype (the explicit structure of the genome that characterizes the particular individual person's genome) is the counterpart of the "existent individuated essence" that connotes the *substance.* The phenotype is the counterpart of the assembly of properties or manifestations of a substance by which it is known to us, termed by Aristotle the *accidence.*

Now, while the genotype and the phenotype vary widely, the genome is highly, although not absolutely, conservative. There is no doubt that—as the result of minor copying errors, for instance—the number of loci is not invariable. But the backbone of individuality consists mainly of the particular permutation of genes rather than the number of loci.

EXAMPLE 16.11. Imagine several car parks built from the same plan in a city by a chain of businesses. They have much the same number of places, the counterpart of the *loci*. The makes of cars parked in them (the *alleles*) may vary widely. Moreover, the number of parking places (the *chromosomal complement*) that the management fits in may vary slightly. In each park, some number of loci will be allocated to the president, vice-presidents, and other administrative staff each of whom will be given a standard company car. The result will be like a genome that is highly conservative in a few places but highly diverse elsewhere.

Over as many generations as any one geneticist is able to study, the complement of loci in the human genome (the number of spaces in the car park) and their allocation to chromosomes cannot be expected to change much. But the behavior over many hundreds of generations becomes a matter for the evolutionist rather than the geneticist; and the format in both the size and the arrangement of the genome may slowly change until quite new species appear. The general belief—pieced together from a great many sources of data—is that the changes are Random and relatively infrequent, and their fate, though partly a matter of chance, is largely determined by how well the resulting phenotype performs in a more or less hostile world, and in the face of competition both within and among species.

While the besetting temptation among genetic evolutionists (and especially the biochemists among them) is to study the genotype to the exclusion of all else, two dissident voices keep them from that false path, each by its own telling viewpoints.

First, the population geneticists insist that while the radical changes lie in the genotype, what determines their fitness and hence the forces of selection is the phenotype; and since one of the major trends in evolution is for mechanisms to be generated (by selection) that drive a deeper and deeper wedge between genotype and phenotype and make the connection between them more and more roundabout, there must be a proper balance between the two claims. The genotype is one matter, and the phenotype is another; and while they are related, nothing but trouble will result if the one is studied without any attention to the other.

Second, both the Medical and the clinical geneticists, ultimately interested as they are in the operation of the organism as a whole, will demand a reasonable hearing not only for genotype and phenotype but also for mechanisms for adaptation, reliability of development in normal ontogeny, and emergent mechanisms that must be understood if the relationship between the genes and corporate behavior of the body is ever to rise beyond the status of a pure black box. Some glimpse of the possible scope for these mechanisms is given by the peculiar and unexpected properties that exist in two loci that interact epistatically (Murphy and Trojak 1981; Trojak and Murphy 1981, 1983). Extension of this line of thought to three and then to many loci is an interesting question that is adumbrated in the studies of Sewall Wright (1969). But it has not attracted the attention and pursuit that it merits.

Normality and Function

The topic of the fitness of a phenotype and how it might bear on well-being calls for some subtlety in analysis. The word *fitness* is floridly ambiguous. But it is neither courteous nor enlightening to harp on the ambiguity to the exclusion of all else. We cannot peremptorily suppose that all using the term are fools who do not look where they are going. However ill identified, the inchoate notion of the fit is not totally devoid of significance. Various writers have taken various tacks with it. We must suspect that they all hold some meaning in common, and it is our business to uncover what that communal meaning may be. It is true that the athlete may see fitness in terms of staying power, which is not the same as the population geneticist's perspective of effective reproduction; or the political theorist's notion of worthiness or dignity (what some of them have lately taken to calling *gravitas*); or the evolutionist's view of fitness as an attribute of the genetic line and its permanent contribution to the species; or the Moral Philosopher's notion of virtue; or the sociologist's view of civic cooperation. These viewpoints and others, seem, and indeed are, diverse. But in general they are not contradictory. They all have in common the recognition that some states are better than others. While the word *better* (being frankly an attitudinal term)[3] is as ambiguous as ever, the fact that in all these verbal transformations their communality of meaning is neither dissipated nor resolved suggests indeed that buried deep in them there is some elusive quality, largely but not wholly in common. Such an aggregation may be explained in various more or less satisfactory ways.[4] Two ways come to mind here.

The first is that the idea we have of fitness is a composite one, essen-

---

3. The cant of the era is to call such terms *value-laden*—a most unhappy phrase, because the word *value* is a bigger hornet's nest of semantic confusion than ever. In the mathematical sense, for instance, *value* could be identified with *quantitation* and would be interpreted in that way by a physicist, Probabilist, Statistician, etc. An epistemologist would think of it perhaps in terms of the quality and the implications of evidence. An auctioneer at Christie's would think of it in terms of purchase price. A Moral theologian would view the latter interpretation with horror.

4. We have a suspicion prompted by an excellent ontological analysis by Ayala (Dobzhansky et al. 1977) that, Probabilistically, basic phenomena in a vital system are either wholly tautologous or else wholly independent (Murphy 1988, 1992, 1997, n.d.-b). Intermediate states encountered empirically are readily intelligible as artifacts due to ambiguity of the sample space. That may ultimately be the mechanism here.

tially residing in multiple dimensions (in the same sense that the stability, or lack of it, of a four-legged table depends on at least four measurements) of which each of the various criteria gives a glimpse; and that the best definition (and therefore conception) would be to reconstruct it in a space of minimum dimensionality, yet to be determined.

The second is that we are really looking at a nest of tautologies that have been obscured by our imperfect and fallacious methods of observation.

EXAMPLE 16.12. Consider, for instance, the phrase "a big man." The rough idea is reasonably clear, but there are endless ways that one might try to define it. Weight, perhaps; but a short man weighing two hundred kilograms would be not big but obese. A man two meters high but cadaveric would be not big but tall. A champion weight-lifter of inconspicuous size would be not big but strong. And so forth. Sherlock Holmes, nothing if not an epistemologist, would identify a big man by the length of his stride and the depth of his footprints. Journalists, perhaps, gauge a big man by his impressive bearing. One might have called Napoleon a great man, but not a big one. All are trying to identify somebody who is physically striking, and in some way physically awe-inspiring.

On the topic of normality itself there has been a modest Philosophical literature on functional fitness and normality. We can give only a sketchy account of it, leaving a full exposition for another time. The key feature of this argument is the assumption that bodily parts have functions that may be examined and analyzed. In the light of how well the function is carried out, we may gauge the organism to be normal or not. Now, we cannot go into arguments in detail. But at a first level of analysis, we can think of four possible warrants under which the notion of function is introduced.

Postulated. It might be that for some reason a writer feels more or less compelled to suppose that function is a necessary idea. But where nothing that amounts to an epistemic warrant is given for this position, it is best viewed as an axiomatic statement. For instance, deists and theists may argue from the notion of a Divine Providence, and they are not bound in that context to declare what reasons they may have for their beliefs. They may merely state a position and see what conclusions it leads to; and there may be all shades of opinion as to how far the function develops through primary causes (such as special creation) and how far by secondary causes (such as Darwinian evolution). Some Darwinians may choose to argue without any assumption of Providence, and their reasons or motives for that position need not be stated or defended. Perhaps their stance is that, whatever the mechanism of mutation may be in detail, the *unit of selection* is not the nucleotide but rather the function that is necessary for survival and therefore driven by selective forces to exist. This might be fairly taken as the construction on function that would be put by such writers as Ruse (1971).

Imputed. The position of imputed function is more difficult to state accurately. It is the position, taken by such writers as Boorse (1973, 1977) and Millikan (1989), that implicitly presumes the wherewithal to read the function into the observed behavior of the biological operation. To call it inference would be too strong, since despite careful talking around the point, no formal epistemic statements are made. In this standpoint, it is reasonable to say that the function of the eye is to see, of the ear to hear, and so forth. There is some not very well defined assumption that claims of this kind not only are reasonable but also have clear meaning. In these terms it is not easy to see how this construction would accommodate structures that have no beneficial effects (always assuming that such structures exist). The Darwinian notion (that cells change Randomly and without purpose, and that should a change be beneficial, it will become common) necessarily supposes that there are many intermediate states that have no easy functional interpretation. One such is the case where the phenotypic evolutionary change from form *A* to form *B* is beneficial; but the change, to be effected, requires that every one of ten nonallelic genes must at some stage simultaneously attain particular forms. The genes will attain these states by mutation. Where nine of the ten mutations have occurred there will be no benefit, and from the standpoint of function the change so far must be without significance. Furthermore, should some of those that have already attained the desired forms be the victim of further drift before other genes have attained their desired forms, the benefit will be further delayed. Note also that while the change may involve no improvement on an old function, it may very well confer a major benefit from taking on a totally different function.

EXAMPLE 16.13. The telencephalon originally functioned as an organ of smell, a major faculty in the fishes, particularly in hunting. But in this organ developed what we now regard as the higher functions of intellect, dexterity, elaborate interpretation of sound and visual imaging, abstraction, language, and all the rest, with massive growth of the brain, though with some considerable depletion of the olfactory sense. It seems unlikely that any of these changes occurred in a few quick strides or warrant any confident claim that the Philosopher would have no difficulty in identifying nascent forms of the eventual function—or, for that matter, in identifying, in the present state, some revolutionary function that may develop in the future.

Whatever these difficulties, there seem to be with us in every generation those who might be termed (not in any technical Philosophical sense) naturalists—that is, astute observers of living nature—who seem to be able to say that a species has such and such characteristics that serve to protect it against X or to further its goal Y. Their method comprises keen observation, imagination, and common sense; but they profess no further formal Philosophy of what they are doing, or how they defend it.

Inferred. The proponents of inferred function are rather more structured in their approach. They frankly read a transcendent purpose into the phenomena of living nature. Some are Paleyites; some (such as Julian Huxley and perhaps Waddington) profess a kind of transcendental pantheism; some, like Teilhard de Chardin (1959), are theistic teleologists. The importance of function-as-inferred to Ethics is that these viewpoints are used both as apologetic arguments and (at the hands of the natural-Law ethicists) as a means of discerning what functions are natural and should be sustained and advanced.

Façon de parler. The term *façon de parler* denotes a "way of speaking." That is, if a statement is said to be a *façon de parler*, its content is to be taken not as a formal proposition but as a vivid or syncopated mode to avoid tedious paraphrases. For instance, to say that sharks developed fins so that they could steer more precisely would, to a strict and formal Darwinian, sound repellently teleological; but it could as well be used as a concise way of phrasing a more proper but much more tortured statement about fins being evolved by the cumulative effects of Random new mutations that were selected for because they enhanced control over steering, which was an advantage in such and such situations, and so on. Ayala (Dobzhansky et al. 1977) constructively explored the possibility of a Darwinian teleology but ending with reservations about its sense.

In the domain of functional analysis Achinstein (1977) seems to have taken something of this stance, using the word *function* in a facultative fashion with three different meanings that he explicitly identifies: (1) *design function,* that for which some artifact was expressly designed by a deliberative mind; (2) *use function,* the actual useful benefit that results from its properties; and (3) *service function,* the current benefit that is derived from its properties. The latter may be diverse or diversified. In the strict Darwinian scheme, the first kind of function would have no representation. The second would include all those mutant processes that turned out to be useful for one purpose or another. The third would include many opportunistic appropriations, as that, for instance, the anterior pituitary gland was once part of the gastrointestinal system, and the genitalia have been developed from the primitive urological system. Also the use function of the femur lies in a means of weight bearing and locomotion; but to it we may add the service function of the femur as a fighting weapon for a dexterous hominid, an appropriation that has also been called *eolithic* (q.v.).

CONCLUSION

The healthy development of Medical Ethics depends on continued activity at the interfaces among Medicine, science, and Ethics. This interchange is imperative but demanding. Scientific knowledge and insight grow apace. The scope of clinical enterprise and the continued deliberations in Ethics call for unceasing mutual adjustment. The sheer growth of data and technique and the benefits of specialization (but also the perils of isolation) are constant sources of tension. This interdisciplinary culture (never a well-cultivated field of scholarship) must be promoted with energy and enthusiasm if the convoluted nature of the data and the techniques are to be adapted to the complex working of health and disease.

Appendix 1
The Unconscious

This very brief account of the unconscious mind is included purely to make more intelligible some of the material in this book. There is much diversity of opinion, and considerable care must be taken over the vocabulary (Ellenberger 1970; R. J. Campbell 1989; Moore and Fine 1990).

DEFINITION OF THE UNCONSCIOUS

The unconscious is the part of the mind (or more properly of the personality) that functions without the person being aware of it at the time, but that can be perceived subsequently, perhaps soon afterward or years later, or perhaps never. Compared with the conscious mind, the unconscious is enormous. In it are deposited all experiences of the past waking and sleeping states with varying degrees of significance to the person.

ACCESS TO THE UNCONSCIOUS

The person's access to his or her unconscious is (by definition and in fact) always retrospective and may occur spontaneously or with professional aid. The psychiatrist keeps in mind the existence of the unconscious and its participation in the making of decisions and the shaping of behavior. While the person remains unaware of its content and functioning at any given moment, the psychiatrist (or other professional) may gain access to the unconscious through diverse avenues: free association, the analysis of dreams, motor and sensory slips of mental functioning, thought blocks, jokes, gestures, mannerisms, tics, and the evaluation of body language expressed in psychophysiologic and psychosomatic reactions. Once reached, information from the unconscious becomes utilized by the conscious mind or becomes stored in the preconscious. Caution has to be exercised as to the meaning of recalled items. The term *preconscious* refers to memory as such, free associations, and the accessed memories from the unconscious. Interaction occurs among the conscious, preconscious, and unconscious parts of the mind.

THE UNCONSCIOUS AND REPRESSION

In the encounters of daily life, an issue that appears overwhelming to the person and threatens to disorganize mental function (including any issue from within the person such as an instinct, urge, or impulse) is repressed into the unconscious. This repression (which is itself at the time an unconscious defense) consigns to a guarded region the entire issue or whatever parts in it are threatening. Then, either spontaneously or with professional help in a healing process (psychotherapy), the repressed material and its derivative defenses become adequately perceived (insight is developed), and they are dealt with so that the issue no longer disrupts personality function.

Repressed issues are stored in the unconscious not merely as topics but accompanied by the psychic energy that would have been expended at the time had it been possible to resolve them in the conscious mind. The accumulation of such unresolved issues and the accompanying energy may in turn threaten the person from within and lead to the formation of complex defenses, like psychophysiologic, psychosomatic, neurotic, or psychotic reactions. The energy in the unconscious may discharge itself in various ways: in the development of insight and normal psychic processes; or by pathologic responses, such as display of abnormal attitudes, organic dysfunction, obsessions, phobias, compulsions, hysteria, delusions, and hallucinations. In the course of the psychologic maneuvering, various defense tactics are used: symbolization, displacement, substitution, regression, denial, acting out, rationalization, and so on.

THE UNCONSCIOUS AND PERSONALITY DEVELOPMENT

The psychodynamics of mental function at conscious, preconscious, and unconscious levels arises from innate and environmental factors involved in the development of the individual's personality toward differing degrees of maturity.

Appendix 2
The Grammar of Voice

In the primitive structure of Indo-European languages, a verb may have various voices. Thus, "I am holding a book" is in the active voice, since the subject (I) is the performer of the act of holding, and the object (a book) is that which is acted on. But "The book is held by me" is in the passive voice, something that is done to the subject of the sentence by an external agent (me). There are other voices. In Greek, for instance, there is a middle voice with diverse interpretations that have in common something like the subject doing something to, for, or on behalf of itself. English grammarians make little of this middle voice; but it is certainly encountered.

EXAMPLE A2.1. Take the verb *to present*. The Medical instructor *presents* a patient to a class of students (active voice). The patient *is presented* to the class by the instructor (passive voice). The patient *presents* with a three-month history of increasingly severe headache (middle voice). The last usage is grammatically and notionally quite authentic. (In an extreme case, the patient might present in a hospital with these complaints even if the hospital turned out to be totally empty—that is, there was nobody to present the complaint to.)

Another form, one that is closely akin to the middle voice, is at least some uses of the reflexive. In the usual grammatical definition, the reflexive is that construction in which the subject and the object of the sentence are the same individual, as when a man shaves himself. But in French and in Spanish, for instance, there is in fact a second form (which operates under the same grammatical rubric) in which the sense is more akin to the Greek middle voice: "I wash myself the hands" ("Je me lave les mains," "Me lavo las manos").

Another grammatical device distinguishes the middle voice by excluding the use of a direct object, by making the verb intransitive. The use of the passive form then either becomes impossible or stilted to the point of ridiculousness.

EXAMPLE A2.2. We can accept the sentence "They put up with their friend's bad temper," but "Their friend's bad temper was put up with by them" is a ludicrous construction.

———

To round this discourse out, we must address one further notion that is both complex and confusing. There is a class of verbs traditionally termed deponent in which the meaning is active but the grammatical form passive. Thus, the Latin verb *conor* (I try), from which the word *conation* is derived, is passive in form, but its meaning is clearly active. One feature of such verbs is that grammatically they have no active voice. So there is the risk of confusing deponent verbs with what are merely mistaken for deponent but are properly defective verbs, that is, verbs for which there are missing parts.

EXAMPLE A2.3. The verb *to go* in English, for instance, is a defective verb. It has no past definite tense. The proponents of synthetic grammar will insist that the past definite tense of *go* is *went*. But that is a pure fiction. The word *went* has etymologically nothing whatsoever to do with the word *go*. It is the past tense of the quite unrelated (and now almost obsolete) verb *to wend*. Again, the Latin verb to go is *ire* and it has a past definite, *ivi*. Like its English counterpart, the Spanish verb *ir* is cobbled together from various sources, a present tense from the quite different Latin verb *vado* and a past definite from the verb *to be,* with which it is identical (*fuí, fuiste,* etc.). It is remarkable that so august an authority as Ramsey (1956: 282–83) merely hints that the current verb *ir* is a botch.

Once the question is raised as to who decides, and how, that a verb is deponent, there are some odd results.

EXAMPLE A2.4. The Latin verb *nascor* (I am born) is classed among the deponent, and not the defective, verbs. But who, one wonders, decided that it is active in meaning, and on what grounds? Surely not English classicists, for in English (and in German) both the meaning and the form are passive. "The child was born": birth is something done to the infant. The mother is the active agent; in somewhat old-fashioned language, she *bore* the child. Now, in Spanish the old Latin deponent becomes an uncompromising active verb: *nací* thus becomes grammatically something like "I undertook birth." It is the very opposite of a deponent verb, being (by English standards, at least) passive in meaning, yet it is active in form. Likewise in the French, *Je naquis* is active.[1] In Russian, the form *ya rodiltsya* is reflexive. So English infants at birth are expelled; Spanish infants simply leave; Russian infants extricate themselves. Whether these grammatical differences make

———

1. The perfect tense, *Je suis né,* is anomalous because it looks passive in form, as (by English standards) it is in meaning. Grammarians, however, have compiled a list of French verbs (many of them verbs of motion) that have this odd form in the past composite (perfect) tense. (In rather old-fashioned English, for instance, one may say "I am gone" instead of the more usual form "I have gone.") But at best that is a grammatical contrivance. To say that something belongs to a list of exceptions does not *explain* anything.

for semantic differences, we cannot say. Again we note that in English the verbs *die, starve,* and *enjoy* are all active (or arguably middle) voice, but in Latin *(mori, fame confici,* and *frui)* they are passive in form and assigned to the deponents.

No doubt the grammarians (whose concerns are different from ours) will see voice in formal terms. For our purposes we do well to attach voice as much to meaning as to grammatical forms. Insofar as the issue is doing or being done by, we should recognize a continuous scale of voice. Some words that in a technical grammatical sense are active may in a semantic sense be almost purely passive. Where an encounter involving action is concerned, we may arrange verbs on a continuous scale from staunchly active to really, or virtually, passive. There is a series of verbs associated with dispute that illustrate the gradation: *seize, extort, demand, exact, agree, accept, undergo, submit, suffer, succumb.* All are active in form; but on the continuous scale of Ethical voice, they extend from strong activity to virtually helpless recipience.

There are yet other verbs that may or may not have voice. The verb *to be* in most languages has no voice (indeed, in Russian it is ordinarily not used at all in the present tense). *To appear, to seem,* and *to simulate* are other instances. Paraphrases of it (like *to find oneself*) are reflexive. The verb *to become* has a curious quality. In spirit it has no voice or, by default, middle voice. In English there are few critical tests of its voice, and they are ambiguous. In Spanish the verb *devenir* and its counterpart in Catalan, *devindre,* are largely avoided. The French form, *devenir,* is certainly used, although much less than in English. In Latin the verb is said to be semideponent: for its present tense there is an active form *(fio, fis, fit)* but for its past tense a passive form from the verb *facere* (to make).[2]

---

2. In principle, the credal Latin form "Et homo factus est" could mean either "And he became man" (an autonomous action) or "And he was made man" (a contingent experience), a curious technical looseness in a formula expressly designed to rebut Arianism!

Appendix 3
A Note on Rights

Here we examine briefly the question of whether Medicine and science can illuminate the formal use of rights in Medical Ethics.

Patients are almost universally accorded respect as persons, conditional freedom from coercion, and conditional choice as to plan of treatment. But there is public concern over these matters. Commonly, statements of the policies of the hospital or medical practice are publicly displayed. Typically such statements simply provide information to the patient (although such display or its contents may in part at least be Legally mandated).

Decisions and policymaking in Medical practice often have consequences that affect several recipients, who compete for the Agent's consideration. The many needs and Medical choices concerning a particular patient may be in conflict. Distribution of medical resources and attention to the various needs of the patient are common points of decision. A further tension exists between the care of individual patients and the demands of public health. A popular notion of how to solve such Ethical problems is the invocation of rights of patients, and perhaps of other parties to decisions. In some instances we may conceive of such rights as a subset of respect (as understood in Chapter 13).

RIGHTS AS A POPULAR NOTION

There is currently much popular interest in rights. People speak of constitutionally guaranteed rights; women's rights; political, civil, and human rights; even rights of pets, of wild animals, of vegetation, and of certain inanimate natural phenomena. The notion in part reflects the current litigious attitude prevalent among the public about settling and forestalling disputes. Moreover, there is a hope that if certain rights were to be recognized or established, then appropriate, advantageous, and useful decisions would be facilitated.

SEMANTICS

The term *right* is used in the sense of entitlement and of authority (*Webster's* 1988: sense 2). The cognate German, French, Spanish, and Italian words *Recht, droit, derecho,* and *diritto* are used in much the same way. Several kinds of right may be distinguished.

There are, for example, *contractual rights,* that is, rights prescribed by the terms of a contract.

A *statutory right* is an entitlement or authority expressed by a code of law.

EXAMPLE A3.1. Statutory rights regulate voting in elections to public office, and access to evidence in actions at law.

An *intrinsic right* is one attaching to the nature of a person or Thing. We note, however, that a narrowly particularized formulation of such a right runs the risk of violating the principle of conterminality.

EXAMPLE A3.2. The first person ever to suffer from AIDS, although confronted with a totally new and unprecedented illness, at least experienced features that resembled and needed to be diagnostically distinguished from well-established diseases. The presumption that this person merited help is not evidently vitiated because he was (at the time) in a unique state in which he was the only source of secure information bearing upon the diagnosis and management of his disease. On the other hand, the lack of reasonable precedent offers no such indulgence to someone who solicits the help of a physician because he cannot get his car started or because he is having bad luck at cards.

Many other sources of rights might be listed (custom, common law, political franchise, etc.) that are of no particular interest to Medical Ethics.

RIGHTS IN HUMAN HISTORY

Before inquiring about a role for rights in Medicine, we need to review some history. Appeal to rights as such has in fact had a limited history, and that chiefly in the political or Legal, not the Philosophical, domain. Indeed, Aristotle, Plato, and Aquinas had nothing to say about rights (Flew 1989).

Hereditary kings in Old Testament times and in medieval Europe claimed their office "by divine right," but this concept had to do with a mandate for rulers, not ordinary people. Even when rights were recognized, protection by law first occurred in very limited ways. Free Roman citizens under the Empire enjoyed certain Legal perquisites. But it was much later that anything resembling a constitution emerged, in fact a contractual instrument.

EXAMPLE A3.3. After the Norwegian immigration to Iceland, to check the use of vendetta as a means of redressing grievances, the landed gentry developed a process of binding agreements. The Icelandic solution was a contractual one, in which violators of agreements lost their protection and could be dispossessed or killed with impunity (Magnusson and Pálsson 1960). A further step, the Magna Carta of 1215, was a political settlement between the English barons and King John that spelled out certain political entitlements for landed citizens.

It was not until the late sixteenth century that political, and to some extent Philosophical, thinkers began to put forward the notion of rights as principles of conduct. Even so, the main point they considered was the legitimacy of various societal institutions (which were soon to undergo reorganization in the American and French revolutions).

Locke and, later, Hobbes postulated that persons possess *natural rights*. For Locke these existed simply as a kind of natural equipment; his concept appears to have stemmed from Hooker's interpretation of the medieval scholastic notion of *natural Law* (Copleston 1948b: 51). Hobbes, instead, visualized a presocietal state in which persons were constantly at war to protect their rights until they agreed to vest them in a society (ibid., p. 56). Helvétius and other French social Philosophers based rights on their utility (Copleston 1967: 17 ff.). Spinoza in his Moral Philosophy derived from the actual existence of power a (natural) authority to put rights effectively into practice; when the power (e.g., of a monarch) weakens so that rights cannot be implemented, the natural authority is forfeited (Copleston 1948b: 258 ff.).

Such arguments in turn became the basis for the political rights that are a feature of constitutional law in America and France, and subsequently in many other countries. Even so, one does well to note that many such instruments originally applied only to narrowly defined segments of the population, and their extension to cover all citizens occurred over an extended period.

EXAMPLE A3.4. In the United States, political rights were not at first accorded to all citizens but only to landholders (as in thirteenth-century England). Slavery persisted until 1865, and women were not enfranchised voters until 1922. Switzerland, which for centuries had been democratized by the institution of government by town meeting, had no women's suffrage until some seventy years later.

———

Nevertheless, since the American and French revolutions, various concepts of rights have come to be embedded in all manner of political, Legal, and religious documents.

RIGHTS IN MEDICAL ETHICS

We regard Medical Ethics as at least an interface, and ideally as an intersection, between Philosophy and Medicine, together with adjuncts in science. A basis for rights in the scope of Medical Ethics thus involves points of contact in Medicine and in Philosophy. In searching for these we have to pay attention to ontology and provenience (qq.v.).

Ontology

As we have seen, proponents of rights have not been agreed as to ontology, whether the rights are intrinsic or acquired (by contract or by statute), and whether they are mutable or not. Nevertheless, let us consider what basis there might be for rights strictly within the context of Medicine. Here we cannot turn to a statutory or contractual source. There must be no hint that legislated privileges may be presumed to constitute any Ethical structure, except indirectly in that law is among the structures to be respected in Ethical discourse. A universal intrinsic right might validly arise from the simple fact of personhood; but particularizing the basis of an intrinsic right runs the risk of violating the principle of conterminality.

It thus appears that few particular rights can be said to exist self-evidently and without explicit warrant. Rather, they are ontologically derivative, even though they may raise deeper questions. Such derivative rights may be conceptually useful at the level of casuistry — that is, at the level of individual cases — rather than in working out a general principle of solution.

Recently the proposition was casually put forward by a prominent British politician that persons have rights to anything that is not forbidden by law. While the statement was not advanced as a profound theoretical principle, nevertheless it was expressed in the public domain by a person in political office, and so can be treated with some seriousness. Leaving aside the question of whether law is the only domain of rights, the definition of rights by default seems to make of rights what would be better seen as the absence of wrongs (or of nonrights). Perhaps this attitude is more commonplace than we had supposed. It has some important implications, however. The general concept of a right as a principle that may be invoked to support a claim that a wrong is being perpetrated is familiar enough. However, the total set of possible courses of action is so enormous that only a minute fraction of them can be constrained in even the most regimented society or the most constricting political principle. A listing of rights then becomes a prodigious task, and inevitably in large part trivial. One would have a defined right to put dried orange peel inside one's grand piano and infinitely more of the same; and inevitably any principle of appeal to a right would become utterly trivialized, and virtually impotent.

Provenience

However, let us imagine attempts to use putative rights-as-such for decision making in Medicine. Problems arise in regarding them as if they were absolute. When two or more patients are involved, their rights may be in conflict. Even where only one patient is involved, that patient's putative rights may conflict with one another (e.g., the right to live and the right to be free of pain). Reasonable resolution will require us to attach *weights* to the conflicting rights. The focus of the resolution then passes from the putatively absolute rights themselves to a means for agreeing upon their respective weights, with all the attendant problems, including the provenience of the evidence. Such a system should receive careful attention. But its warrant for totally overriding the ordinary decision-theoretic means of resolving Medical conflicts, outlined in Chapter 10, is not at all self-evident.

We conclude that in the present state of ontological analysis, rights have no special function in Major or Minor Medical Ethics.

Glossary

This list is intended as an informal set of definitions, for reference and for help-ful commentary. In many cases better and more detailed definitions are to be found at the appropriate section of the text.

ab initio (= from the beginning): The primordial state. In contrast with a priori (q.v.), which denotes the state immediately before a particular proposition is explored.

abstraction: An arbitrary, simplified assembly of characteristics that members of a group share, to be used as the basis for prudent generalizations that may be applied to all of them.

accountability: A feature of responsibility in the individual, who may be subsequently called upon to explain and justify a course of action undertaken or ignored.

accuracy: See *precision* and *bias*.

Act (capitalized): A discrete, deliberative action of high ontological density (q.v.), performed by a human being. Actions in this idealized form may not exist, and are certainly rare.

action: An unconscious activity that involves splanchnic movement.

adaptation: The development, whether purposive or not, of a feature that increases the chance of survival of an organism in a hostile environment.

ad hoc: Applied to a device (term, decision, procedure, etc.) introduced with the purpose of meeting a specific demand. Examples include ——— definitions, rules of procedure, bylaws. See *conterminality, principle of.*

affect: The emotional aspect of psychic function.

Agent (capitalized): The person who acts. The ——— is not merely the subject of the sentence. In the sentence "The man's wife suffered much indignity at the hands of her neighbor," the voice is active and the wife is the subject; but she is not, in the ordinary sense, the ———, who, depending on details, might be the neighbor.

agnosia: The state of not knowing; ignorance. (The word also has a technical, neurological meaning.)

allegiance: Used especially in the scholarly sense that if there are two or more conflicting, nontrivial objectives in an inquiry, the scholar may, without loss of esteem, choose one over all others: for example, a pragmatic solution rather than one in principle.

allele: One of two or more forms of the gene that may occupy a single genetic locus.

amicus (for *amicus curiae* = friend of the court): A nonparticipating witness in the external phenomenology of responsibility (q.v.).

analysis: The breaking down of a complex structure (chemical, physical, conceptual, Psychological, etc.) into simpler components. Also, the result of such a process. The word also has less obvious meanings, for example, in Philosophy and mathematics.

anaplastic: Mostly used to denote cancerous cells that have reverted to a primitive, undifferentiated form. Hence, metaphorically, primitive, primordial, unstructured, undifferentiated, regressive.

apodictic: In the ontological sense, certainly true as a necessity of thought (e.g., the existence of existence); in the epistemic sense, cogently demonstrated beyond cavil or dispute.

a posteriori: Used of a proposition that is asserted (usually with a specified Probability) to be true as a conclusion from an analysis.

a priori: Used of a proposition that is asserted with a specified Probability to be true before an argument is put forward. Used without Probabilistic qualification, it is taken to mean that the proposition is certainly true. What is an ——— statement in one proposition may be an a posteriori (q.v.) statement from another (antecedent) argument.

arbitrary: Used of a decision about terms of meaning, action, classification, and so forth that is arrived at by reasonable and amicable means, typically for practical purposes rather than as a rational inference or deduction from solidly established principles. There is to be no element of caprice in this term; either it shall be agreed upon by all parties to a dispute, or statements made under it are to be treated as contingent. An ethicist, for instance, may call the amputation of a leg, even a therapeutic amputation, a mutilation. A surgeon might not use the word *mutilation* in that sense; and disputants may agree to treat the word as a technical term in Ethics. ———— usages are tolerated because there is no better decision available. They are promptly replaced in the light of better understanding.

artifact: Used in two quite different senses. (1) **Medical:** An appearance or presence that is generated by the methods of observation or inference and in no way related to what is being observed (e.g., an accidental mark on a chest X-ray or a stain on a slide that has been improperly washed). (2) **Archaeological:** An object made or shaped by a human being.

ascertainment: The process whereby an entity or an event is brought preferentially to the attention of a scholar (typically an investigator). For instance, in genetics an entire family of subjects with a genetic disorder may be discovered because one member, the proband or propositus (qq.v.), is seen and diagnosed, and, because of the familial character of the disorder, the other members too are examined. ———— **bias:** Because the proband is (tautologously) affected, the proportion of the family being affected is higher than would be expected from Mendelian segregation ratios (q.v.). Appropriate adjustments must be made in segregation analysis.

assertion: An emphatically stated proposition that in general implies a confident belief because of firm Logic or coercive empirical evidence.

assumption-of-convenience: An assumption made, not because it is believed, but because it makes the ultimate solution of a problem easier. Classical uses are in the proof by reductio ad absurdum in which the ———— is shown to lead to absurd conclusions and therefore its contrary must be true; and as the null hypothesis (q.v.) in Neyman-Pearson (q.v.) hypothesis testing.

atresia: A congenital defect of anatomy in which a structure, properly hollow (e.g., the intestine, a blood vessel, or the cerebral aqueduct) lacks any lumen.

authentic (noun **authenticity**): Genuine; corresponding to that-which-is, to reality; true. The word is necessary because such words as *true, real,* and *actual* have all been the victims of doctrinaire manipulations by more or less implicit Philosophies. The mainstream view of scientific and Medical thought is that whatever the epistemic and conceptual problems, there is at least in principle an inviolable *something* that is a rational object of inquiry which is perhaps unlike any existential theory about it. It is not certain a priori that such a *something* exists. If it does not, the simplest course is to deny that truth exists; hence, science has no meaning and the so-called successes of science are in effect successes of black-box technology. However, many have seen fit to divert the word *truth* to denote a subjective construction of the data of experience. For the mainstream scientist it is a constant struggle to find words to represent the idea that is being constantly eroded by such verbal devaluation.

authentication: An epistemological principle that a proposition may not be said to be false unless it could be shown to be true, if true.

autochthonous: Originating where it is first encountered. Indigenous, native. Not arising as the result of any external mechanism.

autonomous: Self-regulating, although susceptible to information from outside the system (as, e.g., the heartbeat).

average: The mean or expectation (of a Random variable). The three terms are interchangeable, but the term —————— is commonly reserved to denoting the sample estimate (q.v.) of the expectation.

axiom: A statement that is taken for granted as the starting point of an argument, either because it is held to be obvious, or because it rests on a mass of sound evidence, or simply as a formal assumption for reaching contingent conclusions.

Baconian principle: The principle that a sufficiency of good empirical data, collected without prejudice, will eventually lead to the solution of any scientific problem.

balanced polymorphism: A state of a Mendelian locus in which there are two or more alleles with the heterozygotes more fit than the homozygotes. It is a stable dynamic equilibrium in which any perturbation of the frequencies will tend to be corrected to the stable state; hence, it acts against any tendency for an allele to become extinct by the Random variation of family size over (perhaps many) generations (genetic drift).

Bayesian Logic (capitalized): A principle of inference, which eventually came to fill the void left by Hume's demolition of the theory of inductive proof. In it apodictic proof is replaced by Probabilistic affirmations about each of several competing conclusions that in each case comprise the Probabilistic support for it from cumulative previous experience (as the prior or a priori Probability) and the conditional Probability of some additional evidence to yield a posterior or a posteriori Probability. It is to be contrasted with Neyman-Pearson theory (q.v.), in which the prior Probabilities are either inaccessible or ignored. (See Murphy and Chase 1975; Murphy 1982.)

bias (of an estimator): In Statistics a systematic error, the difference between the mean value of an indefinitely large number of estimates each based on a Random sample of fixed size and the quantity being estimated.

binary: A variable attribute that may assume one of two but only two states that are exhaustive and mutually exclusive (e.g., existent and nonexistent).

black box: An image or representation of a structure as a featureless intermediary between an input and an output. The image may take this form out of necessity (because the inner workings of the structure are not known, or perhaps cannot be known); or because the analysis is simplified; or because the analyst is exploring robustness (q.v.). Contrast *white box,* in which all the inner workings of the structure may be explicitly understood and measured. Most working models are of an intermediate shade of gray.

bottleneck: Used to denote a variable quantity at one point in a complicated interaction that limits the rate of operation of the system as a whole. For example, "The strength of a chain is its weakest link." The strength of the chain can be improved only by improving that of the weakest link. (The identity of the ——— may vary from one system to another, depending on the specifications.)

canonize: *Webster's* (1988) gives us "to treat as illustrious, preeminent, or sacred" (sense 5). In our context it means to single out one feature, property, or characteristic of a thing or quality that designates its essence. The metal mercury has various properties, among them density, conductivity, specific heat, melting and boiling points, and chemical affinities. But mercury exists in various (isotopic) forms, and the details of its behavior vary with conditions such as temperature and pressure. Because of almost ideally high ontological density, the atomic number of mercury (80), which is invariant among all its isotopes and in all its physical and chemical states, is ———d or singled out as the identifying feature of mercury. No other element has this atomic number, and all substances indistinguishable from mercury have that atomic number. Much of the struggle for a coherent formulation of Medicine is a quest for canonical features.

cardinality: The number of distinct elements in a set. For a continuous set (e.g., the set of all possible heights), the ——— is infinite. See *dimensionality.*

casuistry: The practice of applying the principles of Minor Ethics to individual cases (see *Ethics, Minor*). (It will include many particular details in mitigation, special pleading, etc.)

categorization: The process of putting a population comprising the realizations of experience (empirical qualities, the results of experiment, intrinsic properties, etc.) into distinct, mutually exclusive, and exhaustive classes or groups or sets or categories. This definition does not imply that the contents of any category are homogeneous; rather, it implies that the ———— has disposed of an important fraction of the total variation in the class in a way that is conceptually illuminating and heuristic in its implications.

certainty: A state of consensual assurance about some proposition or prediction. Where the issue is in principle Random, ———— corresponds to a Probability of 1. Contrast *Certitude*.

Certitude (capitalized): A state of nonconsensual (e.g., personal) assurance about some proposition or prediction. Contrast *certainty*.

Chaos (capitalized): In mathematics, a dynamic system that, among other features, cannot be decomposed and has behavior that is exquisitely sensitive to the initial conditions in the system. Although it is a deterministic system, so long as any error of measurement occurs, it will be unpredictable.

Charcot joint: Also called neuropathic joint. A progressive destruction of the gross anatomy of a joint by repeated injuries that, because of defective sensation, pass unnoticed and hence are inadequately healed. Once a common feature of tabes dorsalis, it is now a rare condition seen mostly in diabetic neuropathy.

Chinese box: A toy comprising a nest of boxes of graduated size fitting successively one inside another. Hence, by analogy, any Logical or ontological system in which each level of operation (and hence analysis) derives its warrant from a higher level, and so perhaps in infinite regress.

clinical genetics: That branch of clinical Medicine that deals with clinical aspects (diagnosis, prognosis, prevention, and management) of disorders that have important and variable hereditary components in their etiology. See *Medical genetics* and *human genetics*.

clinician: Any person (dentist, gynecologist, midwife, nurse, obstetrician, physician, psychiatrist, Psychologist, surgeon, veterinarian, etc.) who exercises professional skill in matters of health, from direct contact with individual patients in matters involving their diagnosis, prognosis, treatment, management, or preventive care.

cognition: That aspect of psychic activity dealing with knowledge, perception, reflection, reasoning, and so on. Contrast *affect* and *conation*.

cohort: A term (originally denoting a walled garden and later a division of the Roman army) now used in epidemiology to signify a defined population of subjects who undergo a diachronic (q.v.), usually prospective, study and typically having some simultaneously experienced event (birth, disease, operative procedure) in common, and in this respect are homogeneous.

commensurable: Capable of being compared by a common scale of measurement.

commensurate: Used of entities that are at best imperfectly commensurable (such as labor and pay). The word ———— implies that there is a reasonable relationship between the entities, at least a monotonic one, and arguably a proportional one (twice as much labor earning twice as much pay).

complexity (of a structure): The number and nature of instructions that are needed to reconstitute the structure. Repetitive structures (such as a crystal) have low ———— and conversely.

compromise: A pragmatic and arbitrary outcome of a dispute, in which certain concessions in principle are made by all without any guarantee that differences in principle have been adequately resolved. See *consensus* and *resolution*.

conation: The striving aspect of psychic activity (e.g., the urge to run away when afraid). See *affect* and *cognition*.

confounding: A symmetrical relationship between two entities (like inertia and mass; or two causes or two effects) in which in general or in particular there are no methods, theoretical or empirical, by which they may be analytically separated. There are degrees of incomplete confounding. See *redundancy; symmetry; tautology*.

consensual: Characteristic of any conclusion that has been reached by consensus (q.v.). ———— **Ethics:** Ethics that is based on ———— conclusions.

consensus: An academically sound outcome from a dispute in which a single set of coherent principles adequately accommodates all coherent arguments and criticisms that have been advanced by at least one disputant. Not to be confused with compromise or majoritarian view. (Truth is not democratic.) ———— is perpetually at the mercy of future knowledge and understanding.

consequentialism: A form of Ethics that proposes that the appropriateness of an Act is to be gauged solely by its foreseeable consequences.

consistential: Used of the demand that a sound truth is approached by, and must eventually satisfy, all reasonable considerations germane to it, for instance, the *theoretical* and the *empirical* (qq.v). Thus, Newton showed theoretically that the speed of sound at sea level should be about 960 feet per second. Empirical studies showed it was about 1,100 feet per second. Laplace by the theory of adiabatic expansion arrived at a ———— answer.

consultand: A technical term in the theory of genetic counseling (Murphy and Chase 1975) designating a person about whose present or future progeny the risks of inheriting a particular gene or genes are to be determined. The ———— may or may not be personally affected and may be concerned about the gene available in the other spouse. But note that a person inquiring about grandchildren, nephews, cousins, and the like is not a ————.

contagion of belief: The process of the spread of a belief, not by independent, individual, scholarly assessment of its merits, but on the weight of the authority of revered individuals.

conterminality (adjective **conterminous**): Having coinciding limits. Washington and the District of Columbia (D.C.) are conterminous: any part of the one is (by Legal definition) inside the other. Hence, all arguments from ———— are purely a matter of definition and are logically trivial. The **principle of** ———— is that—inasmuch as one quest for scholarship is to reach conclusions that are fewer and more compact than the facts they are to encompass and hence lead to the benefits of corroboration—a conclusion must have a wider domain of application than any particular problem that occasioned it. To say that the U.S. Congress must be inside Washington because it is inside D.C. offends against this principle, whereas to say that it must be inside the United States because D.C. is in the United States does not offend.

contingent: At least partially dependent on specified anterior factors. Event *A* is ———— on event *B* if (for whatever reason) the Probability of *A* is affected by the occurrence of *B*.

continuity: The quality of being uninterrupted. The term has several quite different meanings in the context of inference. ——— in a mathematical function may be defined in several ways, of which the simplest is that its graph can be continuously traced by a pen on a surface without the pen being at any stage raised off the surface.

continuous: That which has the property of continuity. A ——— Random variable is one such that although (as for all distributions) the Probability of the whole set of values is 1, the Probability of any particular value for the outcome is 0. It is a common mistake, especially in genetics, to suppose that a ——— distribution is one such that all the possible values lie within a single connected domain: if there are interruptions so that the domain is divided into two or more clearly separate groups, the distribution is "discontinuous." (Some geneticists regard the latter as a technical term. But in Probability theory *discontinuous* is a solecism to be put on the same level as the word *disregardless*.)

counterirritant: A medication applied to irritate the skin in the neighborhood of a deep-lying pain, which, it has been found empirically, alleviates the pain.

Darwinism: The broad surmise that (in modern terms) all species are descended from primitive forms by Random change (mutation) and preferential survival (selection) of certain forms on their merits in confronting the environment (adaptation). The theory expressly supposes that the changes are pure random drift, not in any way directed to any endpoint.

data: Collective information furnished by empirical observation and experimentation.

decision: A critical point of Ethics in which speculation and the analysis of evidence change to purpose and action. In most problems in Medicine (as contrasted with operative surgery) the ontological density of the decision is much lower than the traditional image supposes.

density: A term used in various ways, all in one way or another connoting compactness, thickness. In physics it denotes specific gravity; in writing, conciseness; in a continuous Probability distribution, the degree to which a Random variable is concentrated in particular neighborhoods of the domain; in ontology, the decisiveness with which the boundaries and form of an entity may be discerned.

deontology: The study of Moral obligation.

desideratum (plural **desiderata**): An optative term denoting a property (e.g., of a method) that is to be desired and will be appropriately fostered (e.g., efficiency and unbiasedness in estimators).

deus ex machina (= a god from the machine): A contrivance in the theater that allows an actor portraying a god to appear from on high, perhaps to rescue from danger the favored character. Hence, fancifully extended to any ad hoc device designed to extricate an investigator from an intractable problem. Typically it is incorrigibly particular and not falsifiable. (A notorious example is the so-called principle in evolutionary theory of the "survival of the fittest" when *fitness* means the capacity to survive. The principle reduces to the tautology "survival of the survivors.")

diachronic: Used of an empirical study of a process essentially over a period of time, as opposed to a synchronic study, which deals with an instantaneous state of the system. The former is often informally called longitudinal and the latter cross-sectional.

diagnosis: Used to denote two ideas. (1) The conclusion about the category of disease from which a patient is suffering. (2) The process whereby that decision is made (better called the diagnostic process). Throughout this book, the latter meaning is denoted by an upper-case letter.

dialogue: A discussion on a topic among disciplines in which the rules of procedure are symmetrically applied. In a ———— between physicians and lawyers, the rules of disputation shall not be imposed by either side but be agreed upon by both; there shall be no distinction between witnesses and advocates so that both may be freely examined and cross-examined; if there is to be sworn testimony, all members (including the procedural chairmen) shall be sworn.

differentiation: The process of expansion of a property of a primordial cell at the expense of other properties (e.g., of muscle cells to contract but with the loss of the capacity that the liver cell has to detoxify). Contrast *anaplastic.*

dimensionality (of a variable): The number of values that are required to specify the state fully. Contrast *cardinality.* The centimeter-gram-second system has three dimensions; but the cardinality of any one Random realization of them may be much larger, even infinite.

discrete: Used of a set of Things that are each clearly separable without intermediate transitional forms. If quantitative, the number of values they may assume is at most countable. In a ——— Random variable, each possible value has a Probability greater than zero. Contrast *continuous*.

disease: A loose, poorly defined term used to denote a lack of well-being, or a state of physical or mental impairment, or the preliminary stages of what in time may be expected to lead to such a state. The term is arbitrary, arguably unnecessary, and only in extreme cases does it lead to useful conclusions.

disjoint: Used of two events, states, or the like that are mutually exclusive. The states "over seven feet tall" and "under three feet tall" are ———. However, the terms *tall* and *obese* are not.

distribution function (DF): The proportion of a Random variable, X, assuming a value equal to or less than a particular (non-Random) value x as a function usually written f(x).

dogmatic: Used of a proposition that is stated with high precision and hence is readily falsified if false. The Watson-Crick model is an excellent example, and it has been widely and correctly (although we suspect facetiously) referred to as "the dogma." The use of the term ——— to mean *assertive* is widespread but to be deplored. (See Murphy 1981c.)

domain: A general term to denote any area, space, topic, subject matter, or the like, the limits of which are explicitly defined. Its chief merit is to provide escape from irrelevant semantic associations and imagery.

dominant: A phenotype due to a single allele that obscures or occults the phenotype due to another allele (i.e., gene at the same locus). Contrast *recessive; epistatic; hypostatic.*

dynamic system: A recursive mathematical system in which the outcome from the current step is the argument for the next step. The trivial example $x_n = x_{(n-1)} + 1$ generates the positive integers. A ——— may be rich in form even when not complicated in formulation.

eliminative materialism: The doctrinaire Philosophy that sentiments and experiences (belief, desires, hopes, fears, etc.) do not exist, cannot be investigated, and have no meaning.

embedded: Placed in a specific context. In mathematics, for instance, a straight line may be ——— in an infinite straight line, in a plane, in a space, and so on, in each of which it has a slightly different meaning that leads perhaps to different inferences. Two Random samples containing precisely the same data may be —— in two quite different sample spaces.

emergence: The existence of properties in complicated systems that exhibit no trace in any part of simpler systems and cannot be predicted from them. (In the empirical world the corresponding phenomenon is commonly called property ——).

empirical: A method of seeking truth by experience, experiment, and observation rather than by formal deduction from sound premises. The term is often but falsely used as disparaging. The mathematical constant π has been computed to many millions of decimal places on a theory assuming Euclid's axioms. But —— observation has shown that in the world of physics Euclid's theory is only approximately true.

endpoint: Some agreed event (in time, space, dosage of a drug, etc.) that is empirically accepted as denoting the completion of a process or state. Typical ——s are death, maturity, the limit of a desert, the disappearance of pain. The ideal, so-called **hard** —— is binary (e.g., moment of death). Often, and usually for technical or Ethical reasons, there is said to be a **soft** ——, either indefinite (such as the cure of depression) or bearing a questionable relationship to the trait of interest (as in substituting the level of blood cholesterol for atherosclerosis). Sometimes the —— is made hard artificially, as in substituting the median lethal dose of a drug for the minimal lethal dose; the former is much less sensitive to sample size than the latter.

enthymeme: A syllogism in which a premise or the conclusion is absent but implied. "George parked his car opposite a fire hydrant. He will therefore be fined." (The second premise "To park opposite a fire hydrant is punishable by a fine" is implied but not stated.)

eolith (= dawn stone): A crudely chipped flint. Metaphorically, the opportunistic use of a structure for a purpose for which it is accidentally apt but otherwise unrelated (e.g., use of a long bone as a weapon).

epistemic (also **epistemological**): Pertaining to epistemology (q.v.). —— **tension:** The clash between the robustness of a model and the power of a test used to falsify it. A robust model is one that will predict the outcome accurately in a particular application even if the assumptions underlying the model are not strictly met. A powerful test of goodness-of-fit will detect discrepancies between the assumptions of the model and the data. Clearly these desiderata in a test are antithetical. If the model fits the data, we expect the data to fit the model.

epistemology (adjective **epistemic** or **epistemological**): The study of sound design and interpretation of evidence. Logic may be regarded as a highly formalized subdivision of ———.

estimate: The result of applying an estimator (q.v.) to a set of data.

estimation: The problem of making formal guesses with known and desirable properties, about some feature of a Random variable (its parameters, moments, domain, percentiles, etc.) from a finite, properly constructed sample of realizations (data).

estimator: An invariant formal procedure to be applied to a sample of data in order to obtain an estimate (q.v.) of some parameter or other characteristic of a distribution. There are many forms of ———s that differ in their simplicity, efficiency, asymptotic properties, and so on. (See Murphy 1982.) Each may yield its distinctive estimate. Note that an ——— is a prescription for manipulating data, so that if the data are Random, so is the ———.

Ethics (capitalized): The study of the relationship between facts and arguments, on the one hand, and the explicit courses of action to attain a specified end, on the other. **Billiard-ball** ———: ——— based on the assumption that the operations consist exclusively of indecomposable Acts applied to indecomposable Things and their consequences. **Confrontational** ———: ——— that consists of displaying all the Logical relationships among the facts and the possible courses of actions and their consequences, and leaves the decision up to the ethicist without further constraint. **Consistential** ———: A form of ——— in which the deductions from the axioms are in full agreement with the experience and wisdom of its consequences. ——— **of exceptions:** A provision (akin to equity in law) to redress anomalies in traditionalist and systematic ———. The supposition that they can be formulated argues that the systems they are overriding could be reformulated to include them. (See *phronesis* and *illation*.) **Major** ———: The fundamental conceptual structures of ———. **Minor** ———: The principles of applying Major ——— to concrete classes of problems of ——— (e.g., mutilation or consent). **Nihilistic** ———: The extreme view that neither the discipline nor the content of ——— serves any purpose in making decisions. **Situation** ———: The extreme view that the details of the particular case are of such overwhelming importance to the analysis that the other aspects (organized Ethical theory and traditional ———) may be ignored. See *casuistry*.

etiology: The science of identifying and studying the causal components of an outcome, especially a disease. Also the enumerating of the same. Contrast *pathogenesis*. Metaphorically, the ——— of a cake is the list of ingredients; the pathogenesis is the recipe for making the cake from them.

eugenics: A semitechnical word not in great favor in either Medicine or genetics because of the abuses that have been associated with it in the past. There are two quite distinct meanings depending on the two meanings in Classical Greek (namely, *nobly born* and *born well*). (1) The policy of manipulating human stock in which certain characteristics arbitrarily reckoned to be excellent will be promoted. (2) The search for the causes of birth defects that can be foreseen and anticipated.

evidence: The raw material of debate that is evident (i.e., that is a matter of naive experience and not the result of elaborate processing, manipulation, or inference). If there is a challenge that a datum is indeed evident, then it must be analyzed at the appropriate depth to meet that challenge. For instance, the statement that a person has been bitten by a gila monster may be challenged as not evident because the term *gila monster* is not a naive statement but a (more or less) zoological inference from certain features that should replace the statement. In turn, these features may themselves be challenged as not ———.

exhaustion: A method of demonstrating the truth of a proposition by establishing that it is individually true in every possible case. The method is tedious, but when all else fails it may be used with confidence. A recent example is the proof by computer of the so-called four-color problem (Appel and Haken 1977; Appel, Haken, and Koch 1977; Tymoczko 1979; Swart 1980), that all the closed, nonoverlapping regions in a plane may be individually painted by at most four colors such that no two regions sharing a common border are of the same color.

existents: Objective entities in the empirical world that science is concerned to discover and explore.

existentialism: A system of Philosophy that affirms that existence is ontologically anterior to essence, as opposed to the contrary essentialism of Plato and his theory of ideal forms. On this radical metaphysical proposition has been based a wilderness of special meanings, attitudes, and ethical practices that are difficult to grasp coherently. In practical terms the word *existential* has come to denote that which is rooted in past and current experience. From the standpoint of the epistemology of science, neither stance can usefully be treated as preferred: the growth and understanding of science depend on an unceasing interplay between coherent theory and inalienable respect for experiment and empirical observation.

exoteric: Readily available to the nonspecialized public.

expectation: The mean or average of a Random variable (q.v.) or of a function of it. Note that this term is not a statement of what (in the ordinary sense) is to be expected. The ——— for family size in a population may be 2.37, but we do not ever expect that there will be families with 2.37 children.

façon de parler (= way of speaking): An expression that is not intended to be taken literally and perhaps has no literal sense. It is used to convey some subtle perspective on what is being discussed. For example, "As winter approaches the sun sets earlier and farther to the south." The sun does not literally set, nor does it literally move south in winter.

false dichotomy: A choice between beliefs that are apparently incompatible but in fact are compatible.

falsifiability: An epistemic (especially a positivistic) principle of the authenticity of a statement: namely, that if the statement were false, it could be proved to be false.

fardel: A schematic representation of the burden (pain, disability, Medical care, financial cost, embarrassment, etc.) imposed by a disorder (usually genetic) as a function of time. The total cost is then the area under the graph of this abstract function. A ——— or its equivalent is at least implicitly involved in decision theory. (See Murphy and Chase 1975.)

fitness: A term of such ambiguity that it is best avoided altogether in the Medical context. Its principal meanings are as follows. (1) The state of well-being (**clinical** ———). (2) Mean effective fertility (**genetic** ———) (Murphy 1978b). (3) Probability of permanent descendance (**evolutionary** ———). (4) Worthiness of responsible office (**moral** ———). (5) State of physical conditioning (**athletic** ———). Great confusion results from mixing these various meanings.

Fisherian inference: An assumption-of-convenience that in Statistical analysis, whether estimation or testing of models, the only pertinent issues are the data under immediate consideration and some specific surmise or assumption. Prior convictions, published data, alternative hypotheses, and the like are ignored, at least for the present. (See Hacking 1965.)

Flew's principle (of permutation): If two premises lead to a valid conclusion that offends the illative sense (q.v.), we may reverse the argument and declare at least one of the premises false. (See Flew 1989.)

forensic Medicine: That branch of scholarship that addresses the overlap of Medicine with the (juridical) law. It comprises two major branches: the contribution that Medical knowledge and principles may make to a Legal investigation (especially Legal trials); and that branch of law that bears on the licit conduct of Medical practice both in civil and in criminal matters. —— is much the same as Medical jurisprudence. The latter, however, is mainly used to denote the overlap as viewed from the Legal standpoint.

fractal: A set of points for which the Hausdorff-Besicovitch dimension strictly exceeds the topological dimension (see Mandelbrot 1977: 15). The —— is encountered in dynamic processes, iterative geometrical constructions like the Koch snowflake and the Mandelbrot set. Many claim that diverse phenomena in the real world (e.g., the answer to the question "How long is the coast of Britain?"; the structure of the pulmonary tree) can only be dealt with as ——s. A characteristic feature of ——s is self-similarity (i.e., no matter how much the scale is enlarged, the general pattern remains the same).

freedom: The absence of constraint either physical, Logical, mathematical, or Moral.

full-thickness: A term used in skin grafting to denote a specimen that is not made from a superficial layer of epidermis and dermis only but also of subcutaneous tissues. It provides an irresistible metaphor to describe concerns that take all the details appropriate to an analysis into consideration and not merely a superficial and convenient abstraction.

Galton-Fisher theory: The principal model in classical quantitative genetics, which shows that additive, independent, stochastic contributions of components to a trait, all of about the same magnitude, will account for genetic traits that are measurable rather than categorical, and that the distribution of such a trait will be multivariate Gaussian. (See Fisher 1918.)

Gaussian distribution: A limiting pattern in the theory of linearly additive Random variables, the exclusive theory of classical quantitative genetics. —— does not accommodate such important physiological and ontogenic phenomena as homeostasis, Chaos, fractals, complexity, homeorrhesis, and general systems theory, which have been almost wholly neglected. Gauss, a major mathematician (who died in 1855), was not a party to the genetic theory.

gene: The hereditary code for the irreducible phenotypic component.

genetic linkage: The relationship of two loci such that the Probability that genes at each locus inherited from a particular parent will part company in meiosis is strictly less than 0.5. If it equals 0.5, the loci are said to be unlinked.

genome: The full complement of genetic material present in a typical person.

genotype: The genetic constitution of a typical person. ——— may be applied to a single locus or some larger aggregate. Contrast *phenotype*.

gold standard: Used metaphorically, in biology and Medicine, to denote a referent that is either tautologously or (most often) virtually the trait of interest, used to judge how far a simpler and more convenient test may lead to misclassification. Thus, if the caseating lesion and acid-fast mycobacteria are to be the ——— of pulmonary tuberculosis, we could judge the diagnostic specificity and sensitivity of pulmonary X-ray findings.

hardware: In computer terminology, the permanent electronic components of a computer. Contrast *software*.

hard-wired: By analogy with computers, used of a function or process that is not ordinarily optional. For instance, in a species as a whole the particular alleles present at a genetic locus are not ———, since several varieties may exist. But the alleles present in a particular member of the species are inexorably fixed at conception. The machinery for segregation of genes seems at present to be ——— over most of the animal kingdom.

hazard: The instantaneous risk that an entity undergoes a specific Random change to some other state (e.g., decay of an atom detected in a particle counter). For lethal events, the ——— is a statement about those members of the population who are still alive. The ——— for a myocardial infarction at age fifty usually supposes that the risks exist only in the living, so the denominator is the survival rate at that age. Thus, the instantaneous age-specific risk is an unbiased estimate of the ———. Contrast *Probability density*, for which the denominator is unity.

heuristic: Used in two senses. (1) Demonstrated informally rather than apodictically, as in "a ——— proof." (2) A line of thought, usually imaginative and speculative, that turns out to be rich and illuminating. Darwin's theory of natural selection is ——— in both senses.

high resolution (ontological and epistemic): Denotes that which by its nature or accessibility may be stated and studied in precise terms. See *resolution*.

homeostasis (adjective **homeostatic**): A physiological process, essentially cybernetic, in which important, quantitative, bodily variables (e.g., temperature, blood pressure, blood glucose) are continually monitored, and when they stray beyond acceptable limits (either spontaneously or by environmental perturbations), processes that redress the change are called into play.

homonymous: An optical term denoting those parts of the two retinae that are receiving light stimuli from the same source.

hull: An informal term to denote the confines of an object of high ontological density.

human genetics: That branch of genetics that deals with human beings as a species. Contrast *clinical genetics* and *Medical genetics*.

hypallage (= an exchange): A device, commonly deliberate in poetry, in which an adjective or its equivalent is attached to the wrong one of two or more nouns. It is a common minor unintentional mistake in science. For example, in Statistics the significance level ("the p value") is not an attribute of a parameter (such as the mean) but an attribute of the sample (conditional on some conjectured value of the parameter).

hypostasis (adjective **hypostatic**): Used in two radically different senses. (1) **Genetic** ———: The state of a genotype at one locus, the phenotypic effects of which are obscured or occulted by the effects of another locus. (2) **Philosophical** ———: The attribution of entity to something the existence of which is strictly a conjecture or an inference.

identity: Denotes in the strict sense (which we wish to preserve) the same individual (q.v.). Two individual Things are not identical simply because they are indistinguishable even on the most minute scrutiny. In this sense, *identical twins* used for *monozygous twins* is a misnomer. Properly we may not claim that a Thing and its properties, or two properties of the one Thing (like thunder and lightning), are identical.

illation (adjective **illative**): A high level of cognitive criticism that judges and may reject the conclusion of a Logical argument. For instance, the acceptance as valid of the principles of Logic cannot itself be a Logical conclusion and is ———. As a recent example, the objections to the proof of the four-color theorem (see *exhaustion*) are pentheric and illative. In the cognitive field ——— resembles phronesis (q.v.) in the Ethical and Moral fields.

immanent: Residing within, latent, inherent.

imminent: Impending, threatening.

imperative: The mood of a verb that urges to action, that exhorts, commands.

incommensurable: Used of quantitative properties of two or more entities that cannot be compared on any common scale (e.g., the color of a shirt and the price of potatoes).

incommensurate: Not commensurate (q.v.).

independent: Used in two main senses. (1) In informal language it usually means *disjoint* (q.v.). (2) In Probability theory (and often explicitly assumed in Statistics), two events A and B are (stochastically) ——— if and only if the Probability of the one occurring is the same whatever the outcome for the other. The Probability that a card picked from a regular deck is a seven is the same whatever its suit and, hence, whether or not the suit is known or even ignored. The outcome of the suit and denomination are thus ——— events.

indicative: That mood of a verb that simply asserts fact.

individual (= that which cannot be divided without loss of its identity): That unit of being that, because of some principle of unity, is distinguished from the rest of existence. Though on a coarser scale, it is thus precisely analogous to the Greek word *atomic*. The atom is not unsplittable in the physical sense, but when split, it loses its identity. Likewise, the human being can be divided up but beyond a certain stage can no longer be called a human being.

inform: As well as the usual meaning (to impart factual matter), ——— also means "to contribute to the terms in which a proposition is formulated." For example, the theory of genetic linkage is ———ed by Mendel's Laws of genetic segregation.

instinct: A spontaneous and nonreflective response or attitude, especially that characteristic of action taken at short notice, particularly in nonhuman animals.

integrity: Wholeness, and hence related to the cognate words *wholesome, hale, healthy.* The quality of not being corrupted even in parts. The term is often used as rhetorical applause for unimpeachable morality.

intent: Plan or purpose; intention. **Constructive** ———: The consensual interpretation of the aims of a particular Act. **Idiosyncratic** ———: A personal ——— not amenable to the ordinary canons of objective adjudication.

intention: Purpose; goal; the object of one's consideration or concentrated attention.

interaction: The process and consequences when two individual entities come into apposition. For example, a chemical ———; social ———. These processes are hypostatized, although details may be extremely elaborate. In Statistical theory, however, ——— is a purely formal statement about nonadditivity of the effects of two efficient causes; hence, it may be an artifact generated by the inadequacy of the model or the means of observation and remedied by reforming them (e.g., by transformation of the variables).

intentionality: A common (some suppose indispensable) phenomenon of awareness that demands an object upon which the awareness is fixed. The view that it is wholly indispensable implies that awareness cannot exist without an object (i.e., in the intransitive state).

intersection of sets: The set of events, outcomes, decisions, and so on that belong to each of the sets concerned. The king of hearts is the only card that belongs to both the hearts and the kings. It therefore is the intersection of hearts and kings. See *union of sets.*

Klein bottle: A hypothetical bottle which, like the Möbius strip (q.v.), has a single surface that cannot be orientated.

know-nothing: The assumption-of-convenience in any analysis that no evidence outside the current domain of discussion is pertinent. It may be viewed as a general epistemic stance analogous to Fisherian inference (q.v.) in Statistics.

lag time: In a homeostatic process (q.v.), the interval between the receipt of a signal by a sensor and the execution of the cybernetic response by the effector organ.

likelihood: A technical term in Statistical inference (Murphy 1982; Hacking 1965; Edwards 1992). A formula for the Probability of a particular outcome from an experiment involves a mathematical form; a set of parameters; and a particular outcome. Seen as a prediction from known parameters, the formula is a Probability statement about a particular, but uncertain, outcome or set of outcomes. Seen as a statement after the event from the known outcomes, it is a ——— statement about the unknown parameters.

Logic (capitalized): That branch of formal reasoning concerned with making valid inferences from given premises. Known also as Minor ———, deductive or Aristotelian ———.

Logical positivism: An epistemic theory that all statements that have meaning are either analytic (i.e., redundancies or definitions) or empirically verifiable.

longevity: Remarkably prolonged survival. The term obviously implies a contrast with most of the other members of a cohort. No such comparison is involved in the wholly neutral term *survivorship* (q.v.), for which ——— is commonly misused.

lumen: The continuous hollow interior of a vessel, open at both cut ends.

machine noise: Minute contaminants of data introduced by the operation of a computer, for the most part due to the fact that only a finite number of decimal places are preserved in storage and intermediate calculations, resulting in the rounding of numbers by methods that vary from one computer to another. It may be a major effect in special cases, for instance, in Chaos and in operations of matrices with determinants close to zero.

malapropism: Use of a word somewhat similar in sound to, but differing in meaning from, what is intended (e.g., "The patient's recovery was a *fortuitous* outcome," where the word intended is *fortunate*).

manipulation: A change due to intervention from outside the components and specifications of the system. Any demonstrable consequences not found in (nonmanipulated) controls cannot then be readily ascribed to spontaneous changes within the system itself.

mean: The average or expectation (qq.v.).

Medical genetics: That branch of genetics that deals with the explicit workings of mechanisms whereby variation in genotypes leads to varying phenotypes that have a bearing on health and disability. It bears to clinical genetics the relationship that pathology bears to clinical Medicine.

Medical jurisprudence: See *forensic Medicine.*

metanoia: A change of disposition or attitude. It is a recognition that not only was some particular course of action deplorable but that it resulted from an attitude or way of thinking that is itself faulty and needs to be amended. For example, a major goal of treating alcoholism and drug addiction is to effect a ———, not merely to rely on prohibitive barriers against the temptation to relapse.

metaphor: A familiar image or example that, because of its vividness or its insights, may be used as a token expression for what may otherwise be difficult to grasp. Such would be the use of the computer term *hard-wired* to denote a structure that is part of a system and not merely an optional adjunct to it. Unlike an analogy, a ——— supposes familiarity with both terms. *Genotype* and *phenotype* may be used as an analogy, but not as a ———, for the Philosophical terms *substance* and *accident*.

metathesis: A Spoonerism, or interchange of two sounds in a word (as lar*nyx* for lar*ynx* or phago*sotize* for phago*cytose*).

metonymy: A rhetorical device in which one item is substituted for another with which it is associated. The word *melancholy* ("the black bile") is commonly used metonymously for *depression* because of a (now discredited) theory of its cause.

mitigation: The perception that although a decision, Act, or the like is Morally deplorable or Ethically inadequate, nevertheless it is to be judged less opprobrious for some identified reason (e.g., it was a mistake made in good faith, or it was undertaken hastily because of extraordinary urgency). It is thus always a modification not of a judgment but of the moral, juridical, or social response to it. As such, it falls outside the scope of this book. But any attempt to redress an evaluation (of the Act in question) that is *in principle* unsound (e.g., because the evaluation is inadequate) is outrageous. The proper recourse in the latter case is to amend the criteria of evaluation.

Möbius strip: A planar strip twisted once about its main axis with the ends joined into a closed ring (see Figure 14.1). Any two points on the strip can be joined by a pencil line without either lifting the pencil or crossing the edge.

model: An abstraction of an actual or putative phenomenon in which details not deemed relevant to some line of inquiry are eliminated or ignored. What is retained may be mathematical, or pathological, or clinical, or other, and the ——— qualified accordingly (e.g., the linear ——— in Statistics or the genetic mouse ——— of diabetes mellitus).

Monte Carlo trials: A way of circumventing the fact that formal investigation of the properties of a Probabilistic or (especially) Statistical procedure may prove intractable. In ———, the investigator devises a method of generating many separate outcomes from artificial data in which the appropriate Random component has been incorporated, and then treats the outcomes as real data from which the counterparts of such properties as bias, variance, efficiency, and distribution function may be calculated by the usual methods.

mood: A grammatical term denoting the nature and purpose of a sentence, whether to communicate what is fact or thought to be fact (**indicative** ——); desire (**optative** ——); command (**imperative** ——); or contingency (**subjunctive** ——).

motive: The impelling force that converts a judgment of the intellect into an action of the will. Often, and deplorably, confused with reason (q.v.). A group of investigators may publish a fraudulent account of an experiment they have not done. Their —— for so doing is fame and glory. Their reason is that they think the fraud will go undetected.

multilocal: Used of a trait or phenotype that is influenced to a nontrivial degree by genes at many loci. Contrast *unilocal* (or Mendelian).

multiple-hit process: A process operating over time in which a sufficient accumulation of damage from Random insults leads to failure of a system. The traditional example from folklore is the nine lives of the domestic cat.

mutation: A change in the structure of genetic material that arises in the formation of either somatic cells or germinal cells. The —— may involve segments of widely variable size, from a nucleotide to an entire haploid set.

mutational debt: A concept pertaining to classical genetic population dynamics, according to which every harmful mutation will eventually lead to genetic death of the ensuing genetic line. The current body of unpurged harmful genes constitute the ——.

naturalist: A person who studies plants and animals by acute but uncomplicated observations with little appeal to sophisticated science or theoretical speculation.

Neyman-Pearson theory: A system of Probabilistic proof of a hypothesis that dismisses the contrary or null hypothesis as an implausible account for the evidence being considered. It is an expedient to deal with Bayesian Logic (q.v) when the prior Probabilities cannot be specified. Unlike Bayesian Logic, —— does not treat the competing hypotheses symmetrically but assigns to the investigator the onus of demolishing the null hypothesis, which, when the data are scarce, is a severe challenge.

noise: Those aspects of data that are supposed to contain no information about, and throw no light on, some preassigned topic. This judgment is usually contingent on what is decreed by some accepted theory about the topic, and is hence a prior, but arbitrary, judgment.

nominalism: The theory that all existent entities are incurably particular. As a result, the cardinality and the dimensionality (qq.v.) of nature are equal and identical. There is thus no useful reduction of empirical reality into general categories that may be mutually enlightening.

normal: A word with powerful and uncontrolled overtones of emotion and moral indignation that is so ambiguous and in most cases so ill defined as to serve no useful purpose. It is a fund of cautionary exercises in spurious Logic and Ethics. Any specific usage is best handled by some more focused term.

nosology: The formal study of distinguishing and classifying diseases.

null hypothesis: A surmise about what the outcome of a Random process should be, against which the observed outcome may be compared. Sometimes (e.g., in Mendelian genetics) the ——— is a model, which may be vindicated by the goodness-of-fit resulting. Sometimes (typically in epidemiological inquiry and in therapeutic trials) the ——— is seen as an assumption-of-convenience (q.v.) (that the treatment has no effect), and rejection is taken, by default, to be proof of a significant effect (etiological or therapeutic, as the case may be).

objectivity: The supposition that a certain class of empirical phenomena may be represented in such a way that there is a consensus about their existence and properties that owes nothing to the subjective viewpoint of any particular observer.

odds: An alternative and strictly equivalent way of representing the relative Probabilities of two events. In a single roll of a die, the Probability of getting a six is 1 in 6 and that of getting some other result is 5 in 6. The ——— are 1 to 5 of getting a six or of 5 to 1 against getting a six. Quoting ——— for three or more competing events becomes untidy.

ontogeny: The entire process whereby a fertilized ovum develops into a mature adult.

ontology: That branch of Philosophy that deals with being as being, the intrinsic nature and relationships of the primary elements of discourse.

ontological density: A term borrowed by analogy from *Probability density* (q.v.). Suppose that the limits of a Thing are defined by reference to one or more coherently measurable scales (e.g., distance, time, rigidity, compression). The Thing is then said to have high —————. For a diamond, there is a very abrupt transition from being outside it to being inside it. By contrast, in astronomy, Barnard's star is composed solely of gas. Observers approaching it would find that the compactness of the star changes very slowly with distance, and there is no point at which there is any convincing evidence that their journey had changed from being outside the star to being inside it, or from entering it to leaving it. We therefore say that the diamond has a very high ————— with respect to distance and Barnard's star has a very low one. In the same way, a flash of lightning and the twilight in midsummer just south of the Arctic circle have very high and very low ————— with respect to time.

optative: The mood of a verb that addresses matters to be desired.

Oracle of Delphi: A soothsayer of Classical antiquity who gave forecasts with content so ambiguous that they could be claimed successful whatever the outcome. In scientific inference, the term is applied metaphorically to a system of predictions that frustrates any criterion of falsifiability (q.v.). For example, a useful, but not compelling, test that a process of selection is Random might be that the numbers of men and women in the sample are nearly equal. But knowing that this criterion is to be used, the sampler might constrain the selection so that equal numbers of the two sexes are chosen but still without using Random sampling.

organ: A set of bodily cells specialized to carry out a coordinated function in an individual organism.

organization: The process whereby a set of components are induced to operate coherently so as to promote some purpose not severally available to the components.

pain: An ambiguous term denoting (1) a physiological process of communicating information about harmful stimuli that specific sense organs detect (sense of —————); (2) a disagreeable and distressing sensation associated with the same, the highest central representation being in the thalamus; (3) a metaphorical appropriation of the foregoing to denote any distressing experience such as grief or social or spiritual trial.

paradigm: A clear example of an archetypal pattern to be used as a structure in a scholarly analysis. The common grammatical example is the declension of a verb. In recent years ——— has been used in a bewildering variety of meanings, mostly obscure.

paraphrasis: The restatement of a proposition in terms that do not change the level of its complexity (e.g., translation into another language). **Epistemic** and **ontological** ——— or transversal: The strategy that the analysis of a complicated system may be facilitated by viewing the same structures and relationships from a different standpoint not evident in a purely formal statement.

parochial: Concerned with matters of purely local (as opposed to cosmic or global) importance.

parsing: The grammatical discipline of identifying the components of a sentence and the relationships among them. **Epistemic** and **ontological** ———: Top-down analysis. The strategy for exploring a complicated process by identifying its components and their relationships one to another; and so recursively until the whole has been coherently decomposed into its elements.

pathogenesis: The process whereby a disease is generated from its causal components. Contrast *etiology.*

pathogenetics: That branch of Medical genetics concerned with a whitebox (q.v.) account of how mutation is translated into the actual detail of genetic disease (e.g., how the mutation from hemoglobin A to hemoglobin S leads to impaired resistance to pneumococcal infections, stunted growth, recurrent sickle-cell crises, etc.).

patient: Used in two senses. (1) A person more or less directly receiving or requiring clinical attention or assistance. (2) In the domain of responsibility, the person who is the recipient of some experience at the hands of the Agent.

penetrance: A loose term, abhorred by exact geneticists, to denote that a genotype, suspected to be Mendelian, has a phenotypic impact in some proportion of members of a genetically homogeneous population, that is, for all dominants or hemizygotes, or in homozygous recessives. If this proportion is 100%, the trait is "fully penetrant"; otherwise it is "incompletely penetrant" or "nonpenetrant." (Except in those rare usages where a testable mechanism is proposed to account for non———, the attribution is meaningless. There are other explicit, well-known mechanisms, e.g., hypostasis, extreme Lyonization, the absence of an environmental challenge, etc., that may reduce the proportion of affected cases.)

pentheric: Exacting from a proposed solution to a problem some desideratum neither explicitly stated nor reasonably implicit in its formulation before the fact.

perseveration: Continuation of an Act, response, or the like beyond the point at which it serves any further useful purpose.

phenotype (adjective **phenotypic**): The total set of properties of a genotype. Amorphic or null genotypes lack any positive ———.

phronesis: An attitude that reserves the right to override the conclusion of a formally sound argument. To ensure that consistency is not undermined, the exercise of ——— must involve either a rejection of the validity of the argument or an argument that the formulation of the issue is inadequate (e.g., because its structure is oversimplified or, by application of Flew's principle that one or more of the premises or data must be false). In the Ethical sphere, ——— is analogous to illation (q.v.) in the inferential field.

pleiotropy: The expression of a single gene in multiple, disparate phenotypic manifestations. The mechanism may be by changes in a material (e.g., calcium ions) that take part in many reactions. (This is sometimes called a "pedigree of causes.") Sometimes the gene may have two or more identifiable regions that after translation have quite different spheres of action. (See Pyeritz 1989.)

point d'appui (= a fulcrum): A point of legitimate and unforced engagement between disparate fields. For example, phenotyping in the light of Mendel's Laws of inheritance have a ——— in lawsuits concerning disputed paternity.

positivism: The epistemic theory that knowledge is conterminous with formalized empirical studies of natural phenomena.

postulate: An assumption specified at the start of a coherent system of reasoning. Traditionally it is distinguished from an axiom (q.v.), which is an assumption about fact, whereas a ——— is an assumption about the admissibility of an operation or maneuver. For instance, in the empirical testing for causality, the assumption (right or wrong) that investigators have free will is an axiom, whereas the appeal to manipulation is a ———. The two terms are now used interchangeably. (A recent trend, which we deplore, is to use the word ——— to mean a surmise or conjecture after the data have been examined.)

power: The Probability in Statistics that the null hypothesis will be rejected when it is false. A perfect test would have a ——— of 100% at a significance level of 0%.

pragmatic: Practical. The word commonly carries pejorative overtones of substituting the Baconian principle for reflective thought. However, as with the word *empirical,* this attitude is supercilious prejudice. Since abstraction almost always involves dismissing as irrelevant some detail, unreflecting use of the result may lead to gross incongruities (as in Chaos). The ——— experience may act as a consistential safeguard.

precision: In a procedure for estimating an unknown quantity, a form of refinement in which multiple determinations give results that agree closely with each other (i.e., have a relatively small variance). Contrast *accuracy,* which is a quality of estimation that in a very large sample gives a mean close to the quantity being estimated (i.e., the bias is small).

prescind: In an argument involving multiple terms, to treat of a term or terms while expressly setting aside inquiry into the others. Thus, a historian might deal with the economic consequences of the slave trade while ———ing from moral issues of slavery.

preventive: Pertaining to that branch of Medicine that is concerned not with the cure or the resolution of disease but with the anticipation of its pathogenesis (q.v.). There is ambiguity wherever the critical change from possible or latent or subclinical states to authentic disease is inadequately defined. What some may regard as prevention of atherosclerosis might by others be regarded as the arrest of the early stages of disease. The ambiguity is most striking in so-called secondary prevention (e.g., the use of drugs, diets, physical exercise, restriction of smoking, etc. to prevent further damage in those who have already had manifest vascular disease).

principle: An appeal to a fundamental relationship (e.g., a universal Law) from which wide deductions may be made.

Probability (adjective **Probabilistic**) (capitalized): An open, measured, scale from 0 to 1 representing a judicious degree of assurance about some particular outcome of a Random experiment. Various pragmatic criteria have been put forward for discovering the appropriate ———, such as well-founded theories (as in Mendelian genetics); the limiting value of the empirical proportions in *n* replications of the process, as *n* goes to infinity; actuarial assessments; and so on. ——— may assume various ontological forms: objective, subjective, and personal.

Probability density: A refinement needed to adapt Probability to continuous variates. The Probability of a human being dying at an age of x years exact to an infinite number of decimal places, $f(x)$, is zero. Thus, $f(100) = 0$. Also $f(60) = 0$. But that does not mean that they are equally plausible claims. We make this statement exact by saying that for any positive small amount h, the Probability of dying between 60 and $(60 + h)$ years is much greater than the Probability of dying between 100 and $(100 + h)$ years. The ratio of the former Probability to h that is approached as h becomes smaller is the ——— $f(60)$.

proband: That person exhibiting a trait by whom the attention of an investigator (e.g., geneticist or epidemiologist) is called to the existence of the trait in others, especially relatives and colleagues. (Tautologously, the ——— is always affected.)

propositus (female **proposita**, plural forms **propositi** and **propositae**): Proband (q.v.).

provenience (adjective **provenient**): The study of the sources of empirical data, sampling, soundness of technical methods, and so on involved in the conversion of raw experience into sound empirical data. It may be regarded as that component of epidemiology that is under the auspices of some discipline (science, history, mathematics, etc.) other than Philosophy.

purview: The scope of authority or domain of inquiry in a discourse. The ——— of this book is neither Philosophy nor Ethics.

quiddity (= whatness): That which is seen as the nub, the gist, the point of the point of something. An informal version of *essence* (that in a Thing which makes it what it is).

Random (capitalized): Used of a system or process in which the outcome of any realization (q.v.) cannot, even in principle, be predicted with certainty but follows a Probability distribution. A necessary feature of ———ness in a variable is that, scaled, the ordered outcomes from realizations will come arbitrarily close to that for the distribution function as the sample size increases without limit.

Random variable: In Statistics, a variable to which no value may be arbitrarily assigned but that is assumed in a realization (q.v.) of a Random process with fixed Probability or Probability density.

realization: A term having (apart from lay usages) a technical meaning in science to denote that a conjectured process takes place. For instance, in tosses of a coin, the type of each toss is a ———. In the process the outcome changes from a Random variable to a datum.

reason: The cognitive process whereby one reaches a broad judgment on the merits of an evaluation or decision. It is not to be confused with motive (q.v.). ——— is broader than Logic, comprising elements of judgment (illation, phronesis, intuition, speculative arguments, and half-truths).

recessivity (adjective **recessive**): A genetic phenomenon in which the phenotype due to one gene is obscured or occulted by a different allele at the same locus. Contrast *hypostasis.*

recipient: Patient. In the context of responsibility, the person or Thing for which the Agent is responsible.

redundancy: A formulation in which there are more pieces of information available than are necessary to arrive at a unique solution.

reductionism: (1) Ontologically, an attitude to scientific inquiry that a full comprehension of a finite set of indecomposable fundamental principles provides a sufficient basis for understanding all the observable phenomena of the sensible universe. (2) Epistemically, ——— means that parsing will eventually lead to that sufficient set of principles. (3) Scientifically, ——— implies that the epistemic endeavor will run into no insuperable Logical problems such as Chaos or unbounded emergence.

refinement: A general term to denote the degree of exactitude with which a quantitative statement is made. It embraces accuracy, precision, and resolution (qq.v.). In general the overall ——— is given by whichever of these three quantities is least exact. Thus, an estimate, however precise, of the mortality in a disease where the data are collected from necropsies is so biased as to make precision of no importance. A measurement of height made on a scale calibrated in centimeters may be anywhere within 1 cm of the true value. Here it is the resolution that determines the ——— of the measurement.

reflex action: An involuntary response to a peripheral stimulus (e.g., tapping a tendon, a cutaneous stimulus, shining a bright light) transmitted through an afferent path to the spinal cord or the lower centers of the brain, exciting a local and nondeliberative response that issues through an efferent path leading to a response. The response may occur at a site not necessarily close to the stimulus.

reflexive: Used of that which relates to itself, especially by acting on itself. A grammatical term to describe a verb in a sentence in which the subject and the object are conterminous.

regression: Decline from a higher to a lesser state of fullness, maturity, or excellence. **Psychological** ———: An unconscious defense manifested as a return to an earlier pattern of solution for a problem, and perceived by a qualified observer or the consensus of a group of observers, as inappropriate although under stress it would be accepted as appropriate. **Statistical** ———: The systematic component of the relationship between a Random variable and some other variable. For example, height and weight are related in some imperfectly understood way. The line showing the estimated mean weights for all particular heights in the domain of height is the ——— of weight on height. The ——— may take a wide variety of mathematical forms.

reliability: Used of a process that attains a required end with a characteristic precision and Probability. High ——— is a quality of overwhelming Darwinian importance in ontogeny.

replicate: Used of a multiplicity of realizations (q.v.) of the same process. A generalization of the word *duplicate*. It may be applied to assays from aliquots of one specimen; or multiple Monte Carlo trials; or groups of animals given an identical diet or other treatment. A common intent of obtaining ———s is to study how much of the variation in a process is due to pure experimental error (as distinct from that due to unidentified covariables).

representative sampling: A method of inquiry into a whole population by taking a sample in which the Probability of any set being chosen is specified in advance. This skilled technique is not to be lightly invoked by the amateur. (The sample is not representative of any subgroup, e.g., women, if they have a Probability of zero of being included.)

resolution (or **resolving power**): The degree of refinement allowed by the nature of an entity (**ontological** ———) or the nature of the means available for studying it (**epistemic** ———). Thus, the ontological resolving power of the size of a sibship is ordinarily 1, since the number of children is an integer. A sibship with 2.37 members has no ordinary meaning. The epistemic ——— of studies by a light microscope is $0.2\,\mu m$, which is a function of the wavelength of visible light. ——— is not to be confused with Random error (see *Random*), which is encountered in stochastic systems only.

respect: Consideration and esteem (in various senses of both; see Chapter 13) shown by one person to another.

responsibility: A word with several interlocking meanings (see Chapter 14). It has three facets of major importance: accountability, available special skills, and quality of behavior.

richness: The extent and variety of the possible realizations (q.v.) of a multi-partite system.

rights: In the Ethical treatment and manipulation of persons, certain constraints deemed inherent in the essence of being human, and supported and guaranteed by society. The epistemology of such claims is often tenuous, and no ontology at all may exist. (See Appendix 3.)

robustness: A property, whether of a structure, of a model, or of formal inference by estimation or hypothesis-testing, in which the reliability of the conclusions is little affected by minor departures from the formal assumptions. Contrast *Chaos.*

rule of thumb: A concise, often grossly oversimplified, means of making practical decisions that are good approximations to what might be attained by deep reflection (e.g., "When in Rome do as the Romans do"). The ——— has use when many decisions have to be made rapidly, but it has no standing as a method of solving any problem in principle.

sample estimate: The result of applying an estimator (q.v.) of a parameter to a sample of data.

sample space: The set of all possible outcomes of an inquiry. Also termed "the universe" or "the population of reference."

scientific revolution: A term used by Kuhn (1970) to denote what he perceived as selected critical stages in science in which the strain of accumulated scientific discoveries demands that existing canons of thought be replaced. Examples are heliocentric cosmology, Newtonian mechanics, Mendelism, and relativity physics. Darwinism, although revolutionary, has been historical in tenor and is only now beginning to acquire the sharpness and refinement required of a scientific theory.

segregation: The process in the formation of a germinal cell by which, of the two alleles present at a locus in a parent, one or other is transmitted, but not both. ——— **ratio:** The proportion of phenotypes in the offspring of a specified type of mating.

selection: In population dynamics, the diachronic (q.v.) impact on the fate of a particular genotype of its absolute or relative fitness.

set: An abstract assembly of entities (points or elements) that have in common some quality or qualities, and for certain purposes of discourse may be treated as subjects of Logical generalizations.

sign: See *symptom.*

skepsis: That intellectual discipline driven by unbelief that seeks stringently to refine scientific statements of truth and to protect them from flawed Logic, inference, and provenience.

skepticism: An attitude of militant disbelief with no constructive intent that supposes the goal of science is to demolish a belief for the sake of demolishing it, regardless of merits.

slippery slope: A vivid metaphor for the concern that once any attenuation of an adamantine principle, however small, is allowed, the principle will be progressively eroded.

software: In a computer, optional and movable components (operating systems, programs, files, etc.) that may be interfaced with the hardware (the permanent parts of the computer).

solipsism: The extreme subjective view that one's perception and analysis of the universe and the formulation of behavior are so personal that input from others is useless, without weight, and even wholly figmented.

splanchnic: Visceral. In physiology the word denotes that the muscular and other functions involved are under the control of the autonomic nervous system and hormones, and not accessible to the influence of the somatic (voluntary) nervous system.

Statistics (adjective Statistical) (capitalized): A branch of scientific formalism concerned with the organization and analysis of data that are either measurable, ordered, or categorizable. The prevailing formal theory is Probabilistic, but other theories (e.g., the classification of atoms, Chaos, and fractals) may come within the purview of the field. The popular use of the term to mean any set of numerical data whatsoever is in this book denoted by the lower-case equivalent. (The form Statistic is a noun denoting a condensation of a set of data, e.g., the use of the sample mean as an estimate of the true mean.)

strategy: In the conduct of war, the art of preparing an army to conduct war and to contrive a venue that will put one's army at best advantage. Contrast *tactics,* which is the art of fighting the resulting battle. These two terms are used metaphorically in Medicine. A surgical operation would be tactical. The decision to operate, the preoperative care, and the choice of the right time to operate would be strategic.

stochastic (adjective **stochastically**): Aleatory, Random, Probabilistic. Typically used of dynamic processes.

suffering: A state of distress that suffuses the whole individual, often but not necessarily associated with pain (q.v.), that draws its being as much from the implications of the cause of distress as it does from the pure perception.

survivorship: The complement of the distribution function of a Random variable as a function of time. The proportion of a cohort that is still alive as a function of time.

syllepsis (or zeugma): A rhetorical figure in which a word is used of two adjacent terms in a sentence, one literal and the other metaphorical (e.g., "He devoured the contents of the book and a large pizza").

symmetry: A form generated by a fixed relationship of a geometrical feature with respect to a given axis or point of ———. In **lateral** ———, one half is the mirror image of the other. **Radial** ——— is exhibited by a bowl made on the potter's wheel. Metaphorically, ——— is often used of a mutual or reciprocal relationship. If A is the mirror image of B, then B is the mirror image of A, and there is no adequate preference between them. Where one state is preferred for at best trivial ontological reasons, conclusions that are asymmetrical must be suspect. For instance, the right-handed person has no obvious argument that left-handed persons are abnormal; and conversely. Confounding of effects of manipulations is symmetrical. It is correct to say, "The effects of A and B are confounded." The form "A is confounded by B," though widespread, is Logically incorrect.

symptom: A traditional distinction is made in Medicine between information resulting from examining the patient (a *sign*) and information offered by the patient (a *symptom*). The clinician may be unable to corroborate the symptom for various reasons: because it is subjective (as in tic douloureux); because it was transient and had disappeared before the clinician could corroborate it (e.g., a cardiac arrhythmia); because it is a hysterical conversion; because there is a defect in the patient's perception (e.g., color-blindness); because it is a fabrication; and so on. Uncorroborated symptoms may often be given little weight by the clinician; but there are somatic disorders in which there are no corroborating signs (e.g., migraine).

synchronic: See *diachronic.*

syncrisis: The process whereby the entire contents of two or more lines of thought are compared, reconciled, and compounded into a single coherent set. It has something of the same meaning as conflation or, in set theory, union of two sets.

syntaxis: The discipline of studying the effects of composing ("putting together") two or more components. In grammar, ———— corresponds to syntax. **Ontological** and **epistemic** ————: Bottom-up analysis, the strategy of exploring a complicated process by successively building from appropriate elements (atoms, amino acids, etc.) primitive components that are in turn composed into more elaborate components and so recursively until the completed object of inquiry has been synthesized.

system: An assemblage of distinct and distinguishable components that operate together with corporate effects not discernible from any subset of the components operating in isolation.

t statistic (also Gosset's or "student's" *t*): The distribution about some conjectured value of the true mean of a Random sample expressed as multiples of the method-of-moments estimate of the standard deviation based on the same sample. The ———— is a measure of the Probability of the sample mean contingent on some hypothesis about the true mean. Exact interpretation of the result is usually based on the assumption that the data follow a Gaussian distribution.

taboo: Social pressure to prohibit certain behaviors. Our use of the word here refers to what is outlawed from measured discussion of the nature and fundamentals of strong ethical sentiments (e.g., cannibalism, racism, genocide).

tactics: See *strategy.*

tautology: A defining statement such that the term and its definition are interchangeable. "A quadruped is an animal with four feet" is a definition. "All quadrupeds have four feet" is the ———— "All animals with four feet have four feet."

teleology: The study of ends and purpose. Darwinism expressly excludes ———— as a component of the development of species and hence of individuals in particular. **Darwinian** ————: An oxymoron used nevertheless as a concise *façon de parler* denoting that mutations tend to lead to enhanced survival because that ensures their capacity to survive.

Thing (capitalized): An element of existence, or an aggregate of such elements that because of some unifying principle (e.g., corporate purpose) is arbitrarily hypostasized. In general a term of convenience rather than a fundamental concept in its own right.

transversal: See *paraphrasis.*

triviality: A statement that is sound and true but is of no importance. An Ethical ——— is some proposition about behavior that has negligible content. The fact that the content may be negligible does not at all mean that it has no importance in principle (e.g., as a basis for analogy or as an educative device).

truth: That which is. The term is used with a wide variety of meanings. In this book, as in orthodox science, it is supposed that truth exists whether it is known or not, or even if it cannot be known. Denied this assumption, the entire scientific enterprise seems to be quite pointless.

uncanny: That which cannot be known or understood.

unilocal (or Mendelian): Used of a genetic trait that is determined by the genotype at a single locus and is little influenced by the rest of the genome. Contrast *multilocal.*

union of sets: All those particular points or examples (as the case may be) that belong to at least one of the sets concerned. A person will be admitted to the baseball game on producing a season ticket, *or* paying the entrance fee, *or* being a friend of the manager. But fulfilling two of these requisites or even all three will also suffice. Compare *intersection of sets.*

validity: The formal soundness of a Logical syllogism. It is neither a necessary nor a sufficient condition for the content of the conclusion to be true.

value-laden: Used of a system of Philosophical analysis in which value is an essential structure. Since quantitation is of the essence in almost all scientific thought and inquiry, the term ——— throws a heavy burden on the distinction (if indeed there is one) between value and quantity.

variable: Any quantity that is not a constant. A **mathematical** ——— is a quantity in a formula that may be assigned any of a set of values. The relationship between ambient temperature on the centigrade and Fahrenheit scales is given by a formula (which may be graphed) showing all possible values of both; the intercept (32 degrees Fahrenheit) and the slope (1.8 degrees Fahrenheit for every 1 degree centigrade) are not variables but constants. See *Random* ———.

variance: The mean of the square of the difference between a Random variable (q.v.) and the mean of its distribution. Commonly but incorrectly identified with *variation* in the Random variable. (Every nondegenerate Random variable may assume diverse values and must have a distribution, but its ——— may not be definable.)

veridical: Veracious, authentic, correctly stated. We apologize for this pompous word. The simple Anglo-Saxon word *true* (= tree, that which is rooted in reality) has been taken over by Philosophers of all shades of opinion and has become so festooned with arbitrary technical meanings and associations that in self-defense we have to use strange vocabulary.

verifiability: A quality of propositions that allows them to be corroborated by observation or testing.

verification: (1) The process whereby the truth of a statement has been consensually corroborated. (2) An epistemic criterion of the truth of some proposition.

voice: A term used in the grammar of verbs according as the subject of the sentence is the effector or the recipient of the activity implied in the main verb. Conventionally, there are three ———s: active ("The physician *presented* the patient to the students"); passive ("The patient *was presented* to the students"); and middle ("The patient *presented* with a sore throat"). In nicer usage, ——— is better seen as a continuous scale of active participation.

whole-thickness: See *full-thickness.*

white box: An image of the understanding of a structure or process that explicitly lays out the connection between input and output. All the intermediate steps are available for exhaustive study. Contrast *black box.*

References

Abrahamsen, A. F. 1968. Platelet survival studies in man with special reference to thrombophlebitis and atherosclerosis. *Scand. J. Haematol. Suppl.* 3:1-53.

Achinstein, P. 1977. Function statements. *Philosophy of Science.* 44:341-67.

Albert, D. A.; Munsen, R.; and Resnik, M. D. 1988. *Reasoning in Medicine: An Introduction to Clinical Inference.* Baltimore: Johns Hopkins University Press.

Allison, A. C. 1954. Protection afforded by sickle-cell trait against subtertian malarial infection. *Brit. Med. J.* 1:290-94.

Appel, K., and Haken, W. 1977. Every planar map is four-colorable. Part 1: Discharging. *Illinois J. Math.* 21:429-90.

Appel, K.; Haken, W.; and Koch, J. 1977. Every planar map is four-colorable. Part 2: Reducibility. *Illinois J. Math.* 21:491-567.

Autenrieth, G. 1876. *A Homeric Dictionary.* Translated by R. P. Keep. New edition 1958. Norman: University of Oklahoma Press.

Ayer, A. J. 1946. *Language, Truth, and Logic.* London: Gollantz.

Bartlett, J. 1962. *Familiar Quotations.* 13th ed. London: Macmillan.

Bateson, G. 1972. *Steps to an Ecology of Mind.* New York: Ballantine.

Baum, L. F. 1900. *The Wizard of Oz.* Reprinted 1983. Edited by M. P. Hearn. New York: Shocken.

Bayes, T. 1763. An essay towards solving a problem in the doctrine of chances. *Phil. Trans. Roy. Soc.* 53:370-418. Reprinted 1958 in *Biometrica* 45:296-315.

Beauchamp, T. L., and Childress, J. F. 1989. *Principles of Biomedical Ethics.* 3d ed. New York: Oxford University Press.

Beebe, G. W. 1981. The atomic bomb survivors and the problem of low-dose radiation effects. *Amer. J. Epidemiol.* 114:761-83.

Belcher, E. H.; Berlin, N. I.; Eernisse, J. G.; Garby, L.; Glass, H. I.; Heimpel, H.; Lee, M.; Lewis, S. M.; McIntyre, P. A.; Mollison, P. L.; Murphy, E. A.; Najean, Y.; Pettit, J. E.; and Szur, L. 1977. Recommended methods for radioisotope platelet survival studies: A report by the Panel on Diagnostic Application of Radioisotopes in Haematology of the International Committee for Standardization in Haematology. *Blood* 50:1137-44.

Bell, E. T. 1937. *Men of Mathematics.* New York: Dover.

Bentley, E. C. 1912. *Trent's Last Case.* Reprinted 1952. Harmondsworth, Middlesex: Penguin.

Bernard, C. 1872. *De la physiologie générale.* Paris: Hachette.

Bernstein, F. 1930. Fortgesetzte Untersuchungen aus der Theorie der Blutgruppen. *Z. indukt. Abstamm. und Vererbungslehre* 56:233-73.

Blackwell, D., and Girshick, M. A. 1954. *Theory of Games and Statistical Decisions.* New York: Wiley.

Bohm, D. 1957. *Causality and Chance in Modern Physics.* Philadelphia: University of Pennsylvania Press.

Bonica, J. J. 1990. *The Management of Pain.* 2d ed. Vol. 1, pp. 85–86. Malvern, Pa.: Lea and Febiger.

Boorse, C. 1973. On the distinction between disease and illness. *Philosophy and Public Affairs* 5:49–69.

———. 1977. Health as a theoretical concept. *Philosophy of Science* 44:542–73.

Borgaonkar, D. S., and Shah, S. A. 1974. The XYY chromosome: Male or syndrome? *Progress in Medical Genetics* 10:135–222.

Breitner, J. C. S.; Gau, B. A.; Welsh, K. A.; Plassman, B. L.; McDonald, W. M.; Helms, M. J.; and Anthony, J. C. 1994. Inverse association of anti-inflammatory treatments and Alzheimer's disease: Initial results of a co-twin control study. *Neurology* 44:227–32.

Brock, R. C. 1948. Pulmonary valvulotomy [*sic*] for the relief of congenital pulmonary stenosis. *Brit. Med. J.* 1:1121–26.

Bronowski, J. 1951. *The Common Sense of Science.* London: Spottiswoode, Ballantyne.

Buchan, J. 1935. *The House of Four Winds.* Reprinted 1993. Stroud: Alan Sutton, Pocket Classics.

Buerger, L. 1908. Thromboangiitis obliterans: A study of the vascular lesions leading to presenile spontaneous gangrene. *Amer. J. Med. Sci.* 136:567–80.

Bugra, D. 1992. Psychiatry in ancient Indian texts: A review. *Hist. Psychiatr.* 3:167–86.

Bury, R. G., trans. 1929. *Timaeus.* In *Plato with an English Translation.* Vol. 7, pp. 101 ff. New York: Heinemann.

Bussey, H. J. R. 1975. *Familial Polyposis Coli: Family Studies, Histopathology, Differential Diagnosis, and the Results of Treatment.* Baltimore: Johns Hopkins University Press.

Butzow, J. J., and Eichhorn, G. L. 1968. Physical chemical studies on the age changes in rat tail tendon collagen. *Biochim. Biophys. Acta* 154:208–19.

Butzow, J. J.; Eichhorn, G. L.; and Shin, Y. A. 1990. Interaction of DNA and RNA with metal ions. In *Landolt-Börnstein, New Series, Group VII: Biophysics,* edited by W. Saenger. Vol. 1c, pt. 4.4., pp. 277–445. Berlin: Springer.

Butzow, J. J.; Lee, L. V.; Garland, C.; and Eichhorn, G. L. 1997. Specificity of an *Escherichia coli* RNA polymerase-associated NTPase. In preparation.

Butzow, J. J., and Stankis, R. G. 1992. Identification of a component separated on Mono Q purification of *Escherichia coli* RNA polymerase as an NTPase. *FEBS Lett.* 330:71–72.

Campbell, M. 1963. Death rate from diseases of the heart, 1876–1959. *Brit. Med. J.* 2:528–35.

Campbell, R. J. 1989. *Psychiatric Dictionary.* 6th ed. New York: Oxford University Press.

Cannon, W. B. 1932. *The Wisdom of the Body.* New York: Norton.

Cantore, E. 1977. *Scientific Man: The Humanistic Significance of Science.* New York: ISH Publications.

Capron, A. M. 1972. Genetic therapy, a lawyer's response: The law of genetic therapy. In *The New Genetics and the Future of Man*, edited by M. P. Hamilton. Grand Rapids, Mich.: Eerdmans.

Carnap, R. 1966. *Philosophical Foundations of Physics*. New York: Basic Books. Reprinted 1995 as *An Introduction to the Philosophy of Science*. New York: Dover.

Carroll, L. [C. L. Dodgson.] 1872. *Through the Looking Glass*. Reprinted 1991. New York: Random House.

Caspari, R.; Friedl, W.; Mandl, M.; Möslein, G.; Kadmon, M.; Knapp, M.; Jacobasch, K.-H.; Ecker, K.-W.; Kreißler-Haag, D.; Timmermans, G.; and Propping, P. 1994. Familial adenomatous polyposis: Mutation at codon 1309 and early onset of colon cancer. *Lancet* 343:629–32.

Cassell, E. J. 1982. The nature of suffering and the goal of medicine. *New Eng. J. Med.* 306:639–45.

———. 1991. *The Nature of Suffering*. New York: Oxford University Press.

Cerasi, E.; Efendic, S.; and Luft, R. 1973. Dose-response relation between plasma insulin and blood glucose levels during oral glucose loads in prediabetic and diabetic subjects. *Lancet* 1:794–97.

Chargaff, E. 1951. Structure and function of nucleic acids as cell constituents. *Fed. Proc.* 10:654–59 (and references cited therein).

———. 1952. On the desoxypentose nucleic acids from several microorganisms. *Biochim. Biophys. Acta* 9:402–5.

Chesterton, G. K. 1906. O lord of earth and altar. In *The English Hymnal*. Oxford: Oxford University Press.

Chodak, G. W.; Thisted, R. A.; Gerber, G. S.; Johansson, J.-E.; Jones, G. W.; Chisholm, G. D.; Moskovitz, B.; Livine, P. M.; and Warner, J. 1994. Results of conservative management of clinically localized prostatic cancer. *New Eng. J. Med.* 330:242–48.

Churchland, P. M. 1984. *Matter and Consciousness: A Contemporary Introduction to the Philosophy of Mind*. Cambridge, Mass.: MIT Press.

Clark, E. B. 1984. Functional aspects of cardiac development. In *Growth of the Heart in Health and Disease*, edited by R. Zak. Pp. 81–103. New York: Raven.

Cohen, J., and Stewart, I. 1994. *The Collapse of Chaos*. New York: Viking, Penguin.

Cohen, M.; Nagel, T.; and Scanlon, T., eds. 1981. *Medicine and Moral Philosophy*. Princeton: Princeton University Press.

Cohen, M. L. 1991. Chronic pain and clinical knowledge: An introduction. *Theor. Med.* 12:189–92.

Collman, R. D., and Stoller, A. 1962. A survey of mongoloid births in Victoria, Australia, 1942–1957. *Amer. J. Public Health* 52:813–29.

Copleston, F. 1948a. *A History of Philosophy*. Vol. 1, pt. 1. New York: Doubleday, Image.

———. 1948b. *A History of Philosophy*. Vol. 4. New York: Doubleday, Image.

———. 1967. *A History of Philosophy*. Vol. 8, pt. 2. New York: Doubleday, Image.

Costa, P. T., and McCrae, R. R. 1992. Four ways, five factors are basic. *Pers. Individ. Diff.* 13:653–65.

Dante Alighieri. 1300. *La Divina Commedia. Inferno* translated 1939 by J. D. Sinclair as *Dante's Inferno with Translation and Comment*. New York: Oxford University Press.

DeGroot, M. H. 1970. *Optimal Statistical Decisions*. New York: McGraw-Hill.

Descartes, R. 1637. *Discourse on Method*. Translated 1968 by F. E. Sutcliffe. Harmondsworth, Middlesex: Penguin.

Devaney, R. L. 1989. *An Introduction to Chaotic Dynamical Systems*. 2d ed. New York: Addison-Wesley.

Devereux, R. B., and Horan, M. J. 1992. Proceedings of the sixth US-USSR symposium on arterial hypertension: Introduction and overview. *Amer. J. Hypertension* 5, pt. 2:107S-109S.

Dickens, C. 1837. *Pickwick Papers*. Reprinted 1996. London: Westminster.

———. 1839. *Sketches by Boz*. Reprinted 1957. London: Oxford University Press.

———. 1844. *The Life and Adventures of Martin Chuzzlewit*. Reprinted 1975. London: Oxford University Press.

———. 1860. *Great Expectations*. Reprinted 1994. Stamford, Conn.: Longmeadow.

Dilman, V. M. 1981. *The Law of Deviation of Homeostasis and Diseases of Aging*. London: John Wright.

Dobzhansky, T.; Ayala, F. J.; Stebbens, G. H.; and Valentine, J. W. 1977. *Evolution*. San Francisco: Freeman.

Dornhorst, A. C. 1951. The interpretation of red cell survival curves. *Blood* 6: 1284-92.

Doyle, A. C. 1890. *The Sign of Four*. Reprinted 1974. Garden City, N.Y.: Doubleday.

Durham *v* United States, 214 F.2d 862-876 (D.C. Cir. 1954).

Eddington, A. S. 1928. *The Nature of the Physical World*. London: Cambridge University Press.

Edelman, G. M. 1988. *Topobiology*. New York: Basic Books.

———. 1992. *Bright Air, Brilliant Fire*. New York: HarperCollins.

Edwards, A. E. W. 1992. *Likelihood*. Revised and expanded. Baltimore: Johns Hopkins University Press.

Eichhorn, G. L.; Chuknyisky, P. P.; Butzow, J. J.; Beal, R. B.; Garland, C.; Jansen, C. P.; Clark, C.; and Tarien, E. 1994. A structural model for fidelity in transcription. *Proc. Natl. Acad. Sci. U.S.* 91:7613-17.

Ellenberger H. F. 1970. *The Discovery of the Unconscious: The History and Evolution of Dynamic Psychiatry*. New York: Basic Books.

Elstein, A. S.; Shulman, L. S.; and Sprafka, S. A. 1978. *Medical Problem Solving*. Cambridge, Mass.: Harvard University Press.

Emerson, R. W. 1841. Self reliance. Reprinted 1987 in *Essays of Ralph Waldo Emerson*, edited by A. R. Ferguson and J. F. Carr. Cambridge, Mass.: Harvard University Press.

Emery, A. E. H. 1976. *Methodology in Medical Genetics: An Introduction to Statistical Methods*. Edinburgh: Livingstone.

The Encyclopedia of Philosophy. 1967. New York: Macmillan.

Engelhardt, H. T., and Callahan, D., eds. 1976. *Science, Ethics, and Medicine*. Hastings-on-Hudson: Institute of Society, Ethics, and the Life Sciences.

Feinstein, A. R. 1967. *Clinical Judgment*. Baltimore: Williams and Wilkins.

Feynman, R. P., with R. Leighton and E. Hutchings. 1989. *Surely You're Joking, Mr. Feynman!* New York: Bantam.

Fisher, R. A. 1918. The correlation between relatives on the supposition of Mendelian inheritance. *Trans. Royal Soc. Edinburgh* 52:399-433.

―――. 1958. *The Genetic Theory of Natural Selection.* Rev. ed. New York: Dover.

Fleck, L. 1935. *Entstehung und Entwicklung einer wissenschaftlichen Tatsache: Einführung in die Lehre vom Denkstil und Denkkollektiv.* Basel: Benno Schwabe. Translated 1979 by F. Bradley and J. Trenn as *Genesis and Development of Scientific Fact.* Chicago: University of Chicago Press.

Fleming, C.; Wasson, J. H.; Albertson, P. C.; Barry, M. J.; and Wennberg, J. E. 1993. A decision analysis of alternate treatment strategies for clinically localized prostate cancer. *J. Amer. Med. Assn.* 269:2650–58.

Flew, A. 1989. *An Introduction to Western Philosophy: Ideas and Argument from Plato to Popper.* Rev. ed. New York: Thames and Hudson.

Fordyce, W. E. 1988. Pain and suffering: A reappraisal. *Amer. Psychologist* 43:276–83.

Fries, J. F. 1980. Aging, natural death, and the compression of morbidity. *New. Eng. J. Med.* 303:130–35.

Gavrilov, L. A., and Gavrilova, N. S. 1986. *Biologiia prodolzhitelnosti zhizni: Kalichestvenniye aspekty.* Moscow: Nauka. Translated 1991 by J. and L. Payne as *Biology of Life Span: A Quantitative Approach.* Chur, Switzerland: Harwood Academic Publishers.

Genouvrier, E.; Desirat, C.; and Horde, T. 1977. *Nouveau dictionnaire des synonymes.* Paris: Larousse.

Giardiello, F. M.; Krush, A. J.; Petersen, G. M.; Booker, S. V.; Kerr, M.; Tong, L. L.; and Hamilton, S. R. 1994. Phenotypic variability of familial adenomatous polyposis in 11 unrelated families with identical APC gene mutation. *Gastroenterology* 106:1542–47.

Gleick, J. 1987. *Chaos.* New York: Penguin.

Glesby, M. J., and Pyeritz, R. E. 1989. Association of mitral valve prolapse and systemic abnormalities of connective tissue: A phenotypic continuum. *J. Amer. Med. Assn.* 262:523–28.

Gödel, K. 1931. Über untendscheinbare Sätze der Principia Mathematica und System I. *Monatsh. für Math. und Physik* 38:173–98.

Gray, T. 1750. Elegy written in a country churchyard. Reprinted 1968 in *The Poem: An Anthology,* edited by S. B. Greenfield and A. K. Weatherhead. Pp. 143 ff. New York: Appleton-Century-Crofts.

Grüneberg, H. 1963. *The Pathology of Development: A Study of Inherited Skeletal Disorders in Mice.* Oxford: Blackwell.

Hacking, I. 1965. *Logic of Statistical Inference.* London: Cambridge University Press.

Hadamard, J. 1954. *The Psychology of Invention in the Mathematical Field.* Princeton: Princeton University Press.

Hamerton, J. L. 1976. Human population cytogenetics: Dilemmas and problems. *Amer. J. Human Genet.* 28:107–22.

Harbage, A., ed. 1969. *Macbeth.* In *William Shakespeare: The Complete Works.* Rev. ed. Pp. 1107–35. Baltimore: Penguin.

Hardy, G. H. 1967. *A Mathematician's Apology.* Cambridge: Cambridge University Press.

Hart, B. H. L. 1936. *The World War in Outline, 1914–1918.* New York: Faber and Faber.

Heidegger, M. 1967. *Die Frage nach dem Ding.* Tübingen: Max Niemeyer. Translated 1967 by W. B. Barton and V. Deutch as *What Is a Thing?* South Bend, Ind.: Gateway.

Heinlein, R. A. 1970. *I Shall Fear No Evil.* New York: Putnam.

Herrnstein, R. J., and Murray, C. 1994. *The Bell Curve: Intelligence and Class Structure in American Life.* New York: Free Press.

Hill-Zobel, R. L.; Pyeritz, R. E.; Scheffel, U.; Malpica, O.; Engin, S.; Camargo, E. E.; Abbott, M. H.; Guilarte, T. R.; Hill, J.; McIntyre, P. A.; Murphy, E. A.; and Tsan, M. F. 1982. Kinetics and biodistribution of ^{111}In-labeled platelets in homocystinuria. *New Eng. J. Med.* 307:781–86.

Hirsch, M. W., and Smale, S. 1974. *Differential Equations, Dynamical Systems, and Linear Algebra.* New York: Academic Press.

Holmes, O. W., Jr. 1881. *The Common Law.* 48th printing 1923. Boston: Little, Brown.

Hook, E. B. 1975. Geneticophobia and the implications of screening for the XYY genotype in newborn infants. In *Genetics and the Law,* edited by A. Milunsky and G. J. Annas. New York: Plenum.

Hovis, R. C., and Kragh, H. 1993. P. A. M. Dirac and the beauty of physics. *Scientific American* 268(5):104–9.

Hume, D. 1739. *A Treatise of Human Nature.* Book 1, *Of the Understanding.* Reprinted 1898 in *The Philosophical Works of David Hume,* vol. 1, edited by T. H. Green and T. H. Grose. Pt. 3, *Of Knowledge and Probability;* pt. 4, *Of Sceptical and Other Systems of Philosophy.* Darmstadt: Scientia Verlag Aalen.

Iansik, R. 1986. The effect of reflex path length on clonus frequency in spastic muscles. *J. Neurol. Neurosurg. Psychiatry* 48:1122–24.

Ingle, D. J. 1976. *Is It Really So? A Guide to Clear Thinking.* Philadelphia: Westminster.

Jonsen, A. R.; Siegler, M.; and Winslade, W. J. 1986. *Clinical Ethics: A Practical Approach to Ethical Decisions in Clinical Medicine.* 2d ed. New York: Macmillan.

Jung, C. G. 1921. *Psychologische Typen.* Zurich: Rascher Verlag. Translated by H. G. Baynes as *Psychological Types.* Revised 1971 by R. F. C. Hull. Princeton: Princeton University Press.

Kagan, H. M., and Trackman, P. C. 1991. Properties and function of lysyl oxidase. *J. Amer. Resp. Cell. Mol. Biol.* 5:206–10.

Keane, P. S. 1984. *Christian Ethics and Imagination.* Mahwah, N.J.: Paulist Press.

Keats, J. 1819. Ode on a Grecian urn. Reprinted 1968 in *The Poem: An Anthology,* edited by S. B. Greenfield and A. K. Weatherhead. Pp. 143 ff. New York: Appleton-Century-Crofts.

Kellermann, G.; Shaw, C. R.; and Luyter-Kellermann, M. 1973. Aryl hydrocarbon hydroxylase inducibility and bronchogenic carcinoma. *New Eng. J. Med.* 289:934–37.

Kelly, D. D. 1981. Somatic sensory system IV: Central representations of pain and analgesia. Chap. 18 in *Principles of Neural Science,* edited by E. R. Kandel and J. H. Schwartz. New York: Elsevier/North-Holland.

Kelly, T. E. 1986. *Clinical Genetics and Genetic Counseling.* 2d ed. Chicago: Year Book.

Khouri, R. E.; McKinney, C. E.; Slomiany, D. J.; Snodgrass, D. R.; Wray, N. P.; and McLemore, T. L. 1982. Positive correlation between high aryl hydrocarbon hydroxylase activity and primary lung cancer as analyzed in cryopreserved lymphocytes. *Cancer Res.* 42:5030–37.

Kipling, R. 1892. The winners. In *Barrack Room Ballads.* New York: Macmillan.

Koestler, A. 1960. *The Watershed.* New York: Doubleday.

Koizumi, K., and Brooks, C. M. 1980. The autonomic system and its role in controlling body functions. Chap. 33 in *Medical Physiology,* edited by V. B. Mountcastle. St. Louis: Mosby.

Kuhn, T. S. 1970. *The Structure of Scientific Revolutions.* 2d ed. Chicago: University of Chicago Press.

Kurnit, D. M.; Aldridge, J. F.; Matsuoka, R.; and Matthysse, S. 1985. Increased adhesiveness of trisomy 21 cells and atrioventricular canal malformations in Down syndrome: A stochastic model. *Amer. J. Med. Genet.* 20:385–99.

Kyburg, H. E., and Smokler, H. E. 1964. *Studies in Subjective Probability.* New York: Krieger.

Landsteiner, K. 1901. Über Agglutinationserscheinungen normalen menschlichen Blutes. *Wien. Klin. Wschr.* 14:1132–34.

Lewis, C. S. 1946. *That Hideous Strength.* Reprinted 1990. New York: Macmillan.

———. 1947. *The Abolition of Man.* New York: Macmillan.

———. 1955. *Surprised by Joy.* New York: Harcourt, Brace, and World.

Lewis, T. 1946. *Diseases of the Heart Described for Practitioners and Students.* 4th ed. London: Macmillan.

Lewitus, Z., and Neumann, J. 1957. On the distribution of coronary thrombosis attacks. *Amer. Heart J.* 53:339–42.

Li, C. C. 1970. The incomplete binomial distribution. In *Mathematical Topics in Population Genetics,* edited by K. Kojima. Pp. 337–66. New York: Springer-Verlag.

Libby, R. T.; Nelson, J. L.; Calvo, J. M.; and Gallant, G. A. 1989. Transcriptional proofreading in *Escherichia coli. EMBO J.* 8:3153–59.

Liddell, H. G. 1889. *An Intermediate Greek-English Lexicon.* Oxford: Clarendon.

Lindeman, F. J., and Mcintyre, D. M., eds. 1961. *The Mentally Disabled and the Law.* Chicago: University of Chicago Press.

Livingstone, I. R., and Sequeiros, J. 1984. Machado-Joseph disease in an American-Italian family. *J. Neurogenet.* 1:185–88.

Loewy, E. H. 1989. *Textbook of Medical Ethics.* New York: Plenum.

Lonergan, B. J. F. 1957. *Insight: A Study of Human Understanding.* New York: Longmans.

Lorenz, E. N. 1963. Deterministic, non-periodic flow. *J. Atmos. Sciences* 20:130–41.

Lu-Yao, G. L.; McLerran, D.; Wasson, J.; and Wennberg, J. E. 1994. An assessment of radical prostatectomy. *J. Amer. Med. Assn.* 269:2633–36.

McCluskey, I., and Horizonte, B. 1994. Thalidomide's return. *Time,* June 13, p. 67.

McCormick, R. A. 1977. *Ambiguity in Moral Choice.* Milwaukee: Marquette University Press.

McCullough, D. 1992. *Truman.* New York: Simon and Schuster, Touchstone.

Macdonald, G. 1895. *Lilith.* Reprinted 1969. New York: Ballantine.

Macdonald, N. 1978. *Time Lags in Biological Models.* New York: Springer.

McDougall, W. 1924. *Outline of Psychology.* New York: Scribner.

McHugh, P. R., and Slavney, P. R. 1983. *The Perspectives of Psychiatry.* Baltimore: Johns Hopkins University Press.

McKusick, V. A. 1975. *Mendelian Inheritance in Man.* 4th ed. Baltimore: Johns Hopkins University Press.

———. 1994. *Mendelian Inheritance in Man.* 10th ed. Baltimore: Johns Hopkins University Press.

McKusick, V. A.; Egeland, J. A.; Eldridge, R.; and Krusen, D. E.; 1964. Dwarfism among the Amish 1: The Ellis–van Crevald syndrome. *Bull. Johns Hop. Hosp.* 115:306–36.

McKusick, V. A., and Harris, W. S. 1961. The Buerger syndrome in the Orient. *Bull. Johns Hop. Hosp.* 109:241–91.

Magnusson, M., and Pálsson, H. 1960. *Njal's Saga.* Baltimore: Penguin.

Makeham, W. M. 1860. On the law of mortality and the construction of annuity tables. *J. Inst. Actuaries* 8.

Manasek, F. J.; Kulikowski, R. R.; Nakamura, A.; Nguyenphuc, Q.; and Lactis, J. W. 1984. Early heart development: A new model of cardiac morphogenesis. In *Growth of the Heart in Health and Disease,* edited by R. Zak. Pp. 105–30. New York: Raven.

Mandelbrot, B. B. 1977. *The Fractal Geometry of Nature.* Updated and augmented. New York: Freeman.

Maugham, W. S. 1938. *The Summing Up.* New York: Doubleday.

Merton, T. 1948. *The Seven-Story Mountain.* New York: Harcourt, Brace.

Meyerowitz, E. M. 1994. The genetics of flower development. *Scientific American* 271(11):56–65.

Miller, A. I. 1987. *Imagery in Scientific Thought.* Cambridge, Mass.: MIT Press.

Millikan, R. G. 1989. In defence of proper functions. *Philosophy of Science* 56:288–302.

Mills, J. N. 1946. The life-span of the erythrocyte. *J. Physiol.* 105:16–17.

Moore, B. E., and Fine, B. D., eds. 1990. *Psychoanalytic Terms and Concepts.* New Haven: American Psychoanalytic Association and Yale University Press.

Moore, G. E. 1903. *Principia Ethica.* New York: Macmillan.

Moore, P. S., and Broome, C. V. 1994. Cerebrospinal meningitis epidemic. *Scientific American* 271(5):38–45.

Morales, A. J.; Murphy, E. A.; and Krush, A. J. 1984. The bingo model of survivorship II: Statistical aspects of the bingo model of multiplicity 1 with application to hereditary polyposis of the colon. *Amer. J. Med. Genet.* 17:783–801.

Mountcastle, V. B. 1980. Pain and temperature sensibilities. In *Medical Physiology,* edited by V. B. Mountcastle. St. Louis: Mosby.

Murphy, E. A. 1966. A scientific viewpoint on normalcy. *Perspec. Biol. Med.* 9:33.

———. 1972. The normal and the perils of the sylleptic argument. *Perspec. Biol. Med.* 15:566–82.

———. 1978a. Eugenics: An ethical analysis. *Mayo Clin. Proc.* 53:655–64.

———. 1978b. Genetic and evolutionary fitness. *Amer. J. Med. Genet.* 2:51–79.

———. 1979a. Genetic intervention: Strategy and tactics. In *Service and Education in Medical Genetics,* edited by I. H. Porter and E. B. Hook. Pp. 3–9. New York: Academic Press.

———. 1979b. *Probability in Medicine.* Baltimore: Johns Hopkins University Press.

———. 1979c. Where are we going? In *Genetic Analysis of Common Disease: Ap-*

plications to Predictive Factors in Coronary Disease, edited by M. Skolnik and C. Sing. Pp. 2–23. New York: Alan Liss.

———. 1981a. Detection of genetic effects of environmental agents. *Envir. Health Perspec.* 42:127–36.

———. 1981b. Exhaustive partition and incomplete penetrance: Two precarious tautologies. *Amer. J. Med. Genet.* 8:275–79.

———. 1981c. *Skepsis, Dogma, and Belief: Uses and Abuses in Medicine.* Baltimore: Johns Hopkins University Press.

———. 1982. *Biostatistics in Medicine.* Baltimore: Johns Hopkins University Press.

———. 1985. *Companion to Medical Statistics.* Baltimore: Johns Hopkins University Press.

———. 1987. A geneticist's approach to psychiatric disease. *Psychological Medicine* 17:805–15.

———. 1988. The diagnostic process, the diagnosis, and homeostasis. *Theor. Med.* 9:151–66.

———. 1990. Dynamics of quantitative homeostasis VIII: Processes that oscillate finitely many times. *Amer. J. Med. Genet.* 35:552–60.

———. 1992. Critique of diagnostic formalism. In *The Ethics of Diagnosis*, edited by J. L. Peset and D. Gracia. Pp. 255–67. Dordrecht: Kluwer.

———. 1997. *The Logic of Medicine.* 2d ed. (1st ed. 1976.) Baltimore: Johns Hopkins University Press.

———. n.d.-a. Angular homeostasis XI. Unpublished studies.

———. n.d.-b. Covariance. Unpublished studies.

———. n.d.-c. Genetic selection against a linear homeostatic system with one retreat loop. Unpublished studies.

Murphy, E. A., and Berger, K. R. 1987. The dynamics of angular homeostasis I: General principles. *Amer. J. Med. Genet.* 26:457–72.

———. 1991. Angular homeostasis VII: Non-monotonic correction systems. *Amer. J. Med. Genet.* 39:486–92.

Murphy, E. A.; Berger, K. R.; Pyeritz, R. E.; and Sagawa, Y. 1990. Angular homeostasis VI: Threshold processes with bivariate liabilities. *Amer. J. Med. Genet.* 36:115–21.

Murphy, E. A.; Berger, K. R.; Trojak, J. E.; and Rosell, E. M. 1989. Angular homeostasis IV: Polygonal orbits. *Theor. Med.* 10:355–65.

Murphy, E. A.; Berger, K. R.; Trojak, J. E.; and Sagawa, Y. 1988. Angular homeostasis V: Some issues in genetics, ontogeny, and evolution. *Amer. J. Med. Genet.* 31:963–79.

Murphy, E. A., and Chase, G. A. 1975. *Principles of Genetic Counseling.* Chicago: Year Book.

Murphy, E. A., and Francis, M. E. 1971. The estimation of blood platelet survival II: The multiple hit model. *Thromb. Diath. Haemorrh.* 25:53–80.

Murphy, E. A.; Krush, A. J.; Dietz, M.; and Rohde, C. A. 1980. Hereditary polyposis coli III: Genetic and evolutionary fitness. *Amer. J. Hum. Genet.* 32:700–713.

Murphy, E. A.; Meyers, D. A.; and Rohde, C. A. 1987. Genetic ascertainment with heterogeneous risk. *Amer. J. Med. Genet.* 27:669–82.

Murphy, E. A., and Pyeritz, R. E. 1986. Homeostasis VII: A conspectus. *Amer. J. Med. Genet.* 24:735–51.

————. 1996. Pathogenesis of genetic disease. In *Principles and Practices of Medical Genetics,* edited by D. E. Rimoin, J. M. Connor, and R. E. Pyeritz. 3d ed. Pp. 359–70. New York: Churchill Livingstone.

Murphy, E. A., and Renie, W. A. 1984. The dynamics of quantifiable homeostasis IV: Zero-order homeostasis. *Amer. J. Med. Genet.* 18:99–113.

Murphy, E. A.; Rosell, E. M.; and Rosell, M. I. 1982. Deduction, inference, and illation. *Theor. Med.* 7:329–53.

Murphy, E. A., and Trojak, J. E. 1981. The human mutational debt: How is it paid? In *Population and Biological Aspects of Human Mutation,* edited by I. H. Porter and E. S. Hook. New York: Academic Press.

Murphy, E. A.; Trojak, J. E.; Hou, W.; and Rohde, C. A. 1981. The bingo model of survivorship 1: Probabilistic aspects. *Amer. J. Med. Genet.* 10:261–77.

Myers-Briggs, I., with Myers, P. B. 1980. *Gifts Differing.* Palo Alto: Consulting Psychologists.

Nagan, N., and Kagan, H. M. 1994. Modulation of lysyl oxidase toward peptidyl lysine by vicinal dicarboxylic amino acid residues: Implications for collagen crosslinking. *J. Biol. Chem.* 269:22366–71.

Newman, J. H. 1865. *The Dream of Gerontius.* Reprinted 1964 in *A Newman Reader,* edited by F. X. Connolly. P. 453. Garden City, N.Y.: Doubleday, Image.

————. 1870. *A Grammar of Assent.* Reprinted 1955. New York: Doubleday, Image.

Nugent, K. P.; Philips, R. K. S.; Hodgson, S. V.; Cottrel, S.; Smith-Ravin, J.; Pack, K.; and Bodmer, W. F. 1994. Phenotypic expression in familial adenomatous polyposis: Partial prediction by mutation analysis. *Gut* 35:1622–23.

Ober, W. B. 1975. Swinburne's masochism: Neuropathology and psychopathology. *Bull. Menninger Clinic* 39:500–555.

Ogata, K. 1970. *Modern Control Engineering.* Englewood Cliffs, N.J.: Prentice-Hall.

Ogden, C. K., and Richards, I. A. 1960. *The Meaning of Meaning: A Study of the Influence of Language upon Thought and the Science of Symbolism.* New York: Harcourt, Brace, and World.

Olefsky, J. M. 1976. The insulin receptor: Its role in insulin resistance of obesity and diabetes. *Diabetes* 25:1154–62.

————. 1984. Insulin antagonists and resistance. In *Diabetes Mellitus,* edited by M. Ellenberg and H. Rifkin. Pp. 151–78. New Hyde Park, N.Y.: Medical Examination Publishing.

Onghera, P., and Vanhoudenhove, B. 1992. Antidepressant-induced analgesia in chronic non-malignant pain: A meta-analysis of 39 placebo-controlled studies. *Pain* 49:205–19.

Oxford English Dictionary [*The Concise Oxford Dictionary of Current English*]. 1976. Oxford: Oxford University Press.

Pardue, M. L.; Feramisco, J. R.; and Lindquist, S. 1988. *Stress-Induced Proteins.* New York: Liss.

Passmire, J. A. 1966. *A Hundred Years of Philosophy.* Rev. ed. New York: Basic Books.

Pauling, L., and Corey, R. B. 1951a. Atomic coordinates and structure factors for two helical configurations of polypeptide chains. *Proc. Natl. Acad. Sci. U.S.* 37:235–40.

———. 1951b. The pleated-sheet: A new layer configuration of polypeptide chains. *Proc. Natl. Acad. Sci. U.S.* 37:251-56.

———. 1951c. The polypeptide-chain configuration in hemoglobin and other globular proteins. *Proc. Natl. Acad. Sci. U.S.* 37:282-85.

———. 1951d. The structure of feather radius keratin. *Proc. Natl. Acad. Sci. U.S.* 37:256-61.

———. 1951e. The structure of fibrous proteins of the collagen-gelatin group. *Proc. Natl. Acad. Sci. U.S.* 37:272-82.

———. 1951f. The structure of hair, muscle, and related proteins. *Proc. Natl. Acad. Sci. U.S.* 37:261-71.

———. 1951g. The structure of synthetic polypeptides. *Proc. Natl. Acad. Sci. U.S.* 37:241-50.

Pellegrino, E. D., and Thomasma, D. C. 1993. *The Virtues in Medical Practice.* New York: Oxford University Press.

Penrose, R. 1989. *The Emperor's New Mind.* New York: Oxford University Press.

———. 1994. *Shadows of the Mind: On Consciousness, Computation, and the New Physics of the Mind.* Oxford: Oxford University Press.

Platt, R. 1965. Letter to the editor. *Lancet* 2:1125.

Poincaré, H. 1913. *Foundations of Science.* Translated by G. Bruce Halstead. P. 387. New York: Science Press.

Polya, G. 1954. *Mathematics and Plausible Reasoning.* Vols. 1 and 2. Princeton: Princeton University Press.

Popper, K. R. 1959. *The Logic of Scientific Discovery.* London: Hutchinson.

———. 1963. *Conjectures and Refutations: The Growth of Scientific Knowledge.* New York: Harper and Row.

Price, J. L. 1990. Olfactory system. In *The Human Nervous System,* edited by G. Paxinos. Pp. 979-88. New York: Academic Press.

Priest, C. 1983. *The Affirmation.* London: Faber and Faber.

Pyeritz, R. E. 1989. Pleiotropy revisited: Molecular explanations of a classic concept. *Amer. J. Med. Genet.* 34:124-34.

Pyeritz, R. E., and Murphy, E. A. 1989. The genetics of congenital heart disease: Perspectives and prospects. *J. Amer. Coll. Cardiol.* 13:1458-68.

———. 1991. Genetics and congenital heart disease: Perspectives and prospects. Chap. 16 in *Cardiovascular Medicine,* edited by S. B. Knoebel and S. Dack. New York: Elsevier.

Raiffa, H., and Schlaifer, R. 1962. *Applied Statistical Decision Theory.* Boston: Harvard Business School.

Ramsey, M. M. 1956. *A Textbook of Modern Spanish.* Revised by R. K. Spalding. New York: Holt, Reinhart, and Winston.

Reiser, S. J.; Dyck, A. J.; and Curran, N. J. 1977. *Ethics in Medicine.* Cambridge, Mass.: MIT Press.

Renie, W. A., and Murphy, E. A. 1983. The dynamics of quantifiable homeostasis II: Characterization of linear processes. *Amer. J. Med. Genet.* 15:637-53.

Reznek, L. 1987. *The Nature of Disease.* London: Routledge and Kegan Paul.

Robitscher, J. B. 1966. *Pursuit of Agreement: Psychiatry and the Law.* Philadelphia: Lippincott.

Roe *v* Wade, 410 U.S. 113, 93 S.Ct. 705, 35 L. Ed 2d 147 (1973).

Ruse, M. E. 1971. Functional statements in biology. *Philosophy of Science* 38:87–95.

Russell, B. 1940. *An Inquiry into Meaning and Truth.* London: Unwin.

Samkoff, J. S., and Jacques, C. H. M. 1991. A review of studies concerning effects of sleep deprivation and fatigue on residents' performance. *Acad. Med.* 66:687–93.

Schaefer, K. E.; Hensel, H.; and Brady, R., eds. 1977. *A New Image of Man in Medicine.* Vol. 1, *Towards a Man-Centered Medical Science.* Mount Kisco, N.Y.: Futura.

Schiødt, E. 1938. On the duration of life of the red blood corpuscles. *Acta Med. Scand.* 95:49–79.

Schrödinger, E. 1935. Die gegenwärtige Situation in der Quantenmechanik. *Naturwissenschaften* 23:807–12, 823–28, 844–49. Translated 1980 by J. T. Trimmer in *Proc. Amer. Phil. Soc.* 124:323–38.

Schwartz, L. 1995. The art historian's computer. *Scientific American* 272(4):106–111.

Searle, J. R. 1983. *Intentionality: An Essay in the Philosophy of Mind.* Cambridge: Cambridge University Press.

———. 1992. *The Rediscovery of the Mind.* Cambridge, Mass.: MIT Press.

Selye, H. 1936. A syndrome produced by diverse nocuous agents. *Nature* 138:32.

———. 1956. *The Stress of Life.* New York: McGraw-Hill.

Selzer, H. S.; Allen, E. W.; Herron, A. L.; and Brennen, M. T. 1967. Insulin secretion in response to glycemic stimulus: Relation of delayed initial release to carbohydrate intolerance in mild diabetes. *J. Clin. Invest.* 46:323–35.

Shaffer, J. A. 1993. The philosophy of mind. In *The New Encyclopaedia Britannica.* Vol. 24, pp. 152–61. Chicago: Encyclopaedia Britannica.

Sheldon, C. A.; Williams, R. D.; and Fraley, E. E. 1980. Incidental carcinoma of the prostate: A review of the literature and critical reappraisal of classification. *J. Urol.* 124:626–31.

Shelley, M. 1818. *Frankenstein; or, the Modern Prometheus.* Reprinted 1893. New York: Mershon.

Shelley, P. B. 1819. Ode to the west wind. Reprinted 1968 in *The Poem: An Anthology,* edited by S. B. Greenfield and A. K. Weatherhead. P. 196. New York: Appleton-Century-Crofts.

Shipley, J. T. 1984. *The Origins of English Words.* Baltimore: Johns Hopkins University Press.

Smith *v* United States, 36 F.2d 548, 551, 70 A.L.R. 654 (D.C. Cir. 1929).

Smith-Ravin, J.; Pack, K.; Hodgson, S.; Tay, S. K. S.; Philips, R.; and Bodmer, W. 1994. APC mutation associated with late onset of familial adenomatous polyposis. *J. Med. Genet.* 31:888–90.

Stanley, M. S. 1996. *Children of the Ice Age: How a Global Catastrophe Allowed Humans to Evolve.* New York: Crown.

Stebbing, L. S. 1944. *Philosophy and the Physicists.* Harmondsworth, Middlesex: Penguin.

Stevenson, A. C.; Davison, B. C. C.; and Oakes, M. W. 1970. *Genetic Counselling.* Philadelphia: Lippincott.

Stevenson, R. L. 1881. Walking tours. In *Virginibus Puerisque.* Reprinted 1904. London: Chatto and Windus.

Strahan, N. V.; Murphy, E. A.; Fortuin, N. J.; Come, P. C.; and Humphries, J. O. 1983. Inheritance of mitral valve prolapse syndrome: Discussion of a three-compartmental penetrance model. *Amer. J. Med.* 74:967–72.

Swart, E. R. 1980. The philosophical implications of the four-color problem. *Amer. Math. Monthly* 87:697–707.

Teilhard de Chardin, P. 1959. *The Phenomenon of Man.* New York: Harper.

Thom, R. 1972. *Structural Stability and Morphogenesis: An Outline of a General Theory of Models.* Translated by D. H. Fowler. Reading, Mass.: Benjamin.

Thomson, J. A. K., trans. 1955. *The Ethics of Aristotle: The Nicomachean Ethics.* London: Penguin.

Thoreau, H. D. 1854. Conclusion to *Walden.* Reprinted 1971. Edited by J. Lyndon Shanley. Princeton: Princeton University Press.

Title 10, C.F.R. pt. 20 (1994).

Trojak, J. E., and Murphy, E. A. 1981. Recurrence risks for autosomal epistatic two-locus systems: The effects of linkage disequilibrium. *Amer. J. Med. Genet.* 9:219–29.

———. 1983. Paradoxical fixation of deleterious alleles in two-locus systems with epistasis. *Amer. J. Med. Genet.* 16:493–502.

Turing, A. M. 1937. On computable numbers, with an application to the *Entscheidungsproblem. Proc. Lond. Math. Soc.* 42:230–65.

Tymoczko, T. 1979. The four-color problem and its philosophical significance. *J. Philosoph.* 76:57–83.

United States *v* Brawner, 471 F.2d 969, 1039 (D.C. Cir. 1972).

Vácha, J. 1985a. German constitutional doctrine in the 1920s and 1930s and pitfalls of the contemporary conception of normality in biology and medicine. *J. Med. Philos.* 10:339–67.

———. 1985b. Historical roots of the "normal interval" concept in the light of its interpretation today (in two parts). *Scripta Medica (Brno)* 58:35–46 and 419–34.

Vandeveer, D., and Regan, T. 1987. *Health Care Ethics.* Philadelphia: Temple University Press.

Veale, A. M. 1965. *Intestinal Polyposis: Eugenics Laboratory Memoirs, XL.* London: Cambridge University Press.

Veatch, R. M. 1981. *A Theory of Medical Ethics.* New York: Basic Books.

Volloch, V. Z.; Rits, S.; and Tumermann, L. 1979. A possible mechanism responsible for the correction of transcription errors. *Nucleic Acids Res.* 6:1535–46.

Von Mises, R. 1939. *Probability, Statistics, and Truth.* Translated by J. Neyman, D. Sholl, and E. Rabinowitsch. New York: Macmillan.

Waddington, C. H. 1957. *The Strategy of the Gene.* London: Allen and Unwin.

Wallis, Y.; Macdonald, F.; Hultén, M.; Morton, J. E. V.; McKeown, C. M.; Neoptolemos, J. P.; Keighley, M.; and Morton, D. G. 1994. Genotype-phenotype correlation between position of constitutional APC gene mutation and CHRPE expression in familial adenomatous polyposis. *Hum. Genet.* 94:543–48.

Waugh, E. 1964. *A Little Learning.* Boston: Little, Brown.

[*Webster's Ninth New Collegiate Dictionary*]. 1988. Springfield, Mass.: Merriam-Webster.

Weinberg, W. 1912. Methode und Hehlerquellen der Untersuchung auf Mendelsche Zahlen bei Menschen. *Arch. Rass. und Ges. Biol.* 6:694–709.

Whitmore, W. F., Jr. 1956. Symposium on hormones and cancer therapy: Hormone therapy in prostatic cancer. *Amer. J. Med.* 21:697–713.

———. 1994. Management of clinically localized prostatic cancer (editorial). *J. Amer. Med. Assn.* 269:2676–77.

Wiener, N. 1948. *Cybernetics; or, Control and Communication in the Animal and the Machine.* New York: Wiley.

Wilson, A. N. 1990. *C. S. Lewis: A Biography.* London: Collins.

Wittgenstein, L. 1969. *Philosophische Grammatik.* Frankfurt: Suhrkamp. Translated 1978 by Anthony Kenny as *Philosophical Grammar.* Berkeley: University of California Press.

Wright, S. 1969. *Genetics and the Evolution of Populations.* Chicago: University of Chicago Press.

Yallow, R. S., and Bersen, S. A. 1960. Plasma insulin concentrations in non-diabetic and early diabetic subjects. *Diabetes* 9:254–60.

Yanagida, H. 1978. Congenital insensitivity and naloxone. *Lancet* 2:520–21.

Yates, F. E.; Marsh, D. J.; and Maran, J. W. 1980. The adrenal cortex. Chap. 64 in *Medical Physiology,* edited by V. B. Mountcastle. St. Louis: Mosby.

Author Index

Subject Index

patient and public health, 248
Deontology, 21, 94, 134, 142–3, 146,
180, 212, 364, 367
demand for pursuit of accessible
truth, 154
vs. Ethics and vs. Morality, 142–3
and scholarly exactitude, 21n
Diagnostic process, 78
computer in, 49–50, 79
concerns a person, not a population,
49
deceit in, 79
and a new disease, 49
noise in, 78
no sample space for *a priori*, 49
ontology of, 164
optimization of, 91
signs and symptoms distinguished in,
49–50
Dialogue, authentic, 5, 389
Dialysis, renal, 250
Diamond, decisive ontology of, 95–6,
99, 324
Dimensional analysis, 141
Dimensionality, 30, 55–7, 134, 158. *See
also* Cardinality
Discrete processes, 54–5, 128–9, 130,
358
Disease, Chap. 8, 8, 91, 110
as anarchical, 188
definition of, 186–8
distress not essential to, 186–7
dynamic state, 162, 186
early diagnosis and certainty of, 163,
186
vs. health as exhaustive states, 187
and homeostasis, 187–8
as obvious, 162
ontological challenges of, 103, 162
presence of cause insufficient to
diagnose, 186–7
prevention of, 188–9
types of, 187–8
Disjointness, and independence, 60–2
Distribution of survivorship function
(SF), 274
change in, and age, 280–1
as cumulative distribution function
(DF), 275–6
mean survival (average), 276, 287–8;

as area under SF, 276; as inadequate descriptor, 278; and mean
further survival, 278–80
mode, 274
models for, 276–84; blood platelets, 277; competing causes of
death ("bingo"), 277–8; epistemic
weaknesses of, 284; gamma, 286;
general multiple-hit processes,
277; hazard function, 283–4
as Probability density function
(PDF), 274
rectangular, 282–3
variance of, 282–3, 375
Dog breeds, low ontological density of,
163
Double effect, principle of, 115, 237
analogical model of, 125–6
Flew's principle and, 126
lacking existential counterparts, 126
ontology of terms, 115–6
in prostatic cancer, 115
Doubt, epistemic and ontological, 93
Down's syndrome, 53–4
Drift, genetic, 85–6, 182, 184, 398,
414, 419
Dynamic interaction of axioms and
effects, 38–9
Dynamic systems, ontology of, 103

Education, 288, 309, 329
Elastic, meanings of term, 111, 113
Element, and definition by atomic
number, 97
Eliminative materialism, 175
Ellis–van Crevald syndrome (EVCS),
164–5
Empirical fact, 12
and theory, 193, 193n2
End, justifying means, 27, 125
Endpoints, 261, 422
Engineering, as protective insulation,
176
Enthymeme, 137, 148, 271
Environment, 169–70
physical devices to buffer against,
169–76
psychic devices to buffer against,
176–7
Epidemiology, 91